Artificial Intelligence and PET Imaging, Part II

Editors

BABAK SABOURY
ARMAN RAHMIM
ELIOT SIEGEL

PET CLINICS

www.pet.theclinics.com

Consulting Editor
ABASS ALAVI

January 2022 • Volume 17 • Number 1

ELSEVIER

1600 John F. Kennedy Boulevard • Suite 1800 • Philadelphia, Pennsylvania, 19103-2899

http://www.pet.theclinics.com

PET CLINICS Volume 17, Number 1
January 2022 ISSN 1556-8598, ISBN-13: 978-0-323-85013-1

Editor: John Vassallo (j.vassallo@elsevier.com)
Developmental Editor: Karen Solomon

PET Clinics (ISSN 1556-8598) is published quarterly by Elsevier Inc., 360 Park Avenue South, New York, NY 10010-1710. Months of issue are January, April, July, and October. Periodicals postage paid at New York, NY, and additional mailing offices. Subscription prices per year are $262.00 (US individuals), $526.00 (US institutions), $100.00 (US students), $290.00 (Canadian individuals), $552.00 (Canadian institutions), $100.00 (Canadian students), $283.00 (foreign individuals), $552.00 (foreign institutions), and $140.00 (foreign students). To receive student and resident rate, orders must be accompanied by name of affiliated institution, date of term, and the signature of program/residency coordinator on institution letterhead. Orders will be billed at individual rate until proof of status is received. Foreign air speed delivery is included in all Clinics subscription prices. All prices are subject to change without notice. POSTMASTER: Send address changes to PET Clinics, Elsevier Health Sciences Division, Subscription Customer Service, 3251 Riverport Lane, Maryland Heights, MO 63043. **Customer Service: 1-800-654-2452 (U.S. and Canada); 314-447-8871 (outside U.S. and Canada). Fax: 314-447-8029. E-mail: journalscustomerservice-usa@elsevier.com (for print support); journalsonlinesupport-usa@elsevier.com (for online support).**

Reprints. For copies of 100 or more of articles in this publication, please contact the Commercial Reprints Department, Elsevier Inc., 360 Park Avenue South, New York, NY 10010-1710. Tel.: 212-633-3874; Fax: 212-633-3820; E-mail: reprints@elsevier.com.

PET Clinics is covered in MEDLINE/PubMed (Index Medicus).

Contributors

CONSULTING EDITOR

ABASS ALAVI, MD, MD (Hon), PhD (Hon), DSc (Hon)
Professor of Radiology and Neurology, Director of Research Education, Division of Nuclear Medicine, Department of Radiology, Hospital of the University of Pennsylvania, University of Pennsylvania Perelman School of Medicine, Philadelphia, Pennsylvania, USA

EDITORS

BABAK SABOURY, MD, MPH, DABR, DABNM
Chief Clinical Data Science Officer, Oncoradiologist and Nuclear Medicine Physician, Director-Center for Precision Dosimetry and Radiopharmaceutical Treatment Planning, Department of Radiology and Imaging Sciences, Clinical Center, National Institutes of Health, Bethesda, Maryland, USA; Adjunct Professor, Department of Computer Science and Electrical Engineering, University of Maryland Baltimore County, Baltimore, Maryland, USA; Department of Radiology, Hospital of the University of Pennsylvania, Philadelphia, Pennsylvania, USA

ARMAN RAHMIM, PhD, DABSNM
Professor, Departments of Radiology and Physics, University of British Columbia, Senior Scientist and Provincial Medical Imaging Physicist, BC Cancer, BC Cancer Research Institute, Vancouver, British Columbia, Canada

ELIOT SIEGEL, MD, FSIIM, FACR
Diagnostic Radiology and Nuclear Medicine physician, Professor and Vice-Chair, University of Maryland School of Medicine, Department of Diagnostic Radiology; Chief of Radiology and Nuclear Medicine, Veterans Affairs Maryland Healthcare System, Baltimore, Maryland, USA

AUTHORS

ABASS ALAVI, MD, MD (Hon), PhD (Hon), DSc (Hon)
Professor of Radiology and Neurology, Director of Research Education, Division of Nuclear Medicine, Department of Radiology, Hospital of the University of Pennsylvania, University of Pennsylvania Perelman School of Medicine, Philadelphia, Pennsylvania, USA

AMINE AMYAR, PhD
General Electric Healthcare, Buc, France; QuantIF-LITIS EA 4108, University of Rouen, Rouen, France

CHERYL BEEGLE, JD, CRA, R.T. (R)(N) ARRT, CNMT
Department of Radiology and Imaging Sciences, Clinical Center, National Institutes of Health, Bethesda, Maryland, USA

FRANÇOIS BÉNARD, MD, FRCPC
Department of Radiology, University of British Columbia, Vancouver, British Columbia, Canada

KATARINA CHIAM
Division of Engineering Science, University of Toronto, Toronto, Ontario, Canada

MICHAEL T. COLLINS, MD
Senior Investigator, Skeletal Disorders and Mineral Homeostasis Section, National Institute of Dental and Craniofacial Research, National Institutes of Health, Bethesda, Maryland, USA

DONNA J. CROSS, PhD
Associate Professor, Department of Radiology and Imaging Sciences, University of Utah, Salt Lake City, Utah, USA

PIERRE DECAZES, MD
Department of Nuclear Medicine, Henri Becquerel Cancer Center, QuantIF-LITIS EA 4108, University of Rouen, Rouen, France

DAMINI DEY, PhD
Research Scientist, Departments of Imaging and Medicine, Cedars-Sinai Medical Center, Los Angeles, California, USA

LARS EDENBRANDT, MD, DMSc
Department of Clinical Physiology, Region Västra Götaland, Sahlgrenska University Hospital, Professor/Chief Physician, Department of Molecular and Clinical Medicine, Institute of Medicine, SU Sahlgrenska, Göteborg, Sweden

ARMAGHAN FAGHIHIMEHR, MD
Department of Radiology, Virginia Commonwealth University, Richmond, Virginia, USA

FARAZ FARHADI, BS
Department of Radiology and Imaging Sciences, Clinical Center, National Institutes of Health, Bethesda, Maryland, USA

VINCENT C. GAUDET, PhD, PEng
Department of Electrical and Computer Engineering, University of Waterloo, Waterloo, Ontario, Canada

VICTOR H. GERBAUDO, PhD, MSHCA
Department of Radiology, Brigham and Women's Hospital, Harvard Medical School, Boston, Massachusetts, USA

OKE GERKE, MSc, PhD
Professor, Chief Consultant, Biostatistician, Department of Nuclear Medicine, Odense University Hospital, Odense C, Denmark;

Department of Clinical Research, University of Southern Denmark, Odense, Denmark

SEYED MOHAMMAD H. GHARAVI, MD
Assistant Professor of Radiology, Division of Neuroradiology, Virginia Commonwealth University, Richmond, Virginia, USA

PETER GRAYSON, MD, MSc
Chief, Vasculitis Translational Research Program, Associate Director, NIAMS Fellowship Program, National Institute of Arthritis and Musculoskeletal and Skin Diseases, National Institutes of Health, Bethesda, Maryland, USA

STEPHANIE A. HARMON, PhD
Artificial Intelligence Resource Section, Molecular Imaging Branch, National Cancer Institute, National Institutes of Health, Bethesda, Maryland, USA

NAVID HASANI, BS
Pre-doctoral Research Fellow, Department of Radiology and Imaging Sciences, Clinical Center, National Institutes of Health, Bethesda, Maryland, USA; University of Queensland Faculty of Medicine, Ochsner Clinical School, New Orleans, Louisiana, USA

POUL FLEMMING HØILUND-CARLSEN, MD, DMSc, Prof (Hon)
Professor of Clinical Physiology, Head Research, Department of Nuclear Medicine, Odense University Hospital, Odense C, Denmark; Department of Clinical Research, University of Southern Denmark, Odense, Denmark

ELIZABETH JONES, MD, MPH, MBA
Director, Radiology and Imaging Sciences, Department of Radiology and Imaging Sciences, Clinical Center, National Institutes of Halth, Bethesda, Maryland, USA

IVAN S. KLYUZHIN, PhD
Department of Integrative Oncology, BC Cancer Research Institute, Vancouver, British Columbia, Canada

SEISAKU KOMORI
Future Design Lab, New Concept Design, Global Strategic Challenge Center,

Hamamatsu Photonics K.K., Hamamatsu City, Japan

CRAIG S. LEVIN, PhD
Departments of Radiology, Bioengineering, Physics, and Electrical Engineering, Stanford University, Stanford, California, USA

KEVIN MA, PhD
Artificial Intelligence Resource Section, Molecular Imaging Branch, National Cancer Institute, National Institutes of Health, Bethesda, Maryland, USA

ROBERTO MAASS-MORENO, PhD, DABR
Physicist, Nuclear Medicine, Department of Radiology and Imaging Sciences, Clinical Center, National Institutes of Health, Bethesda, Maryland, USA

JONATHAN LEE MEZRICH, MD, JD, MBA, LLM
Assistant Professor, Emergency Radiology, Department of Radiology and Biomedical Imaging, Yale School of Medicine, New Haven, Connecticut, USA

SATOSHI MINOSHIMA, MD, PhD
Professor and Chair, Department of Radiology and Imaging Sciences, University of Utah, Salt Lake City, Utah, USA

ROBERT J.H. MILLER, MD
Cardiologist, Department of Cardiac Sciences, University of Calgary, Calgary AB, Canada

MICHAEL A. MORRIS, MD, MS, DABR, DABNM
Department of Radiology and Imaging Sciences, Clinical Center, National Institutes of Health, Bethesda, Maryland, USA; Department of Computer Science and Electrical Engineering, University of Maryland, Baltimore County, Baltimore, Maryland, USA; Institute for Data Science, Department of Diagnostic Radiology and Nuclear Medicine, University of Miami Miller School of Medicine, Miami, Florida, USA

MOOZHAN NIKPANAH, MD
Department of Radiology and Imaging Sciences, Clinical Center, National Institutes of Health, Bethesda, Maryland, USA

SRIRAM S. PARAVASTU, BA
Pre-doctoral Research Fellow, Department of Radiology and Imaging Sciences, Clinical Center, Skeletal Disorders and Mineral Homeostasis Section, National Institute of Dental and Craniofacial Research, National Institutes of Health, Bethesda, Maryland, USA; University of Missouri-Kansas City School of Medicine, Kansas City, Missouri, USA

ANNE PARISER, MD
Director, Office of Rare Disease Research, National Center for Advancing Translational Sciences, National Institutes of Health, Bethesda, Maryland, USA

REZA PIRI, MD
PhD Student, Department of Nuclear Medicine, Odense University Hospital, Odense C, Denmark; Department of Clinical Research, University of Southern Denmark, Odense, Denmark

ARMAN RAHMIM, PhD, DABSNM
Professor, Departments of Radiology and Physics, University of British Columbia, BC Cancer Research Institute, Vancouver, British Columbia, Canada

MARK ROSCHEWSKI, MD
Clinical Director, Lymphoid Malignancies Branch, Center for Cancer Research, National Institutes of Health, Bethesda, Maryland, USA

SU RUAN, PhD
QuantIF-LITIS EA 4108, University of Rouen, Rouen, France

BABAK SABOURY, MD, MPH, DABR, DABNM
Chief Clinical Data Science Officer, Oncoradiologist and Nuclear Medicine Physician, Director-Center for Precision Dosimetry and Radiopharmaceutical Treatment Planning, Department of Radiology and Imaging Sciences, Clinical Center, National Institutes of Health, Bethesda, Maryland, USA; Adjunct Professor, Department of Computer Science and Electrical Engineering, University of Maryland Baltimore County, Baltimore, Maryland, USA; Department of Radiology, Hospital of the University of Pennsylvania, Philadelphia, Pennsylvania, USA

ELIOT SIEGEL, MD, FSIIM, FACR
Diagnostic Radiology and Nuclear Medicine
Physician, Professor and Vice-Chair,
University of Maryland School of Medicine,
Department of Diagnostic Radiology, Chief of
Radiology and Nuclear Medicine, Veterans
Affairs Maryland Healthcare System,
Baltimore, Maryland, USA

ANANYA SINGH, MSc
Research Scientist, Departments of Imaging
and Medicine, Cedars-Sinai Medical Center,
Los Angeles, California, USA

PIOTR SLOMKA, PhD
Research Scientist, Departments of Imaging
and Medicine, Cedars-Sinai Medical Center
California, Los Angeles, USA

DAVID L. STREINER, PhD, CPsych
Professor Emeritus, Department of Psychiatry
and Behavioural Neurosciences, McMaster
University, St. Joseph's Healthcare, Hamilton,
Ontario, Canada; Professor, Department of
Psychiatry, University of Toronto, Toronto,
Ontario, Canada

RONALD M. SUMMERS MD, PhD
Senior Investigator, Imaging Biomarkers and
Computer-Aided Diagnosis Laboratory,
Department of Radiology and Imaging
Sciences, Clinical Center, National Institutes of
Health, Bethesda, Maryland, USA

ELIZABETH H. THENG, BA
Pre-doctoral Research Fellow, Department of
Radiology and Imaging Sciences, Clinical
Center, Skeletal Disorders and Mineral
Homeostasis Section, National Institute of
Dental and Craniofacial Research, National
Institutes of Health, Bethesda, Maryland, USA;
University of Missouri-Kansas City School of
Medicine, Kansas City, Missouri, USA

BARIS TURKBEY, MD
Artificial Intelligence Resource Section,
Molecular Imaging Branch, National Cancer
Institute, National Institutes of Health,
Bethesda, Maryland, USA

MUHAMMAD NASIR ULLAH, PhD
Department of Radiology, Stanford University,
Stanford, California, USA

CARLOS F. URIBE, PhD
PET Functional Imaging, BC Cancer Research
Institute, Vancouver, British Columbia,
Canada

YANJI XU, PhD
Program Director, Office of Rare Disease
Informatics, Office of Rare Diseases Research,
National Center for Advancing Translational
Sciences, National Institutes of Health,
Bethesda, Maryland, USA

FERESHTEH YOUSEFIRIZI, PhD
Post-doctoral Research Fellow, Qurit Lab,
Department of Integrative Oncology, BC
Cancer Research Institute, Vancouver, British
Columbia, Canada

**KATHERINE A. ZUKOTYNSKI, MD, PhD,
FRCPC, PEng**
Associate Professor, Departments of
Radiology and Medicine, Associate Professor,
Associate Member, School of Biomedical
Engineering, McMaster University, Hamilton,
Ontario, Canada; Adjunct Associate Professor,
The Edward S. Rogers Department of
Electrical and Computer Engineering,
University of Toronto, Toronto, Ontario,
Canada

Contents

Special Topics

> Trust in artificial intelligence (AI) by society and the development of trustworthy AI
> systems and ecosystems are critical for the progress and implementation of AI tech-
> nology in medicine. With the growing use of AI in a variety of medical and imaging
> applications, it is more vital than ever to make these systems dependable and trust-
> worthy. Fourteen core principles are considered in this article aiming to move the
> needle more closely to systems that are accurate, resilient, fair, explainable, safe,
> and transparent: toward trustworthy AI.

> Almost 1 in 10 individuals can suffer from one of many rare diseases (RDs). The
> average time to diagnosis for an RD patient is as high as 7 years. Artificial intelligence
> (AI)-based positron emission tomography (PET), if implemented appropriately, has
> tremendous potential to advance the diagnosis of RDs. Patient advocacy groups
> must be active stakeholders in the AI ecosystem if we are to avoid potential issues
> related to the implementation of AI into health care. AI medical devices must not only
> be RD-aware at each stage of their conceptualization and life cycle but also should
> be trained on diverse and augmented datasets representative of the end-user pop-
> ulation including RDs. Inability to do so leads to potential harm and unsustainable
> deployment of AI-based medical devices (AIMDs) into clinical practice.

> Artificial intelligence (AI) can enhance the efficiency of medical imaging quality con-
> trol and clinical documentation, provide clinical decision support, and increase im-
> age acquisition and processing quality. A clear understanding of the basic tenets of
> these technologies and their impact will enable nuclear medicine technologists to
> train for performing advanced imaging tasks. AI-enabled medical devices' antici-
> pated role and impact on routine nuclear medicine workflow (scheduling, quality
> control, check-in, radiotracer injection, waiting room, image planning, image

acquisition, image post-processing) is reviewed in this article. With the assistance of AI, newly compiled patient imaging data can be customized to encompass personalized risk assessments of patients' disease burden, along with the development of individualized treatment plans. Nuclear medicine technologists will continue to play a crucial role on the medical team, collaborating with patients and radiologists to improve each patient's imaging experience and supervising the performance of integrated AI applications.

Artificial Intelligence (AI) has been rapidly embraced by imaging fields and offers a variety of benefits in nuclear medicine; however, the biggest hurdles to AI in health care will likely not be technological but legal. What happens when an error occurs in the AI setting? A variety of legal causes of action, ranging from medical malpractice, to notions of vicarious liability/agency to products liability may come into play in an AI-related lawsuit. Physicians working with AI need to understand these causes of action, stay abreast of legal developments in AI, and advocate for appropriate guidelines and legislation.

Artificial intelligence (AI) in medical imaging is in its infancy. However, ongoing advances in hardware and software as well as increasing access to ever-expanding datasets for training, validation, and testing purposes are likely to make AI an increasingly prevalent and powerful tool. Of course issues, such as the need to protect the privacy of sensitive health data, remain; nevertheless, it is likely the average imager will need to develop an evidence-based approach to assessing AI in medical imaging. We hope this article will provide insight into just how this can be conducted by applying 5 simple questions, specifically: (1) Who was in the training sample, (2) How was the model trained, (3) How reliable is the algorithm, (4) How was the model validated, and (5) How useable is the algorithm.

Clinical

AI has been applied to brain molecular imaging for over 30 years. The past two decades, have seen explosive progress. AI applications span from operations processes such as attenuation correction and image generation, to disease diagnosis and prediction. As sophistication in AI software platforms increases, and the availability of large imaging data repositories become common, future studies will incorporate more multidimensional datasets and information that may truly reach "superhuman" levels in the field of brain imaging. However, even with a growing level of complexity, these advanced networks will still require human supervision for appropriate application and interpretation in medical practice.

Applications of "artificial intelligence" (AI) have been exponentially expanding in health care. Readily accessible archives of enormous digital data in medical imaging have made radiology a leader in exploring and taking advantage of this technology. AI-assisted radiology has paved the way toward another level of precision in medicine. In this article, the authors aim to review current AI applications in PET imaging of head and neck cancers, beginning with radiomics and followed by deep learning in each section.

The ability of a computer to perform tasks normally requiring human intelligence or artificial intelligence (AI) is not new. However, until recently, practical applications in medical imaging were limited, especially in the clinic. With advances in theory, microelectronic circuits, and computer architecture as well as our ability to acquire and access large amounts of data, AI is becoming increasingly ubiquitous in medical imaging. Of particular interest to our community, radiomics tries to identify imaging features of specific pathology that can represent, for example, the texture or shape of a region in the image. This is conducted based on a review of mathematical patterns and pattern combinations. The difficulty is often finding sufficient data to span the spectrum of disease heterogeneity because many features change with pathology as well as over time and, among other issues, data acquisition is expensive. Although we are currently in the early days of the practical application of AI to medical imaging, research is ongoing to integrate imaging, molecular pathobiology, genetic make-up, and clinical manifestations to classify patients into subgroups for the purpose of precision medicine, or in other words, predicting a priori treatment response and outcome. Lung cancer is a functionally and morphologically heterogeneous disease. Positron emission tomography (PET) is an imaging technique with an important role in the precision medicine of patients with lung cancer that helps predict early response to therapy and guides the selection of appropriate treatment. Although still in its infancy, early results suggest that the use of AI in PET of lung cancer has promise for the detection, segmentation, and characterization of disease as well as for outcome prediction.

Artificial intelligence is an important technology, with rapidly expanding applications for cardiac PET. We review the common terminology, including methods for training and testing, which are fundamental to understanding artificial intelligence. Next, we highlight applications to improve image acquisition, reconstruction, and segmentation. Computed tomographic imaging is commonly acquired in conjunction with PET and various artificial intelligence methods have been applied, including methods to automatically extract anatomic information or generate synthetic attenuation images. Last, we describe methods to automate disease diagnosis or risk stratification. This summary highlights the current and future clinical applications of artificial intelligence to cardiovascular PET imaging.

Positron emission tomography (PET) offers an incredible wealth of diverse research applications in vascular disease, providing a depth of molecular, functional, structural, and spatial information. Despite this, vascular PET imaging has not yet assumed the same clinical use as vascular ultrasound, CT, and MR imaging which provides information about late-onset, structural tissue changes. The current clinical utility of PET relies heavily on visual inspection and suboptimal parameters such as SUVmax; emerging applications have begun to harness the tool of whole-body PET to better understand the disease. Even still, without automation, this is a time-consuming and variable process. This review summarizes PET applications in vascular disorders, highlights emerging AI methods, and discusses the unlocked potential of AI in the clinical space.

This review discusses the current state of artificial intelligence (AI) in ^{18}F-NaF-PET/CT imaging and the potential applications to come in diagnosis, prognostication, and improvement of care in patients with bone diseases, with emphasis on the role of AI algorithms in CT bone segmentation, relying on their prevalence in medical imaging and utility in the extraction of spatial information in combined PET/CT studies.

PET imaging with targeted novel tracers has been commonly used in the clinical management of prostate cancer. The use of artificial intelligence (AI) in PET imaging is a relatively new approach and in this review article, we will review the current trends and categorize the currently available research into the quantification of tumor burden within the organ, evaluation of metastatic disease, and translational/supplemental research which aims to improve other AI research efforts.

Malignant lymphomas are a family of heterogenous disorders caused by clonal proliferation of lymphocytes. ^{18}F-FDG-PET has proven to provide essential information for accurate quantification of disease burden, treatment response evaluation, and prognostication. However, manual delineation of hypermetabolic lesions is often a time-consuming and impractical task. Applications of artificial intelligence (AI) may provide solutions to overcome this challenge. Beyond segmentation and detection of lesions, AI could enhance tumor characterization and heterogeneity quantification, as well as treatment response prediction and recurrence risk stratification. In

Technical

Artificial intelligence (AI) has been widely used throughout medical imaging, including PET, for data correction, image reconstruction, and image processing tasks. However, there are number of opportunities for the application of AI in photon detector performance or the data collection process, such as to improve detector spatial resolution, time-of-flight information, or other PET system performance characteristics. This review outlines current topics, research highlights, and future directions of AI in PET instrumentation.

Artificial intelligence (AI) techniques have significant potential to enable effective, robust, and automated image phenotyping including the identification of subtle patterns. AI-based detection searches the image space to find the regions of interest based on patterns and features. There is a spectrum of tumor histologies from benign to malignant that can be identified by AI-based classification approaches using image features. The extraction of minable information from images gives way to the field of "radiomics" and can be explored via explicit (handcrafted/engineered) and deep radiomics frameworks. Radiomics analysis has the potential to be used as a noninvasive technique for the accurate characterization of tumors to improve diagnosis and treatment monitoring. This work reviews AI-based techniques, with a special focus on oncological PET and PET/CT imaging, for different detection, classification, and prediction/prognosis tasks. We also discuss needed efforts to enable the translation of AI techniques to routine clinical workflows, and potential improvements and complementary techniques such as the use of natural language processing on electronic health records and neuro-symbolic AI techniques.

PET CLINICS

SERIES OF RELATED INTEREST

Advances in Clinical Radiology
Available at: Advancesinclinicalradiology.com
MRI Clinics of North America
Available at: MRI.theclinics.com
Neuroimaging Clinics of North America
Available at: Neuroimaging.theclinics.com
Radiologic Clinics of North America
Available at: Radiologic.theclinics.com

THE CLINICS ARE AVAILABLE ONLINE!
Access your subscription at:
www.theclinics.com

PROGRAM OBJECTIVE
The goal of the PET Clinics is to keep practicing radiologists and radiology residents up to date with current clinical practice in positron emission tomography by providing timely articles reviewing the state of the art in patient care.

TARGET AUDIENCE
Practicing radiologists, radiology residents, and other health care professionals who provide patient care utilizing radiologic findings.

LEARNING OBJECTIVES
Upon completion of this activity, participants will be able to:
1. Review current trends, research, and applications of AI in medical imaging.
2. Discuss core principles and key requirements to enable and promote trustworthy AI systems.
3. Recognize legal developments and the need for appropriate guidelines and legislation in AI.

ACCREDITATION
The Elsevier Office of Continuing Medical Education (EOCME) is accredited by the Accreditation Council for Continuing Medical Education (ACCME) to provide continuing medical education for physicians.

The EOCME designates this journal-based CME activity for a maximum of 15 *AMA PRA Category 1 Credit*(s)™. Physicians should claim only the credit commensurate with the extent of their participation in the activity.

All other health care professionals requesting continuing education credit for this enduring material will be issued a certificate of participation.

DISCLOSURE OF CONFLICTS OF INTEREST
The EOCME assesses conflict of interest with its instructors, faculty, planners, and other individuals who are in a position to control the content of CME activities. All relevant conflicts of interest that are identified are thoroughly vetted by EOCME for fair balance, scientific objectivity, and patient care recommendations. EOCME is committed to providing its learners with CME activities that promote improvements or quality in healthcare and not a specific proprietary business or a commercial interest.

The planning committee, staff, authors, and editors listed below have identified no financial relationships or relationships to products or devices they or their spouse/life partner have with commercial interest related to the content of this CME activity:
Abass Alavi, MD, MD (Hon), PhD (Hon), DSc (Hon); Amine Amyar, PhD; Cheryl Beegle, JD, CRA, R.T. (R)(N) ARRT, CNMT; François Bénard, MD, FRCPC; Regina Chavous-Gibson, MSN, RN; Katarina Chiam; Michael T. Collins, MD; Donna J. Cross, PhD; Pierre Decazes, MD; Lars Edenbrandt, MD, DMSc; Armaghan Faghihimehr, MD; Faraz Farhadi, BS; Vincent C. Gaudet, PhD, PEng; Victor H. Gerbaudo, PhD, MSHCA; Oke Gerke, MSc, PhD; Seyed Mohammad H. Gharavi, MD; Peter Grayson, MD, MSc; Stephanie A. Harmon, PhD; Navid Hasani, BS; Poul Flemming Høilund-Carlsen, MD, DMSc, Prof (Hon); Elizabeth Jones, MD, MPH, MBA; Ivan S. Klyuzhin, PhD; Seisaku Komori; Craig S. Levin, PhD; Kevin Ma, PhD; Roberto Maass-Moreno, PhD, DABR; Jonathan Lee Mezrich, MD, JD, MBA, LLM; Satoshi Minoshima, MD, PhD; Robert J.H. Miller, MD; Moozhan Nikpanah, MD; Sriram S. Paravastu, BA; Reza Piri, MD; Arman Rahmim, PhD, DABSNM; Mark Roschewski, MD; Su Ruan, PhD; Babak Saboury, MD, MPH, DABR, DABNM; Eliot Siegel, MD, FSIIM, FACR; Ananya Singh, MSc; Piotr Slomka, PhD; David L. Streiner, PhD, Cpsych; Ronald M. Summers, MD, PhD; Elizabeth H. Theng, BA; Baris Turkbey, MD; Muhammad Nasir Ullah, PhD; Carlos F. Uribe, PhD; Yanji Xu PhD; Vignesh Viswanathan; Fereshteh Yousefirizi, PhD; Katherine A. Zukotynski, MD, PhD, FRCPC, PEng

The planning committee, staff, authors, and editors listed below have identified financial relationships or relationships to products or devices they or their spouse/life partner have with commercial interest related to the content of this CME activity:
Michael A. Morris, MD, MS, DABR, DABNM: Executive Interest, Ownership, Employee: Advanced Molecular Imaging and Therapy

UNAPPROVED/OFF-LABEL USE DISCLOSURE
The EOCME requires CME faculty to disclose to the participants:
1. When products or procedures being discussed are off-label, unlabelled, experimental, and/or investigational (not US Food and Drug Administration (FDA) approved; and
2. Any limitations on the information presented, such as data that are preliminary or that represent ongoing research, interim analyses, and/or unsupported opinions. Faculty may discuss information about pharmaceutical agents that is outside of FDA-approved labelling. This information is intended solely for CME and is not intended to promote off-label use of these medications. If you have any questions, contact the medical affairs department of the manufacturer for the most recent prescribing information.

TO ENROLL
To enroll in the PET Clinics Continuing Medical Education program, call customer service at 1-800-654-2452 or sign up online at http://www.theclinics.com/home/cme. The CME program is available to subscribers for an additional annual fee of USD 254.00

METHOD OF PARTICIPATION

In order to claim credit, participants must complete the following:

1. Complete enrolment as indicated above.
2. Read the activity.
3. Complete the CME Test and Evaluation. Participants must achieve a score of 70% on the test. All CME Tests and Evaluations must be completed online.

CME INQUIRIES/SPECIAL NEEDS

For all CME inquiries or special needs, please contact elsevierCME@elsevier.com.

Acknowledgment

First and foremost, we wish to thank the distinguished colleagues who contributed to these two volumes dedicated to Artificial Intelligence (AI) and Nuclear Medicine. We deeply appreciate their efforts, their sacrifice of time, and, above all, their generosity to share their perspectives, experience, and expertise.

With sincerity and affection, we acknowledge the guidance of the members of the Society of Nuclear Medicine & Molecular Imaging (SNMMI) AI Taskforce. During the past year, lively discussions at the regular meetings were highly influential in organizing the topics covered in these special AI issues of PET clinics. Specifically, we wish to acknowledge (in alphabetical order): Ronald Boellaard, Tyler Bradshaw, Irène Buvat, Bonnie Clarke, Joyita Dutta, Paul Jacobs, Abhinav Jha, Mathieu Hatt, Prabhat Kc, Quanzheng Li, Chi Liu, Helena McMeekin, Nancy Obuchowski, Peter Scott, Piotr Slomka, Arkadiusz Sitek, John Sunderland, Richard Wahl, and Sven Zuehlsdorff.

We wish to express gratitude to the supporters of this project, Dr. Abass Alavi, Professor of Radiology at the University of Pennsylvania and Dr. Elizabeth Jones, Director of the Radiology and Imaging Sciences at National Institutes of Health (NIH) Clinical Center. These volumes would not have been possible without their trust, encouragement, and support.

There are many others who helped in subtle and not-so-subtle ways. To them, our most sincere thanks indeed.

Finally, we wish to acknowledge the help of publication team, Ms. Karen Solomon, Mr. Vignesh Viswanathan, and Mr. John Vassallo.

Preface

Taming the Complexity: Using Artificial Intelligence in a Cross-Disciplinary Innovative Platform to Redefine Molecular Imaging and Radiopharmaceutical Therapy

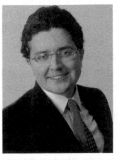 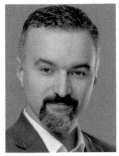 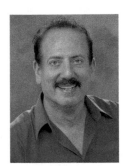

Babak Saboury, MD, MPH, DABR, DABNM

Arman Rahmim, PhD, DABSNM

Eliot Siegel, MD, FSIIM, FACR

Editors

We are on the cusp of a major transformation in medicine. While the latter half of the twentieth century could be considered the *age of computation and connectivity*, the twenty-first century ushered in the era of big data accompanied by the rapidly evolving use of Artificial Intelligence (AI), dominantly in the form of deep learning, to "tame" the complexity associated with the ever-quickening velocity of information, including in molecular imaging and radiopharmaceutical therapy. Advanced AI algorithms have the potential to powerfully capture complex biological data and to be used to make improved predictions.

In the first issue of this collection, our colleagues addressed the use of AI to address complex technical challenges in nuclear medicine and PET imaging, such as improved image reconstruction and enhancement, as well as image segmentation and radiomics, radiopharmaceutical dosimetry, and treatment response evaluation.

The second issue considers practical considerations in the implementation of AI in clinical practice as well as the current state-of-the-art in specific clinical domains.

Saboury and colleagues discuss trustworthy AI in medical imaging, pointing out that AI systems are more opaque than human health care providers and are susceptible to being "fragile and unjust," which could result in breaches of trust in not only AI but also health care in general. They review fourteen core principles and requirements for trustworthy AI systems. In a thematically related article, they point out the critical importance of making AI algorithms aware of rare diseases, which occur in one in ten individuals, but which are rarely included in most image databases that provide training for AI algorithms. They suggest that AI algorithms should be made rare disease "aware" at each stage of their conceptualization and life cycle and should be trained on diverse and augmented data sets, including rare diseases.

To address an important but less explored aspect of AI, Mezrich "demystifies" anticipated medicolegal challenges associated with AI for molecular imaging, suggesting that the biggest hurdles to AI in nuclear medicine may be more legal than technical and advocating for the establishment of guidelines and legislation that he believes are currently poorly delineated.

Critical appraisal of scientific evidence is an important ingredient of a trustworthy AI ecosystem. Steiner and colleagues advocate for

PET Clin 17 (2022) xvii–xix

https://doi.org/10.1016/j.cpet.2021.11.002

1556-8598/21/© 2021 Published by Elsevier Inc.

an evidence-based approach to evaluation of AI in medical imaging using five basic questions, including the training sample, how a model is trained, reliability, validation, and usability.

AI for PET imaging has the potential to help to reinvent workflow, and as Beegle and colleagues suggest, put patients at the center of care. They focus on the application of AI for PET technologists, which they believe will improve communication with patients and allow technologists to replace current "mundane" tasks with more "challenging and satisfying tasks."

This second issue also explores the current state-of-the-art AI applications for PET for eight clinical domains, including **Brain, Head and Neck, Lung, Heart, Vascular System, Bone/Skeleton, Prostate, and Lymphoma**.

Cross and colleagues describe the current state-of-the-art in the most widely written about area of AI in PET imaging, that is, applications in the **brain**. They organize articles about AI and PET into three tiers: workflow/image generation emphasizing quality and dose optimization; cognitive skills emphasizing decision making and progression of disease; and finally, "superhuman" algorithms that provide analysis not currently possible by human experts.

Gharavi and colleagues focus on prediction of response to treatment and tumor markers for **head and neck** cancers, including tumor and nodal segmentation and how to deal with the paucity of head and neck PET/computed tomographic (CT) data sets.

Zukotynski and colleagues review the use of AI in detection and characterization of **lung** nodules and predictive and prognostic biomarkers in patients with lung cancer, including staging, detection of recurrence, and outcome prediction.

Slomka and colleagues describe another area of very active research: **cardiac** PET/CT AI applications, including attenuation correction, dose reduction, and diagnostic and prognostic improvement.

Saboury and colleagues discuss bottlenecks to clinical adoption of PET for **vascular** diseases and predict that AI-based segmentation will bring forth

a revolution in more general applications of PET for quantification and phenotyping of these disorders.

Paravastu and colleagues focus on progress with AI applications in ^{18}F-NaF PET/CT in diagnosis, prognostication, and improvement of care for patients with **bone** diseases.

Prostate cancer imaging using relatively new targeted PET radiopharmaceuticals, such as PSMA, FACBC, and choline, is discussed by Ma and colleagues, who review the current medical literature and predict translation of current research into routine clinical practice using AI.

Hasani and colleagues conducted an extensive scoping review of the current literature on quantification of disease burden in patients with **lymphoma** using AI and PET as well as treatment response and diagnosis and predictions of prognosis. They also review the literature on determination of change over time with an emphasis on going from just the spatial domain to the "spatio-temporal realm."

The second issue concludes with two forward-looking articles. Ullah and Levin describe how AI will improve the design and performance of future PET scanners, from more accurate photon detection to more efficient data correction methods for quantitative imaging. Yousefirizi and colleagues review the concept of "Radiophenomics," a combination of radiomics and analysis of personalized structural and functional patterns of disease or drug response toward detection, classification, and outcome prediction.

We hope that despite the extraordinarily rapidly evolving advances in the application of AI in nuclear medicine, this review of the current state-of-the-art as applied to a variety of diseases and anatomic areas will provide a useful update and guide that will inspire the reader to continue to explore the evolution of AI in PET/CT. The application of machine learning and deep learning for PET/CT will undoubtedly result in major improvements in all aspects of clinical practice by advancing our ability to detect and diagnosis and treat disease more effectively and enhance patient safety and communication. Some have referred to AI as a "genie in a bottle," which speaks to its tremendous power and potential but should also serve as a cautionary metaphor to warn us of the potential dangers and challenges associated with its broad application in nuclear medicine without a well-informed understanding of its limitations and pitfalls.

Babak Saboury, MD, MPH, DABR, DABNM
Department of Radiology and Imaging Sciences
Clinical Center
National Institutes of Health (NIH)
9000 Rockville Pike
Bethesda, MD 20892, USA

Department of Radiology
Hospital of the University of Pennsylvania

Department of Computer Science and
Electrical Engineering
University of Maryland
Baltimore County

Arman Rahmim, PhD, DABSNM
Departments of Radiology and Physics
University of British Columbia
BC Cancer Research Institute
675 West 10th Avenue
Office 6-112
Vancouver, BC V5Z 1L3, Canada

Eliot Siegel, MD, FSIIM, FACR
Department of Radiology
University of Maryland School of Medicine
655 West Baltimore Street
Baltimore, MD 21201, USA

E-mail addresses:
babak.saboury@nih.gov (B. Saboury)
arman.rahmim@ubc.ca (A. Rahmim)
esiegel@umaryland.edu (E. Siegel)

Special Topics

Trustworthy Artificial Intelligence in Medical Imaging

Navid Hasani, BS[a,b], Michael A. Morris, MD, MS, DABR, DABNM[a,c],
Arman Rhamim, PhD, DABSNM[d,e], Ronald M. Summers, MD, PhD[a],
Elizabeth Jones, MD, MPH, MBA[a], Eliot Siegel, MD, FSIIM, FACR[d],
Babak Saboury, MD, MPH, DABR, DABNM[a,c,f,g],*

KEYWORDS

• Trustworthiness • Trustworthy artificial intelligence • Machine learning • Ethics of AI

KEY POINTS

• Trust has been at the heart of the patient-caregiver relationship from humankind's earliest forays into health care.
• Artificial intelligence (AI) systems, rapidly emerging and increasingly used, are complicated and remain largely opaque.
• We are becoming increasingly aware that AI systems might be fragile and unjust.
• Incidences of broken trust by AI systems will be harmful not only to the adoption of AI in medical care but also to general patient trust in medicine and technologies used within this field.
• We discuss 14 core principles and key requirements to enable and promote trustworthy AI systems.

INTRODUCTION

The question is no longer whether artificial intelligence (AI) will impact the future of medicine but instead "by whom, how, where, and when this beneficial or harmful impact will be felt."[1] The rate of development of new and enhanced AI-based technologies is accelerating and permeating every industry. AI has enormous potential to improve human life and the environment around us; however, we must tread carefully ahead in order to realize the opportunities it provides and avoid potential pitfalls.

Acknowledgment of the current and future benefits of AI systems in health care safety, quality,[2] equity, and access[3] is the first step toward developing clear plans to harness its potential. In medical imaging, AI has aided and will be aiding physicians in evaluation of disease progression, prediction, and/or assessment of treatment effectiveness, and tracking disease patterns over time as dicsused by Hasani and colleagues in "Artificial Intelligence in Lymphoma PET Imaging: A Scoping Review (Current Trends and Future Directions)," in this issue. AI also plays an important role in improving the effectiveness of imaging

[a] Department of Radiology and Imaging Sciences, Clinical Center, National Institutes of Health (NIH), 9000 Rockville Pike, Building 10, Room 1C455, Bethesda, MD 20892, USA; [b] University of Queensland Faculty of Medicine, Ochsner Clinical School, New Orleans, LA 70121, USA; [c] Department of Computer Science and Electrical Engineering, University of Maryland, Baltimore Country, Baltimore, MD, USA; [d] Department of Radiology, BC Cancer Research Institute, University of British Columbia, 675 West 10th Avenue, Vancouver, British Columbia, V5Z 1L3, Canada; [e] Department of Physics, BC cancer Research Institute, University of British Columbia, Vancouver, British Columbia, Canada; [f] Department of Radiology and Nuclear Medicine, University of Maryland Medical Center, 655 W. Baltimore Street, Baltimore, MD 21201, USA; [g] Department of Radiology, Hospital of the University of Pennsylvania, Philadelphia, PA, USA
* Corresponding authors. Department of Radiology and Nuclear Medicine, University of Maryland Medical Center, 655 W. Baltimore Street, Baltimore, MD 21201, USA (E.S); Department of Radiology and Imaging Sciences, Clinical Center, National Institutes of Health, 9000 Rockville Pike, Building 10, Room 1C455, Bethesda, MD 20892, USA (B.S).
E-mail address: babak.saboury@nih.gov

PET Clin 17 (2022) 1–12
https://doi.org/10.1016/j.cpet.2021.09.007
1556-8598/22/© 2021 Elsevier Inc. All rights reserved.

workflow and efficiency of time-consuming tasks such as segmentation.[4–6] Yousefirizi and colleagues evaluated the role of AI in segmentation in oncological PET imaging.[7]

At the same time, AI can pose certain risks and a slew of unexpected ethical,[8] legal,[9] and societal[10] challenges that, if not addressed properly, may substantially limit its value. We are becoming increasingly aware that AI systems might be fragile.[11] Graffiti on a stop sign may trick a machine learning (ML)-based classification system into not identifying an stop sign.[12] Additional noise in an picture of a benign skin lesion tricks an AI classification system into identifying the lesion as cancerous.[13] A small section of an image of a cat has been classified as guacamole with 100% confidence by a Google AI-based image recognition algorithm.[14]

So, how can we deliver on the promise of AI's advantages while also dealing with circumstances that have life-or-death repercussions for individuals in medical settings? How can we develop "reliable AI"?

AI progression has been hindered due to limitations in computer performance the complicated nature of AI research including exaggerated claims, confusion, and issues of public trust. This necessitates tight collaboration among scientists at various phases of translational research.[15,16] One topic that continues to be controversial is the trustworthiness of AI. Trust is an important element in the implementation of AI medical devices (AIMDs) into routine practice. One measure of a tool's "trustworthiness" is the desire of physicians and patients to rely on it in a dangerous scenario.[17]

The aviation sector has served as a paragon for safety of its passengers and often inspires efforts to improve patient safety and reduction of medical errors.[18] The recent tragic losses of two Boeing 737 MAX aircraft can teach us lessons on AI systems and how they may be improved as deployed in medical imaging.[19] Such performance failures highlighted the fact that an AI system's output is only as good as its inputs, and therefore the correctness of AI input data is as crucial as the AI's ability to interpret those inputs. The quality assurance and control mechanisms must encompass single or a few isolated algorithms as well as the entire system.[20]

There are presently more than 70 frameworks and lists of AI ethical principles.[21,22] The abundance of such guidelines creates inconsistency and confusion among stakeholders over the most acceptable document.[23] Although the trustworthiness of AI can be an element of ethical principles, not everything related to trustworthiness is a matter of ethics. Specifically, some of the concerns surrounding trustworthiness that are more practical components of clinical practice implementation cannot be addressed in ethical standards and frameworks.

Thus, in this article, we highlight the importance of addressing trustworthiness in the era of medical AI devices, and we suggest a set of essential, but not exhaustive, requirements for an AI system to be considered trustworthy.

TRUST AND TRUSTWORTHINESS FROM THE THEORETIC STANDPOINT

Human interaction is predicated on trust. The entire fabric of our daily lives, of our social order, is based on trust,[24(p443)] and lack of it would paralyze societies and individuals by inaction. Humans are wired with an innate need to trust and to be trusted by those with whom they engage.[25] When trust is misplaced or abused, the trustor may incur significant costs[26]; hence, trusting entails taking a chance and a willingness to be vulnerable.[27,28] In medicine, patients put trust in their physicians and health care providers when the cost may be the difference between life, death, or disability.

Trust is an attitude we have toward people devices, or systems (ie, an AI-based medical software or device) that we believe are trustworthy. Trustworthiness on the other hand is a characteristic, not an attitude. This dichotomy refers to the notion that someone trustworthy may or may not be trusted, and that someone who is trusting may trust someone who is not trustworthy. Trust and trustworthiness are thus distinct notions. In an ideal world, what we trust will also be trustworthy, and those trustworthy will be trusted. To trust someone or something means to (1) be vulnerable to what the trustee does to the extent that interests are entangled with the trustee's performance; (2) rely on the individual or technology to be competent to accomplish the intended goal; and (3) rely on them to be willing to perform the intended task.[17]

Following Annette Baier,[29] a widely shared assumption among philosophers is that to trust someone or something is to rely on them to deliver what was expected.[17,30] However, trust is not mere reliance, as a violation of that trust leads to a sense of betrayal rather than mere disappointment.[31] By trusting, we run the danger of losing precious things we entrust to others, in this case, our health.[17] Karen Jones[32] proposes a different perspective on trust, arguing that there is an emotional component to trust, which means that the attitude central to trust is not simply belief, but also a perceived optimism toward the proposition that the trustee would do what they are trusted to do for the right reasons.

So, *why do we need trust* in society and health care when formal constructs, such as contracts, instructions, and standard operating procedures, are available? These devices and contracts have limitations and are insufficient considering the complex and ever-changing needs of the world, societies, and, on a smaller scale, health care systems. As suggested by the findings of Giddens,[33] the need for trustworthiness does not arise from a lack of driving force but rather a lack of complete information. In addition, a fundamental core of contracts between parties is the element of trust in the counterparties and those engines of enforcement (ie, Food and Drug Administration [FDA], health systems). According to Adam Smith's theory of moral sentiments, people are linked by strong relationships of sympathy, empathy, and trust, and it is on top of this bond that markets and systems within a society may exist.[34]

To address the issue of trust, we must deal with two elements of uncertainty and vulnerability. We can either deal with uncertainty by acquiring more information or by managing the vulnerabilities, which means finding ways to mitigate harm and future actions of the trustee (in this case AI).

IMPORTANCE OF TRUSTWORTHINESS IN ARTIFICIAL INTELLIGENCE–ENABLED MEDICINE: DISSEMINATION AND IMPLEMENTATION SCIENCE

Trust has been at the heart of the patient-caregiver relationship from humankind's earliest forays into health care, when shamans, priests, and medicine practitioners ministered to the sick. People choose to put themselves in the hands of others in their most vulnerable moments, trusting, or at least believing, that they would benefit and be relieved.

Although there is now improved regulation surrounding many medical claims, patient's trust is equally needed in today's scientific and technological environment. The rapid progress in medicine over the past 50 years, especially the exponential increases in the past 25 years, opened possibilities that could not have been conceived a few generations earlier.

AI is advancing at a tremendous speed, with new avenues for its routine application in preclinical, clinical, and administrative health care, as well as promising evidence of its benefits to existing practice. However, these systems are complicated and opaque. Judging and interpreting their outcomes as fair and trustworthy is challenging, and they have shown to be vulnerable to major errors. For example, "heatmaps" corresponding to components of an image that are most important in the decision-making process of an algorithm have demonstrated that AI frequently pays attention to parts of an image that are irrelevant or might be called out as "cheating" by a human (eg, learning the hospital marker and using that knowledge to "predict" pneumonia or using the presence of chest drains to "diagnose" pneumothorax). These kinds of incidents may well be harmful not only to the adoption of AI in medical care, but also to general patient trust in medicine and the technology used within this field.

There are several levels of trust depending on the degree of automation and the risk associated with the work performed. With increased automation and risk involved with the task, a higher level of trust is required. Trusting an algorithm to segment the kidney as a preliminary task for evaluation by a radiologist falls on one end of this spectrum, whereas trusting the algorithm to identify cancer and initiate chemotherapy falls on the other. Therefore, AI-based medical imaging systems can be classified into 5 categories based on their degree of automation, similar to the categorization set forth by Society of Automation Engineers (SAE) for automation of vehicles.[35,36] This 6-layered trust model offers a novel perspective through which the heterogeneity of trust in AIMDs can be realized (**Table 1**).

Furthermore, the distinction between high-risk and low-risk computer-aided device (CAD) is reflected in the law. The FDA distinguishes between two types of CAD used in medical imaging: computer-aided detection (CADe) and computer-aided diagnosis (CADx).[37] The agency distinguishes between CADe, which is designed to simply highlight regions of interest, and CADx, which shows the likelihood of the disease's presence or specifies a disease type.[38] Because CADx presents a greater risk it may be regulated more stringently. Therefore, CADs should adhere to the regulatory and trust standards that are developed based on their category and the risks associated with their task.

There are limited recognized standards or methods to manage and test medical AI systems.[39] It has also been documented that these systems can operate unjustly, resulting in dangerous consequences. Unprepared and inequitable AI adoption and general application in medical services, on the other hand, may bring new obstacles, potentially triggering a chain of skepticism, distrust, criticism, budget reduction, and, ultimately, the third winter of AI. Therefore, appropriate implementation and dissemination of AI in health care necessitate *trustworthy applications*.

Trust is a challenging subject that has inspired several academic arguments in recent years. The conceptualization of what makes AI trustworthy, as of today, remains ambiguous and highly

Table 1
Six levels of automation based on the Society of Automation Engineers (SAE) model and the version appropriate to AI-based medical imaging tools

Levels	SAE Model	Medical Imaging Version
0	**No automation** All driving tasks are carried out by humans.	**No automation** Interpretation/intervention is done solely by the radiologist.
1	**Driving Assistance** The car is equipped with a single automated system (ie, cruise control).	**Physician assistance** The radiologists are in charge of interpretation and intervention, while AI provides secondary oversight (ie, existing CAD software for mammography and lung nodules, worklist prioritization).
2	**Partial driving automation** The vehicle is capable of steering and acceleration. The human is still monitoring all tasks and has the ability to take control at any moment.	**Partial automation** The AI is in responsible for interpretation and intervention, with the radiologist providing secondary monitoring (ie, bone age prediction, chest x-ray pathology detection and report pre-population).
3	**Conditional driving automation** The vehicle is capable of detecting its surroundings. The car can do the majority of driving responsibilities, although human intervention is still necessary.	**Conditional automation** The AI is responsible for the interpretation and intervention only for specific indications, with the expectation that the radiologist will intervene if the results are positive or inconclusive (ie, automated triaging of normal cases where radiologist is expected to intervene if positive but not if negative).
4	**High driving automation** Under specific situations, the vehicle performs all driving tasks. Geofencing is essential. Human intervention is still a possibility.	**High automation** The AI is the lone interpreter/interventionist for a specific indication, with no expectation that the radiologist will intervene. AI can independently reach a differential diagnosis and care plan (ie, AI studies thyroid ultrasound and advises and/or performs a nodule biopsy).
5	**Full driving automation** The vehicle completes all driving duties under all situations. No need for human involvement or attention.	**Full automation** For all indications expected of a radiologist, the AI is the sole interpreter/interventionist. AI can provide a differential diagnosis and make care recommendations on its own (ie, a chest x-ray request indicates "rule out pneumonia" AI reports a bone tumor with a differential diagnosis and recommendations for more imaging/consultation).

Abbreviations: AI, artificial intelligence; CAD, computer-aided design.
Adapted from SAE International Releases Updated Visual Chart for Its "Levels of Driving Automation" Standard for Self-Driving Vehicles. Accessed September 17, 2021. and Jaremko et al. Canadian Association of Radiologists (CAR) Artificial Intelligence Working Group. Canadian Association of Radiologists White Paper on Ethical and Legal Issues Related to Artificial Intelligence in Radiology. Can Assoc Radiol J. 2019 May;70(2):107-118. with permission.

debated in research and practice.[40] To address this need, frameworks and guidelines for *ethical* AI,[10,41] beneficial AI,[42] and trustworthy AI (TAI)[39,40,43] have been set forth to advance AI while minimizing the potential risks associated with it.

The technology sector has been a leader in seeking the implementation of TAI. Microsoft emphasized the significance of trustworthy software in its January 2002 "Trustworthy Computing" message to personnel, users, shareholders, and the rest of the information technology sector.[44] According to an internal Microsoft white paper, security, privacy, dependability, and commercial integrity are the four pillars around which trust is founded.[44]

Others have proposed using the Formal Methods approach of computer science for achieving TAI.[45,46] In this approach, TAI requires a shift away from conventional computer systems' deterministic approach and toward a more probabilistic nature.[47] To create end-user trust, this method uses data science and formal verification in which properties are established over a wide domain for all inputs or behaviors of a particular distributed or concurrent system.[46] On the other hand, the verification mechanism discovers a counterexample, such as an input value for which the program delivers an inaccurate outcome that does not meet the necessary characteristic. This process can provide useful insights for further improving the system. Formal verification provides the advantage of obviating the requirement to test each input value or action one by one, which may be a challenging task for vast (or infinite) state spaces. Similar methods for the development of AIMDs are necessary.

KEY REQUIREMENTS TO PROMOTE TRUSTWORTHY ARTIFICIAL INTELLIGENCE SYSTEMS

When we discuss the topic of the trustworthiness of AI in medicine, it is entirely from the perspective of the patient. For AI to be trustworthy, it needs to be implemented through generalized trust and relational trust. Generalized trustworthiness will encourage the patient to consent to or seek AI-augmented medical care while a relational trust will be developed over time and enables maintenance of trustworthiness after the patient's initial encounter with an AIMD.

Several components can promote the trustworthiness of the AIMD and all processes and individuals who are a part of the AI Ecosystem. In what follows, we list 14 core principles and requirements toward TAI; these are listed in **Fig. 1** and elaborated in the following sections.

Transparency

Transparency promotes informed decision making and is a key component in building trustworthy AI systems. As a result, "black box" AI systems that do not place a strong focus on various indicators of transparency (data use transparency, clear disclosures, traceability, auditability, and understandability) should be avoided in clinical settings as much as possible.

Conceptually there are 2 types of opacity in medical AI systems that can influence trustworthiness: (1) lack of transparency, and (2) epistemic opacity,[48] which we describe next.

Data transparency indicates that data subjects are aware of how their health records are used for AI system profiling and decision-making processes. In this regard, AIMD's public confidence and

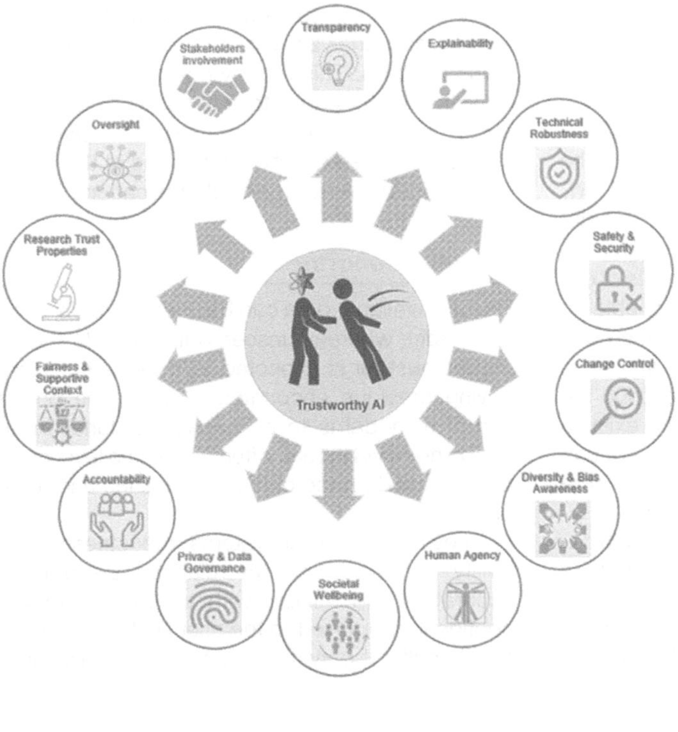

Fig. 1. The 14 core principles and requirements for TAI: the principles are all significant, complement one another, and should be applied and assessed over the entire life cycle of the AI system.

integrity may be jeopardized. Although transparency is essential, one major concern for developers is the risk of harmful usage or patient privacy violations.[49] Vendors should provide the characteristics of the training and testing data used for validation, as well as how an AI system's influence is verified for the labeled claim (purpose, criteria, and limits).

When using a decision support system, a clear distinction must be made on what is conveyed by the AI and the information communicated by the clinician. AI systems should have mechanisms for recording and identifying whether data, AI models, or rules were utilized to generate certain AI outcomes (auditability and traceability). To provide a mechanism to assess and challenge AI system outputs, the influence of the input on the output must be reported in such a manner that medical professionals and patients can understand the relationship.

Epistemic opacity refers to the inability of developers or users (health care providers) to understand how an AI system arrives at a certain outcome. Autonomous systems engage in actions that are difficult to comprehend or predict from users' perspectives, although there is a plethora of tools to probe the algorithm. For instance, Zeiler and Fergus[50] created a visualization approach that provides insight into the function of intermediate feature layers and classifier operations in a convolutional network model. Yet, reducing epistemic opacity and understanding internal rules used in the decision-making processes of evolving AI systems continues to be a challenge. This aspect of AI's black box nature can complicate quality assurance and interpretability or restrict clinician and patient input in the decision-making process.[51]

Explainability

The issue of explanatory opacity refers to the inability to understand and elucidate how and why the system made a particular decision.[48] This differs from epistemic opacity because not only do users need to comprehend technical aspects of decision making, but they should also be able to explain them in plain terms.[10] But does one need a deep grasp of data science, physics, statistics, and epidemiology to understand and describe the residual bias and confounding that may exist in AIMDs? At the very least, there must be enough training materials and disclaimers for health care workers on how to use the system properly.

Amann and colleagues[52] conducted an ethics-based assessment utilizing the Principles of Biomedical Ethics (beneficence, no-maleficence, autonomy, and justice) to establish the necessity for explainability in AI systems used in healthcare. Reportedly, to maximize the well-being of patients (beneficence) and prevent harm (nonmaleficence) as well as trustworthiness, physicians should generally understand and be able to explain the AI decision-making processes. The issue of explainability may not be equally important in different industries; the stakes are far greater in the health care industry, as explainability allows physicians to assess a system's suggestions based on their clinical judgment and expertise. Thus, an explainable system would empower physicians and patients, promoting autonomy, trust, and informed decision-making. Otherwise, parties or physicians may not fully trust the AIMD suggestions and outcomes, especially when their own opinion is different from that of AI.[52]

Transparent mechanisms of risk management and accountability should be in place in case of any adverse events. According to the principles of safety-critical systems, vendors and physicians should be accountable for their claims and the extent that AIMD is involved in patient care. For an AI system to be just, clinicians and operators need to be able to explain and understand the system, as they are ultimately accountable and therefore responsible for addressing if an AI system is for some reason unjust or biased.[53]

Clinicians around the world representing diagnostic radiology and nuclear medicine must advise the scientific community and industry to commit to moving toward "explainable AI" as much as possible. Necessary resources should be allocated to prioritize this aim as a component of AIMD products.[54–57] One strategy to achieve this is by creating a second AI system that tries to explain and analyze what the first AIMD decision was based on. This AI may not be able to explain how the AIMD came to the decision, but it can show what factors were weighed. Overall, a concerted research effort is needed in the frontier of explainable AI for medical applications.

Technical Robustness

Readily available data can be used to train and test the model, whereas unseen data are data that the model must (or is expected to) operate on without having previous encounters with it. The primary aim of a model is to be capable of function and analyzing novel inputs, often with some level of certainty, based on the data it was trained and tested on.

A key aspects of AI systems' robustness is their ability to reproduce the claimed performance accurately and reliably with a certain degree of confidence reported to the user (ie, the physician). Additionally, the system must be generalizable to the claimed user population. These aspects of AI's technical robustness must be regularly monitored through various standardized quality control measures.

Safety and Security

AI-based medical devices and systems in health care must incorporate strategies to minimize any potential harm due security breaches according to the principles of safety-critical systems.[58,59] As such, AIMDs must comply with all existing cybersecurity requirements, and their inherent vulnerabilities, such as model evasion or data poisoning, should be thoroughly evaluated prior to clinical deployment. Health systems and vendors must be transparent regarding the measures taken to mitigate and resolve potential AI vulnerabilities.[60]

Predetermined Change Control Plan

Machine learning systems can be highly iterative and adaptive which may result in product performance improvement or changes over time. AI developers and vendors should anticipated such alterations and create appropriate change control plans accordingly (ie, developing secondary AI-based control system to monitors and reports the changes of the original AI system). Strategies for controlling performance quality and assessing the robustness and safety of the updated AI system should be clearly anticipated and protocoled. Recommendations for retraining systems, performance evaluation, and procedure updates should be included in a well-documented algorithm change protocol. Such measures will enhance quality control and enable organizational and regulatory oversight.[61]

Diversity, Bias-Awareness, Nondiscrimination, and Fairness

Although AI has many benefits for humanity, one of the most serious issues arising from its increased usage is its potential to entrench and perpetuate prejudice and discrimination.[62] The performance of AI medical devices can be impacted if the input training or testing data is flawed (ie, incomplete or skewed data) or if the performance monitoring methods are suboptimal.[13,63] These factors may result in AI-enabled biases, subsequent prejudices, and unintentional discrimination against a group of patients. As a result, in accordance with the Universal Design Principles, any potential bias that could lead to prejudice should be carefully addressed and eradicated from AI systems during the conceptualization and deployment stages.[64]

Socially created biases are common in current AI-based systems in health care.[53] Another form of bias, in addition to bias in training input data, is an overemphasis of particular features (ie, skin color or locality) by AI model developers.

Developers must openly document any efforts made to minimize, and thereby quantify, unfair effects in their models. Second, regulated firms must develop specific, good faith justifications for the models they eventually embrace.[65] AI system performance should be generalizable to all patients suffering from a particular condition regardless of extraneous personal characteristics.[56,66] Patients who are underrepresented or suffer from rare diseases should not be excluded from AI systems development or evaluation [see Hasani and colleagues' article, "Artificial Intelligence in Medical Imaging and its Impact on the Rare Disease Community: Threats, Challenges, and Opportunities," in this issue]. Appropriate validation testing on standardized sets that include a diverse patient population, including rare or unusual presentations of disease, is critical to evaluate the presence of bias in results regardless of the training data used. In recent months, the US Federal Trade Commission has shown an increased interest in AI fairness, openly suggesting that the agency should broaden its monitoring of potentially biased AI.[67]

AI solutions should be created with clinical settings in mind, as well as designed and implemented to accommodate various cultural and organizational norms. Furthermore, such solutions should consider extending access and including those with disabilities or rare diseases.

Human Agency

AI systems in clinical settings should not only enhance the workflow of the care team but also further enable the patient and the care team to make informed decisions and clearly communicate those decisions with others, as in Freidman's fundamental theorem of informatics.[14,68] This will further empower the autonomy of both parties while limiting potential for automation bias. Patients and physicians should understand the extent to which AIMD is integrated in care delivery and the scope of physicians oversight.

Oversight

Appropriate supervision techniques should be used, which may be accomplished using methodologies such as "humans in the loop," "humans on the loop," and "humans in charge."[39] Such approaches will ensure human values are being considered. According to the World Health Organization, AI systems should be thoroughly regulated post-market by independent professional credentialing authorities in a way similar to the way in which medical practitioners are certified and recertified.[69] The approval and auditing processes should not only consider the level of the risk associated with the AI claim, but also the level of learning[70] (supervised or unsupervised) and characteristics such as explainability, transparency, and accountability. AI systems should be monitored and categorized according to their degree of automation and autonomy. Similar to the AI categories set forth by SAE, medical imaging can categorize AIMDs into categories such as (1) no automation, (2) physician assistance, (3) partial automation, (4) conditional automation, (5) high automation, and (6) full automation.[71]

The investigation and validation process should include the AI technology's assumptions, operating procedures, data characteristics, and output decisions. Regular tests and assessments should be conducted in a transparent manner and with sufficient breadth to account for variances in algorithm performance based on race, ethnic origin, gender, age, and other important human traits. Such testing and assessments should be subjected to rigorous, independent monitoring to verify their safety and effectiveness. Medical institutions, hospital systems, and other related organizations should frequently disclose information regarding how choices concerning the deployment of AI technologies were made and how the technology will be assessed on a periodic basis. Its applications, recognized limits, and degree of involvement in decisions should also be considered, all of which can also permit third-party audits and supervision.

Stakeholder Engagement

A comprehensive collaboration and coordination system involving all stakeholders which may include patients, clinicians, insurers, health systems, research investigators, manufacturers, and regulatory agencies is of paramount importance if our goal is to integrate sustainable and trustworthy AI systems in patient care. Active engagement of all stakeholders will enable and mediate transparency, inclusiveness, trust, and accountability, all of which further enhance long-term sustainability of AI systems in clinical practice. Continuous engagement allows stakeholders to provide regular feedback and voice any potential concern at each stage of design, development, and implementation.

Sustainability of Societal Well-being

Deployment of AI into the health care system must be with careful consideration of its potential impact on the social well-being, trust in the health care system, and the physician-patient relationship.[72,73] As such, AI solutions should strive to enhance social interaction within the care team and between the physician and the patient. To achieve this goal, all health care providers who interact with the AI or are impacted by AI's implementation into their workflow should be given an opportunity have an active voice throughout the life cycle of the AI system. Professional societies and health care training programs should take necessary measures to ensure AI related skills and knowledge is incorporated into the education curricula and board examinations of appropriate health care workers.

Privacy and Data Governance

In 2020, there were 29 million health care records breached,[74] demonstrating the widespread theft of patient electronic Protected Health Information (PHI), social security numbers, and private financial information. Deployment of not fully secured AI systems to this environment could pose a risk. However, AI can also help health systems safeguard against cyber threats. AI should have procedures in place to ensure that patient data are kept secure and private. Safeguarding devices at all stages is critical, especially if intercepting or modifying data may affect device functionality. Additional AI can be added to AIMDs for cybersecurity purposes.[75] Cybersecurity AI has the potential to not only distinguish between regular network traffic and harmful hacker activity but can also respond quickly to stop the attack from spreading. Only the bare minimum of personal information should be used (data minimization). A declaration on the methods used to accomplish privacy-by-design, such as encryption, pseudo anonymization, aggregation, and de-identification should be included.[76] To achieve this goal, standardized protocols and guidelines should be recognized and routinely used to safeguard patient privacy and data handling.[77,78]

Accountability

The model's capacity to justify its judgments to the system's users is referred to as model accountability. This entails accepting responsibility for all decisions taken, regardless of whether they were correct or resulted in errors or unanticipated outcomes. Mechanisms for guaranteeing accountability and redress should be in place when adverse events occur. AI medical device manufacturers must be held liable for the claims made by their AI systems. Additionally, clinicians and health systems should be held accountable for the proper integration and deployment of the AI technology into the workflow and delivery of medical services. According to the principles of safety-critical systems, the capacity to independently audit the root cause of a failure in an AI system is vital. Individuals or groups who report real concerns must be protected in accordance with risk management standards.

Supportive Context of Implementation

Developer protection, customer protection, and legal protection are all important considerations. The "supporting context of implementation" is critical for establishing confidence in the AI ecosystem. Patients should be able to seek legal advice and representation if necessary. This strengthens their feeling of agency, and as a consequence, individuals may be more responsive to the innovative intervention, knowing they would be protected in the event of an unforeseen event. This significantly speeds the spread of novel technology.

To prevent this technology from dying prematurely while it is still in its infancy, governments may adopt methods similar to those utilized decades ago to preserve the vaccine industry. In the 1980s, there were a slew of lawsuits filed against vaccine manufacturers. Because of the general anticipated risks associated with lawsuits, there was widespread anxiety that vaccine developers would leave the field. To entice developers, the US government established a federally regulated financial resource, funded by vaccine taxes, to award judgments for injuries caused by certain adverse responses. Similar supportive strategies for appropriate AI use in health care could not only enforce regulations but also foster innovation and advancement toward safe AI deployment.

Promoting Systems for Experimenting Trustworthiness Properties

Health systems, AI developers, and other key stakeholders must collaborate to improve their grasp of psychological, sociologic, and cultural trustworthiness properties. Cultures across the globe often have a variety of value systems and fundamental beliefs that may contribute to the diversity value systems that deem an AIMD trustworthy. Thus, we must discern and implement trustworthy qualities in AI systems in order for them to function across cultural and socioeconomic differences.

SUMMARY

Trust in AI by society and the development of trustworthy AI systems and ecosystems are critical for the progress and implementation of AI technology in medicine. With the growing use of AI in a variety of medical and imaging applications, it is more vital than ever to make these systems dependable and trustworthy. Fourteen core principles are considered in this article aiming to move the needle more closely to systems that are accurate, resilient, fair, explainable, safe, and transparent—toward *trustworthy AI*.

CLINICS CARE POINTS

- Trustworthy AI is not just based on the trustworthiness of an AI Medical Device; it encompasses the entire ecosystem of AI development, production, implementation, and oversight, as well as all the social institutes protecting the wellbeing and rights of stakeholders.

- The fourteen key concepts and standards for trustworthy AI outlined in this article are all significant, complement one another, and should be implemented and evaluated throughout the AI system's life cycle.

- Addressing the existing and future benefits of AI systems through the lens of trust, safety, quality, fairness, and access is the first step toward devising specific plans to harness the full potential of trustworthy AI in medical imaging.

- Clinicians should understand and be able to explain the AI decision-making processes in general to nurture the trustworthiness of AI and enhance patient well-being (beneficence) and prevent harm (non-maleficence).

- Broken trust by AI systems will be harmful not only to the adoption of AI in medical treatment but also to patient trust in medicine and the technology utilized in the profession.

ACKNOWLEDGMENTS AND DISCLOSURES

This research was supported in part by the Intramural Research Program of the National Institutes of Health (NIH), Clinical Center. The opinions expressed in this publication are the author's own and do not reflect the view of NIH, the Department of Health and Human Services, or the US government.

REFERENCES

1. Floridi L, Cowls J, Beltrametti M, et al. AI4People-an ethical framework for a good AI society: opportunities, risks, principles, and recommendations. Minds Mach 2018;28(4):689–707.

2. Davenport T, Kalakota R. The potential for artificial intelligence in healthcare. Future Healthc J 2019;6(2):94–8.

3. Matheny M, Thadaney S, Ahmed M, et al. Artificial intelligence in health care: the hope, the hype, the promise, the peril. Washington (DC): National Academy of Medicine; 2019. Available at: https://nam.edu/wp-content/uploads/2019/12/AI-in-Health-Care-PREPUB-FINAL.pdf.

4. Kapoor N, Lacson R, Khorasani R. Workflow applications of artificial intelligence in radiology and an overview of available tools. J Am Coll Radiol 2020;17(11):1363–70.

5. Nikpanah M, Xu Z, Jin D, et al. A deep-learning based artificial intelligence (AI) approach for differentiation of clear cell renal cell carcinoma from oncocytoma on multi-phasic MRI. Clin Imaging 2021;77:291–8.

6. Weisman AJ, Kieler MW, Perlman S, et al. Comparison of 11 automated PET segmentation methods in lymphoma. Phys Med Biol 2020;65(23):235019.

7. Yousefirizi F, Jha AK, Brosch-Lenz J, et al. Toward High-Throughput Artificial Intelligence-Based Segmentation in Oncological PET Imaging. PET Clin 2021 Oct;16(4):577–96. https://doi.org/10.1016/j.cpet.2021.06.001.

8. Char DS, Abràmoff MD, Feudtner C. Identifying ethical considerations for machine learning healthcare applications. Am J Bioeth 2020;20(11):7–17.

9. Ganapathy K. Artificial intelligence and healthcare regulatory and legal concerns. TMT 2021. https://doi.org/10.30953/tmt.v6.252.

10. Geis JR, Brady AP, Wu CC, et al. Ethics of artificial intelligence in radiology: summary of the Joint European and North American Multisociety Statement. Radiology 2019;293(2):436–40.

11. Zou J, Schiebinger L. AI can be sexist and racist — it's time to make it fair. Nature 2018;559(7714):324–6.

12. Eykholt K, Evtimov I, Fernandes E, et al. Robust physical-world attacks on deep learning models. arXiv [csCR]. 2017. Available at: http://arxiv.org/abs/1707.08945. Accessed September 26, 2021.

13. Finlayson SG, Bowers JD, Ito J, et al. Adversarial attacks on medical machine learning. Science 2019;363(6433):1287–9.

14. Brown M. A Google algorithm was 100 percent sure that a photo of a cat was guacamole. 2019. Available at: https://www.inverse.com/article/56914-a-google-algorithm-was-100-percent-sure-that-a-photo-of-a-cat-was-guacamole. Accessed September 12, 2021.

15. Kaul V, Enslin S, Gross SA. History of artificial intelligence in medicine. Gastrointest Endosc 2020;92(4):807–12.

16. Toosi A, Bottino AG, Saboury B, et al. A brief history of AI: how to prevent another winter (a critical review). PET Clin 2021;16(4):449–69.

17. McLeod C. Trust. In: Zalta EN, editor. The Stanford encyclopedia of philosophy. Fall 2020. Metaphysics Research Lab. CA, USA: Stanford University; 2020. Availabel at: https://plato.stanford.edu/archives/fall2020/entries/trust/.

18. Helmreich RL. On error management: lessons from aviation. BMJ 2000;320(7237):781–5.

19. Federal Aviation Administration. Summary of the FAA's review of the Boeing 737 MAX. 2020. Available at: https://www.faa.gov/foia/electronic_reading_room/boeing_reading_room/media/737_RTS_Summary.pdf. Accessed September 15, 2021.

20. Mongan J, Kohli M. Artificial intelligence and human life: five lessons for radiology from the 737 MAX Disasters. Radiol Artif Intell 2020;2(2):e190111.

21. AI ethics guidelines global inventory. Available at: https://algorithmwatch.org/en/ai-ethics-guidelines-global-inventory/. Accessed August 23, 2021.

22. Winfield A, Profile V my C. Alan Winfield's Web Log. Available at: https://alanwinfield.blogspot.com/2019/04/an-updated-round-up-of-ethical.html. Accessed August 23, 2021.

23. Floridi L. Establishing the rules for building trustworthy AI. Nat Mach Intell 2019. Available at: https://www.nature.com/articles/s42256-019-0055-y.

24. Rotter JB. Generalized expectancies for interpersonal trust. Am Psychol 1971;26(5):443–52.

25. Hawley K. Trust: a very short introduction. Oxford, UK: OUP Oxford; 2012. Available at: https://play.google.com/store/books/details?id=8KTrSrCfhkIC.

26. Covey SR, Merrill RR. The speed of trust: the one thing that changes everything. New York, NY: Simon and Schuster; 2008. Available at: https://play.google.com/store/books/details?id=31Qe_e61Y10C.

27. Kramer RM. Trust and distrust in organizations: emerging perspectives, enduring questions. Annu Rev Psychol 1999;50:569–98.

28. Misztal B. Trust in modern societies: the search for the bases of social order. Hoboken, NJ, USA: John Wiley & Sons; 2013. Available at: https://play.google.com/store/books/details?id=zfIdAAAAQBAJ.

29. Baier A. Trust and antitrust. Ethics 1986;96(2):231–60. Available at: http://www.jstor.org/stable/2381376.

30. Hawley K. Trust, distrust and commitment. Nous 2014;48(1):1–20.

31. Goldberg SC. Trust and reliance 1. In: Oxfordshire, UK: Taylor, Francis Inc, editors. The Routledge handbook of trust and philosophy. Routledge; 2020. p. 97–108.

32. Jones K. Trust as an affective attitude. Ethics 1996;107(1):4–25. Available at: http://www.jstor.org/stable/2382241.

33. Giddens A. The consequences of modernity. Stanford University Press; 1990. Available at: https://play.google.com/store/books/details?id=oU99QgAACAAJ.

34. Evensky J. Adam Smith's theory of moral sentiments: on morals and why they matter to a liberal society of free people and free markets. J Econ Perspect 2005;19(3):109–30.

35. SAE International releases updated visual chart for its "levels of driving automation" standard for self-driving vehicles. Available at: https://www.sae.org/news/press-room/2018/12/sae-international-releases-updated-visual-chart-for-its-%E2%80%9Clevels-of-driving-automation%E2%80%9D-standard-for-self-driving-vehicles. Accessed September 17, 2021.

36. Jaremko JL, Azar M, Bromwich R, et al. Canadian Association of Radiologists (CAR) Artificial Intelligence Working Group. Canadian Association of Radiologists White Paper on Ethical and Legal Issues Related to Artificial Intelligence in Radiology. Can Assoc Radiol J 2019 May;70(2):107–18. https://doi.org/10.1016/j.carj.2019.03.001.

37. Center for Devices, Radiological Health. CADe devices applied to radiology images and device data - 510(k) Sub. Available at: https://www.fda.gov/regulatory-information/search-fda-guidance-documents/computer-assisted-detection-devices-applied-radiology-images-and-radiology-device-data-premarket. Accessed September 17, 2021.

38. Learning from Experience: FDA's treatment of machine learning. 2017. Available at: https://www.mobihealthnews.com/content/learning-experience-fda%E2%80%99s-treatment-machine-learning. Accessed September 17, 2021.

39. Kaur D, Uslu S, Durresi A. Requirements for trustworthy artificial intelligence – a review. In: Barolli L, Li K, Enokido T, et al, editors. Advances in Networked-based information systems. NY, USA: Springer International Publishing; 2021. p. 105–15. https://doi.org/10.1007/978-3-030-57811-4_11.

40. Thiebes S, Lins S, Sunyaev A. Trustworthy artificial intelligence. Electron Mark 2021;31:447–64. Available at: https://link.springer.com/article/10.1007/s12525-020-00441-4.

41. Kohli M, Geis R. Ethics, artificial intelligence, and radiology. J Am Coll Radiol 2018;15(9):1317–9.

42. Beneficial Artificial Intelligence. Harvard Business Review 2019. Available at: https://hbr.org/podcast/2019/06/beneficial-artificial-intelligence. Accessed August 24, 2021.

43. Bærøe K, Miyata-Sturm A, Henden E. How to achieve trustworthy artificial intelligence for health. Bull World Health Organ 2020;98(4):257–62.

44. Gates B. Gates: Trustworthy Computing. Published January 17, 2002. Available at: https://www.wired.com/2002/01/bill-gates-trustworthy-computing/. Accessed August 26, 2021.

45. Vassev E. Safe artificial intelligence and formal methods. In: Leveraging applications of formal methods, verification and validation: foundational techniques. NY, USA: Springer International Publishing; 2016. p. 704–13. https://doi.org/10.1007/978-3-319-47166-2_49.

46. Trustworthy AI. 2020. Available at: https://datascience.columbia.edu/news/2020/trustworthy-ai/. Accessed August 26, 2021.

47. Rajendran JJV, Sinanoglu O, Karri R. Building Trustworthy Systems Using Untrusted Components: A High-Level Synthesis Approach. IEEE Trans Very Large Scale Integr VLSI Syst. 2016;24(9):2946-2959.

48. Ferretti A, Schneider M, Blasimme A. Opening the new data protection black box. Available at: https://www.forbes.com/sites/korihale/2018/05/22/ai. Accessed September 15, 2021.

49. Pesapane F, Volonté C, Codari M, et al. Artificial intelligence as a medical device in radiology: ethical and regulatory issues in Europe and the United States. Insights Imaging 2018;9(5):745–53.

50. Zeiler MD, Fergus R. Visualizing and understanding convolutional networks. arXiv [csCV]. 2013. Available at: http://arxiv.org/abs/1311.2901. Accessed September 15, 2021.

51. Quinn TP, Jacobs S, Senadeera M, et al. The three ghosts of medical AI: can the black-box present deliver? arXiv [csAI]. 2020. Available at: http://arxiv.org/abs/2012.06000. Accessed September 15, 2021.

52. Amann J, Blasimme A, Vayena E, et al. Precise4Q consortium. Explainability for artificial intelligence in healthcare: a multidisciplinary perspective. BMC Med Inform Decis Mak 2020;20(1):310.

53. Obermeyer Z, Powers B, Vogeli C, et al. Dissecting racial bias in an algorithm used to manage the health of populations. Science 2019;366(6464):447–53.

54. Mudgal KS, Das N. The ethical adoption of artificial intelligence in radiology. BJR Open 2020;2(1):20190020.

55. Currie G, Hawk KE, Rohren EM. Ethical principles for the application of artificial intelligence (AI) in nuclear medicine. Eur J Nucl Med Mol Imaging 2020;47(4):748–52.

56. Currie G, Hawk KE. Ethical and legal challenges of artificial intelligence in nuclear medicine. Semin Nucl Med 2020;11. https://doi.org/10.1053/j.semnuclmed.2020.08.001.

57. Geis JR, Brady AP, Wu CC, et al. Ethics of artificial intelligence in radiology: summary of the Joint European and North American Multisociety Statement. Can Assoc Radiol J 2019;70(4):329–34.

58. Knight JC. Safety-critical systems: challenges and directions. In: Proceedings of the 24th International Conference on Software Engineering. ICSE 2002. 25 May 2002:547-550. doi:10.1109/icse.2002.1007998

59. Grant ES. Requirements engineering for safety critical systems: An approach for avionic systems. In: 2016 2nd IEEE International Conference on Computer and Communications (ICCC);Oct. 14-17, 2016:991-995. doi:10.1109/CompComm.2016.7924853

60. Lathrop B. The Inadequacies of the Cybersecurity Information Sharing Act of 2015 in the Age of Artificial Intelligence. Hastings LJ. 2019;71:501.

61. US-FDA-Artificial-Intelligence-and-Machine-Learning-Discussion-Paper.pdf. Available at: https://www.fda.gov/files/medical%20devices/published/US-FDA-

Artificial-Intelligence-and-Machine-Learning-Discussion-Paper.pdf. Accessed September 15, 2021.

62. Zuiderveen Borgesius F. Discrimination, artificial intelligence, and algorithmic decision-making. 2018. Available at: https://pure.uva.nl/ws/files/42473478/32226549.pdf. Accessed August 26, 2021.

63. Fletcher RR, Nakeshimana A, Olubeko O. Addressing fairness, bias, and appropriate use of artificial intelligence and machine learning in global health. Front Artif Intell 2020;3:561802.

64. Odukoya EJ, Kelley T, Madden B, et al. Extending "Beyond Diversity": Culturally Responsive Universal Design Principles for Medical Education. Teach Learn Med. 2021;33(2):109-115.

65. Burt A. How to fight discrimination in AI. Harvard Business Review. 2020. Available at: https://hbr.org/2020/08/how-to-fight-discrimination-in-ai. Accessed August 26, 2021.

66. Allen B, Dreyer K. The role of the ACR Data Science Institute in advancing health equity in radiology. J Am Coll Radiol 2019;16(4 Pt B):644–8.

67. Aiming for truth, fairness, and equity in your company's use of AI. 2021. Available at: https://www.ftc.gov/news-events/blogs/business-blog/2021/04/aiming-truth-fairness-equity-your-companys-use-ai. Accessed September 19, 2021.

68. Friedman CP. A "fundamental theorem" of biomedical informatics. J Am Med Inform Assoc 2009; 16(2):169–70.

69. Health Ethics & Governance. Ethics and governance of artificial intelligence for health. 2021. Available at:https://www.who.int/publications/i/item/9789240029200. . Accessed July 1, 2021.

70. Angehrn Z, Haldna L, Zandvliet AS, et al. Artificial intelligence and machine learning applied at the point of care. Front Pharmacol 2020;11:759.

71. Driving AI adoption: what radiology can learn from self-driving vehicles. Available at: https://www.radiologytoday.net/archive/WebEx0918.shtml. Accessed September 12, 2021.

72. Cassell P. The Giddens reader. London, UK: Macmillan International Higher Education; 1993. Available at:https://play.google.com/store/books/details?id=0kldDwAAQBAJ.

73. Harvey DL. Agency and community: a critical realist paradigm. J Theory Soc Behav 2002;32(2):163–94.

74. HIPAA Journal. 2020 Healthcare data breach report: 25% increase in breaches in 2020. 2021. Available at: https://www.hipaajournal.com/2020-healthcare-data-breach-report-us/. . Accessed August 26, 2021.

75. AI in healthcare: protecting the systems that protect us. Wired. 2020. Available at: https://www.wired.com/brandlab/2020/04/ai-healthcare-protecting-systems-protect-us/. Accessed September 12, 2021.

76. Parker W, Jaremko JL, Cicero M, et al. Canadian Association of Radiologists White Paper on de-identification of medical imaging: part 2, practical considerations. Can Assoc Radiol J 2021;72(1):25–34.

77. Artificial intelligence — Overview of trustworthiness in artificial intelligence. ISO (the International Organization for Standardization). Available at: https://www.iso.org/obp/ui/. Accessed September 12, 2021.

78. Ethically Aligned Design. The IEEE Global Initiative on Ethics of Autonomous and Intelligent Systems. Available at: https://standards.ieee.org/content/dam/ieee-standards/standards/web/documents/other/ead_v1.pdf. Accessed September 15, 2021.

Artificial Intelligence in Medical Imaging and its Impact on the Rare Disease Community: Threats, Challenges and Opportunities

Navid Hasani, BS[a,b], Faraz Farhadi, BS[a],
Michael A. Morris, MD, MS, DABR, DABNM[a,c], Moozhan Nikpanah, MD[a],
Arman Rhamim, PhD, DABSNM[d,e], Yanji Xu, PhD[f], Anne Pariser, MD[f],
Michael T. Collins, MD[g], Ronald M. Summers, MD, PhD[a],
Elizabeth Jones, MD, MPH, MBA[a], Eliot Siegel, MD, FSIIM, FACR[h],
Babak Saboury, MD, MPH, DABR, DABNM[a,c,i,*]

KEY WORDS

• Artificial intelligence • Rare diseases • Positron emission tomography • Medical imaging

KEY POINTS

- Individually Rare, Together Common: Almost 1 in 10 individuals can suffer from one of many rare diseases (RDs).
- The RD community must be recognized and have a seat at the table of AI stakeholders.
- Physicians are expected to be able to diagnose and treat those with common and rare diseases. A similar expectation must be present for AI solutions.
- There is a significant need to recognize the challenge of data imbalance in RDs and to make concerted efforts to provide technical recommendations and guidelines.
- A nationwide RD data repository is an indispensable prerequisite for a fair AI ecosystem.
- The RD community should be protected from any misuses or abuses of AI systems that lead to discrimination.

[a] Department of Radiology and Imaging Sciences, Clinical Center, National Institutes of Health, 9000 Rockville Pike, Building 10, Room 1C455, Bethesda, MD 20892, USA; [b] University of Queensland Faculty of Medicine, Ochsner Clinical School, New Orleans, LA 70121, USA; [c] Department of Computer Science and Electrical Engineering, University of Maryland-Baltimore Country, Baltimore, MD, USA; [d] Department of Radiology, BC Cancer Research Institute, University of British Columbia, 675 West 10th Avenue, Vancouver, British Columbia, V5Z 1L3, Canada; [e] Department of Physics, BC cancer Research Institute, University of British Columbia, Vancouver, British Columbia, Canada; [f] Office of Rare Diseases Research, National Center for Advancing Translational Sciences, National Institutes of Health (NIH), Bethesda, MD 20892, USA; [g] Skeletal Disorders and Mineral Homeostasis Section, National Institute of Dental and Craniofacial Research, National Institutes of Health (NIH), Bethesda, MD, USA; [h] Department of Radiology and Nuclear Medicine, University of Maryland Medical Center, 655 W. Baltimore Street, Baltimore, MD 21201, USA; [i] Department of Radiology, Hospital of the University of Pennsylvania, Philadelphia, PA, USA
* Corresponding author. Department of Radiology and Imaging Sciences, Clinical Center, National Institutes of Health, 9000 Rockville Pike, Building 10, Room 1C455, Bethesda, MD 20892, USA
E-mail address: babak.saboury@nih.gov

PET Clin 17 (2022) 13–29
https://doi.org/10.1016/j.cpet.2021.09.009
1556-8598/22/

INTRODUCTION

Medicine is the art of compassionate care using scientific wisdom and the best available tools. For a physician, each patient is a unique human being, with particular past history and present manifestation. No patient is a "rare patient" or a "common patient"; each patient is a unique human being.

However, modern nosologic taxonomy makes it inevitable to categorize the constellation of clinical findings into specific diseases or syndromes (phenotyping). Here, we group multiple individuals into a specific category. This is a helpful approach because the understanding of the molecular basis of these phenotypic categories enables suitable treatment discovery and implementation. Most of the pharmaceutical treatments are, by design, appropriate for a "group of subjects with a common denominator (specific molecular pathogenesis)".

The cognitive task for clinical medicine includes attentive observation and careful phenotyping of the patients based on their clinical, physical, biochemical, imaging, histopathological, and genetic findings altogether. The result of this process is the appropriate diagnosis. Here is the core of inherent cognitive dissonance: moving between the "unique human-being" and "grouped disease categories"; separation and connectedness at the same time. This paradoxic situation, if unaddressed, manifests itself in a plethora of "diagnostic cognitive biases."[1]

We want each patient to be considered unique and individual and at the same time as connected and included in the appropriate categories as possible. Recognition of a group of diseases as "rare diseases" is an attempt to facilitate the "inclusion" into an appropriate category when it is needed (facilitate the connectedness). Acknowledgment of individual differences and advocacy for "personalized medicine" is an attempt to enable individuation (facilitate uniqueness). These one attempts, albeit seemingly contradictory, are two sides of one reality.

Herein, we will discuss how the issue of "inclusion" could be affected by the advancement of artificial intelligence (AI) in medicine. We intend to show that the interaction between rare diseases (RDs) and AI technology is an impactful event: a potential for dreadful consequences as well as colossal progression and improvement. Which path is our path? It is difficult to predict the future but with active engagement, the future can be invented.

Suboptimal performance of AI technologies in patients with uncommon conditions can significantly hinder the clinical utility and translation of AI medical devices into routine clinical practice.[2] Hence to appropriately incorporate AI into clinical practice, it is an ethical obligation to address opportunities and concerns related to the diagnosis of RD with AI-based molecular imaging. The societal, economic, and health implications of medical AI for patients with RDs can be 2-fold: (1) through the marginalization and exclusion of those with RDs (discrimination by omission) and (2) through blatant or subtle unregulated postdeployment discrimination or malicious uses of AI technologies (discrimination by commission). This paper aims to explore the medical as well as ethical and societal aspects of using RDs-aware AI in the health care system.

Prevalence and Disease Burden

The Orphan Drug Act of 1983[3] classifies a condition as "rare" if it affects fewer than 200,000 people in the United States (**Fig. 1**).[4] RDs are rare when considered individually, yet collectively they are common; they consist of more than 7000 to 10,000 identified conditions[5] influencing more than 350 million people worldwide.[6] The burden and urgency of the problem have also been investigated recently through the cost-of-illness studies conducted by Everylife FDN[7] and Navarrette-Opazoand colleagues[8] which demonstrate large medical and societal expenses as a proxy for unmet medical demands and severity of illness in patients with RDs. RDs encompass a diverse spectrum of conditions, with more than 85% being single-gene disorders and the remainder being rare malignancies, infections, exposures, and polygenic disorders.[9] PET imaging has shown an important role in the diagnosis and management of several RDs including multiple endocrine neoplasias,[10] Von Hippel–Lindau disease,[11] pheochromocytoma and paraganglioma (PPGL),[12] familial carcinoid syndrome,[13] Erdheim–Chester Disease,[14] and Duchenne muscular dystrophy (DMD).[15]

Enigma of Diagnosis

Individuals suffering from RDs often undergo numerous consultations, imaging studies, workups, and are frequently misdiagnosed before the final diagnosis is made[16] – *diagnostic odyssey*. Additionally, this community suffers from sparse and dispersed medical knowledge, resulting in even fewer effective and approved treatment choices.

Physician's familiarity: Maintaining up-to-date knowledge of particular diagnostic criteria for 7000 various RDs poses a unique challenge for many physicians and specialists. The term "diagnostic odyssey" refers to the time of initial disease symptoms until the final diagnosis of RD, encompassing

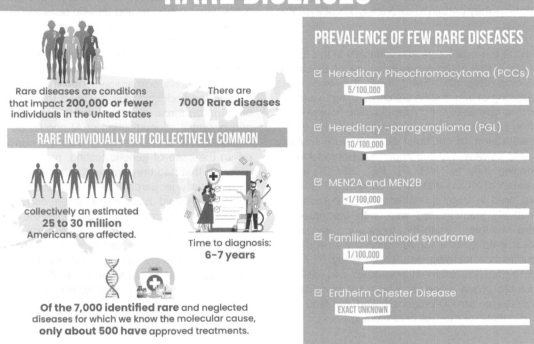

Fig. 1. Individually Rare, Together Common: Statistics related to the epidemiology of RDs and the importance of early diagnosis.

multiple physicians' consults and diagnostic tests.[17] The average living person with *RD endures a 6 to 7 year long diagnostic odyssey in the US.*[18] According to a Belgian survey, the average level of physician awareness regarding RDs is suboptimal.[19] Reportedly, most physicians have the desire to diagnose and treat RDs; however, 40% of general practitioners and 24% of specialists experience a lack of sufficient time to pursue workups necessary to diagnose RD in clinical practice.[20] The situation is made more complicated by the fact that only a small number of clinicians with prior exposure are capable of confirming these rare disorders.

Heterogenous presentation of rare diseases: Another related concern is the heterogeneity of symptoms of each disease and sporadic presentation in the body. These factors lead to underdiagnosis or delayed diagnosis of RD. Even when the patient is suspected of having a RD, there is still a significant chance of misdiagnosis due to overlapping symptoms of many RDs.[21] As a result of these issues, the time-to-diagnosis (TTD) of RDs is significantly prolonged.

A hypothetical solution for this problem, according to Hirsch and colleagues,[22] is a symptom checker mobile application that assesses patient symptoms to compile lists of likely diseases and subsequently gives safe next step advice. An application can provide a list of specialists, genetic testing, remote self-testing, and continuous tele-monitoring of health status, all of which could help lower the TTD of RDs and lower disease burden from this community.[22]

Role of Artificial Intelligence and Medical Imaging

Recent advancements in information technology, particularly machine learning (ML), and AI have shown significant prospects of AI-based medical devices (AIMDs) in diagnosis, management, and pharmaceutical development for various diseases.[23,24] Although these advancements have been less prominent in RDs, AIMDs have demonstrated notable results in several dimensions of common diseases (CDs) diagnosis and prognosis (eg, breast cancers, brain tumors, fractures).[25–27]

One reason for such lack of progress in RDs is the scarcity or heterogeneity of available data on a particular RD. As the success of an AI algorithm is directly correlated with the quality and size of datasets,[28] it is imperative to address these concerns as they pertain to different types of available RD data.

Although text-mining methods may be promising in the near future, the variability in the quality of data, the heterogeneous nature of Electronic Medical Records (EMR), and the incomplete reporting of information are challenging to semantic interoperability.[29,30] *Imaging data*, however, are often standardized, more consistent, and allow the visualization of multiple systems from multiple points of view. We see enormous potential in the imaging data (ie, MR, CT, PET, SPECT) in the training of AI algorithms as images are typically procured in large quantities and processed in a relatively standardized way, with less inter- or intra-observer variability, therefore providing a great data source for AI training.[24] Specifically, multivariate imaging data (Total Body PET (TB-PET)) that are often standardized can visualize multiple organ systems, which are of particular importance for RD diagnosis, and can lend itself particularly well to use in AI training.

Stigma of Diagnosis

Although RD-aware Software-as-a-Medical Device (SaMD) is the first essential step toward better integration of AI in Medicine, our responsibility does not end there and should include the prevention of potential abuses. One must be cognizant of the potential downstream effects and ethical implications of AIMD postdeployment. AIMDs enable continuous and early disease monitoring and detection; while clinically beneficial, this information can be intentionally or unintentionally misused in the context of over-generalizations by health systems, insurance, or even stigmatization against an already vulnerable population.

Similar concerns were raised with the advent of next-generation sequencing (NGS), involving large-scale *whole-exome sequencing (WES) and whole-genome sequencing (WGS)*, which enabled the third-party gathering of large amounts of patient data.[31] Sensitive medical information, when made available to a third party without proper deidentification, could potentially have negative repercussions for a person in terms of future insurance, employment, or health care opportunities. As an example, patient WGS findings have been used by heart and lung transplantation teams to decide whether to list an individual as an organ recipient.[32] Yet, despite the recommendation of the Americans with Disabilities Act (ADA)[33] and Genetic

Information Nondiscrimination Act (GINA)[34] reportedly, many transplant programs across the US continue to be biased and discriminate against those with intellectual and genetic diseases.[35]

Therefore, the issue of data protection and ownership becomes more crucial than ever. It is not far-fetched to assume that many families and patients would have a similar response to AI-based diagnosis or management if they think the results and findings would be used to stigmatize or ostracize them. This foreseeable consequence and potential stigmatization of AI should be disclosed by the team before the testing is conducted. In the case of genetic testing, many families asserted that had they known the results of WGS to potentially jeopardize the transplantation option, they would have never given consent to testing. This argument further supports the notion that the information regarding third-party use of patient data must be a part of the informed consent form. Publicly available informed consent forms can provide substantial benefit and legal protection in court if information is used for discrimination.

RARE DISEASES & ARTIFICIAL INTELLIGENCE OPPORTUNITIES AND CHALLENGES

In this section, we initially explore the bioethics of RDs in AI, and then discuss the reasons why the medical AI industry and the RD community should actively collaborate in this new era of AI in medicine. We begin by outlining the reasons why the AI community should create medical devices that are RD-aware which can diagnose RD with the same accuracy as CDs.

Ethical Considerations Related to Artificial Intelligence-Based Diagnosis and Management of Rare Diseases

a. *Exclusion*: The scarcity of diverse representation in precision medicine and other biomedical research has been a well-known problem.[36] Ethical AI is diverse in its training data and performance outcomes.[37] Lack of inclusion of RDs in AIMDs does not align with bioethical values of *beneficence* and *justice*. For instance, rare genetic variants and uncommon conditions may be overlooked or their association with common, complex diseases can be misinterpreted.[38] The exclusion of patients with RDs at the training stage of the AI system subsequently leads to worse performance due to sampling bias and the absence of generalizability. Additionally, this inclination can create bias in future medical studies conducted based on AI-produced data. To maximize clinical benefits and minimize harm, the SaMD must perform with safety (to prevent injuries and hazards), efficiency (able to effectively solve the problem at a reasonable cost), and equity (that the advantages of the application are shared fairly by all).[39] Thus, the deployment of AI that excludes a subgroup of individuals would diverge from any progress toward the goal of maximizing clinical benefits and addressing health inequities in historically neglected populations.

b. *Stigmatization*: Personal health information (PHI) handled and enhanced by AIMDs must not be used against the patient for insurance, employment, delaying, or denying of medical care.[40] For example, there are differences across transplant programs when it comes to the availability of standards and listing policies for genetic diseases and intellectual disabilities.[35] Confidentiality transgressions with unethical usage of PHI may occur endangering the social fabric of this already disadvantaged community of patients with RDs.

c. *Consent for revealing incidental findings by rare diseases-aware artificial intelligence:* AI can open the door for vast amounts of patient data and sensitive information to play a role in clinical decision making.[41] The chance of incidental findings is inherent in medical imaging studies. Using AI-based detection algorithms can further enhance rates of incidental findings in these studies. The discovery of early signs of RDs could be among incidental findings detected in imaging studies with the assistance of RD-aware detection algorithms. For example, an automatic AI-based whole-body PET/CT ordered for the staging of a tumor can detect a new disease that was not expected at the time of testing. Are we obligated to reveal the new information to the patient? If not, how much information should the clinician reveal to the patient? Revealing the data we did not intend to find to patients has ethical and psychological implications that need to be addressed. Clear communication regarding the use of AI findings is necessary for all patients including those with RDs. This is because the health provider and patients' knowledge of AI capabilities and expectations of use of AI findings may often be different. Regardless of the fact that there is significant discussion regarding what findings should be returned, patients will have vastly diverse experiences based on which physicians and health care professionals they received care from. The same issues were present for NGS.[42] We must learn from the implementation of NGS in clinical practice for the successful translation of AI into precision medicine and RD diagnosis and management.

Why Should the Artificial Intelligence Community Recognize Rare Diseases as One of the Stakeholders?

To achieve the full potential of these technologies and create a sustainable AI ecosystem, AI medical devices should be integrated into an ethical platform that patients and physicians can trust [Navid Hasani and colleagues article, Trustworthy Artificial Intelligence in Medical Imaging, in this issue].[43,44] There are 5 reasons why the AI industry in health care needs to consider the inclusion of RDs:

(1) The Food and Drug Administration (FDA) and the scientific community are aware that the performance of an AI medical device depends on the training data. It is not far-fetched that the effectiveness of an AI trained and evaluated on common conditions will be incapable of use in RDs. Thus, by neglecting RDs at the AI training and development stage, the developer is unable to claim any application of the algorithm for the diagnosis or management of those with RDs.

(2) The RD community is vulnerable and has been historically neglected by researchers, drug developers, medical specialists, and policymakers.[45] There are substantial disease and financial burdens placed on surviving patients diagnosed with an uncommon disease and their families.[46] Therefore, in the era of AI in medicine, it is imperative to use advancements of AI-based medical imaging to appropriately diagnose and manage patients with RDs, minimizing the magnitude of potential harm to this underserved population.[47]

(3) If RDs are neglected and AI is deployed into health care, the potential absence of accurate and consistent RD-related diagnosis may worsen an already devastating situation. This would have significant negative implications for both the RD and the AI community which hinders the society's and medical community's trust in AI. When patients refer to their physician for certain symptoms, they expect an accurate diagnosis. If the physician works with an AI-based medical imaging device system that can assist in the diagnosis of diseases, that device must be accurate in detecting RDs as similarly expected for CDs. Otherwise, when AI encounters an uncommon disorder phenotype it may depict aberrant behavior, categorize the phenotype into a

CD group, or label it as unknown. Diversity in data includes the diversity of ethnic groups, genders, ages, and diseases. In terms of disease diversity in training data, there must be an assorted range of rare and common illnesses that the AIMDs can detect.[48] Inability to do so due to an underrepresentation of uncommon conditions can conceivably induce biases in the performance and evaluation of disease burden.[49] AI developers must be aware of such biases to avoid potential AI-induced discrimination further widening the health disparity gap.[50]

(4) As sustainable growth of AI in society needs the definition of trustworthiness, it is ethical and obligatory to consider RDs. The advent of AI tools and their associated abilities have created a new *ethical* and *social obligation* for intelligent interventions that, if leveraged appropriately, can significantly improve RD-related diagnosis, treatment, and patient support systems. Suboptimal performance of an AI diagnostic tool that disproportionately impacts the RD community would substantially limit translation to clinical practice as well as trustworthiness of AIMDs in health care.[22]

(5) The inclusion of RDs and data diversity Improves the robustness of AI systems and their utility in a variety of clinical settings. Enhanced performance of such systems contributes to a more diverse market, hence more profitable for AI developers. Therefore, the financial and social advantages of accurate and successful AI medical devices would be beneficial for the AI community and developers. Furthermore, studying and gathering data on RDs can provide insights into the intricacies of biological mechanisms underlying many CDs which can be leveraged by the developers to further improve the performance and robustness of future AIMDs.

Why Should the Rare Disease Community Want to Be an Active Stakeholder in the New Era of Artificial Intelligence in Medicine?

Now, let us examine this from the perspective of the RD community and patient advocacy groups. Patients with RDs confront a number of significant challenges: late diagnosis and misdiagnosis, limited disease-modifying therapies, proper response to therapies, valid monitoring tools as well as little private-sector R&D and public health prioritization due to a low number of diagnosed patients in each disease category.[51–53] The power of AI can be used to address these obstacles. As such, the implications of AI in health care are

critical for RD diagnosis and management. This period can be the best or the worst of times for RDs diagnosis and management.

There are great opportunities for the inclusion of RD data into AI-based diagnostic tools, especially considering the growing complexity of medical data (*Big Data*)[54] and advancements in deep learning. AI tools can analyze and learn from large and complex datasets for quantitative assessment purposes[55] such as using PET for objective detection and characterization of neuroendocrine tumors.[56] AI-based decision support systems may be developed to assist clinicians in their differential diagnosis of RD.[21] Other algorithms can assist in therapeutic research and development (i.e. *human-on-a-chip* or *clinical-trial-on-a-chip*).[57,58] Recent AI research in meta-learning has demonstrated unprecedented success in training AI with limited data (to mimic the scenario for RD) using discriminative ensemble learning, fast few-shot transfer learning, and generalized zero shot learning (ZSL) for chest X-ray diagnosis.[59–61] **Table 1** provides a short list of examples of how ML and AI algorithms are currently being used to further advance RD screening, treatment, and research.

At the same time, most efforts in the era of AI in medicine are focused on advancing CD diagnosis and management, neglecting the inclusion of RDs. This is an essential detail because, at a time whereby AIMDs are progressively developed and incorporated into clinical practice, we must highlight the maleficence of using AIMDs not capable of detecting RDs as accurately as CDs. As such, the deployment of AI tools into clinical practice could bear detrimental impacts on patients with undiagnosed RDs. Considering the *automation bias* associated with AI in health care, reliance on AI systems incompatible with RDs may promote misdiagnosis or *prolong the TTD* for undiagnosed patients with RDs.[70] A prolonged TTD not only exacerbates suffering but also can lead to further financial and health debilitation of patients and families.[16]

HOW TO ENABLE THE DEVELOPMENT AND IMPLEMENTATION OF RARE DISEASES-AWARE ARTIFICIAL INTELLIGENCE SOLUTIONS
Outreach and Collaboration with all Stakeholders

In a sustainable AI ecosystem, active collaboration exists between all stakeholders throughout the lifecycle of AIMDs. The recognition and inclusion of RD patient advocacy groups (PAGs) in the circle of stakeholders are important and must be

Table 1
Tangible examples of AI improving RD diagnosis and management

Title	Description
Symptoms checker website	AI-based applications allow patients or physicians to input presenting symptoms to determine the probabilistic differential diagnosis based on various RD databases.[62]
RD diagnosis support using facial features	Gurovich and colleagues[63] proposed a novel facial recognition algorithm called DeepGestalt, powered by FDNA inc., that classifies distinct facial features from photos of individuals with rare neurodevelopmental and congenital disorders. The phenotypic analysis algorithm is trained on 100,000 images and can distinguish between 200 different rare syndromes achieving 91% accuracy in identifying the correct diagnosis in the top 10 suggestions.[63]
AI for RD drug repurposing	Lee and colleagues[121] used the URSAHD (unveiling RNA sample annotation for human diseases) machine learning framework to apply genetic and molecular information from hundreds of complicated conditions to medication repurposing. Similarly, Ekins and colleagues created an end-to-end ML algorithm that leverages [64] large quantities of screening data to predict bioactivities for therapeutic targets and molecular properties with increased levels of accuracy.
AI-based genetic devices	The ML algorithm "Xrare" proposed by Li and colleagues[65] jointly uses phenotypic and genetic evidence for the identification of causative gene variants in RDs and the prioritization of these diagnoses.
AI-based Human-on-a-chip and Clinical-Trial on-a-Chip drug development	Almost 95% of RDs do not have an approved treatment option [66]. Recent AI systems have shown great promise in promoting drug development or repurposing of available therapeutics. For example, the human-on-a-chip (HoaC) or organ-on-a-chip[58,67] is a novel CNN-based model that mimics human organ functionality in interconnected in-vitro bioengineered micro-physiological systems. This medical imaging technology can recapitulate clinical trials on a chip (CToCs)[68] lowering the costs and recruitment barriers related to conducting RD clinical trials (scarce number of RD patients)[57]. This technology promotes research and development of novel PET radioactive tracers for tumor detection and treatment by introducing human phenotypic models early in the drug discovery process.
AI and PET Enables Orphan Drug Development	AI-based PET kinetic modelings have the potential to yield valuable data regarding the pharmacokinetics of investigational pharmaceuticals with a small number of participants.

(continued on next page)

Table 1
(continued)

Title	Description
Radiophenomics: AI-based medical imaging for recognition of rare disease manifestation	TB-PET powered with AI capabilities has enormous potential to identify imaging patterns suggestive of rare diseases phenotypes. Therefore, using image-based phenotyping (radiophenomics) the AI can suggest a possibility of a rare disease pattern to the physician.
AI-based medical imaging management of rare diseases	Pretest probability is the likelihood of having a condition before the results of a diagnostic test are known[69]. AI algorithms can be trained to understand the pre-test probability and incorporate it into screening and management in individuals with rare diseases. The accuracy of the probability scale generated by AI and the ideal threshold used on the image may vary depending on the pre-test probability.

enforced by appropriate regulatory committees. Stakeholders involved and affected (directly or indirectly) throughout the lifecycle of AI include patients, physicians, and all the relevant providers, health care systems, payors, regulatory agencies, professional societies, and patient groups. Inclusive, transparent, and active engagement of these stakeholders throughout the development, design, and postdeployment surveillance of AI systems is needed. Patient advocacy groups specific to each RD are trusted by patients and physicians and can provide substantial assistance in building trust in using AI to diagnose RDs. By active engagement, RD patient leaders and PAGs can communicate concerns related to denying or delaying health care services through discussions with stakeholders and regulatory agencies.

There must be clear and continuous outreach efforts to educate patients regarding AI advancements in RD diagnosis and treatments.[71] Grass-root organizations should educate the RD community and patients on the challenges and opportunities of AI-based RD diagnostic tools while building trust and helping to identify inappropriate adoption of AI in health care. Patient advocacy groups can be used as a liaison between the needs of patients with RDs, physicians, and the AI development industry.

To further advance the utility of AI tools in health care, continuous medical education is necessary. Such efforts directed toward medical professionals can facilitate the timely diagnosis and treatment of patients with RDs in outpatient and inpatient settings.[72] Clinicians should be able to maintain a baseline knowledge of RDs and keep up to date with new treatments and diagnostic tools. PAGs and organizations can convey the current state of art AI-based RD diagnosis to physicians and request that knowledge is transferred from physicians to the patients.

The National Organization of Rare Diseases (NORD), Genetic Alliance (GA), the Chan Zuckerberg Initiative[73] are instrumental in increasing the capacity of RD patient groups, issuing policies, and incentivizing industry for more efforts toward diagnosis and treatment of RDs.[72,74] NORD now consists of more than 2000 and the GA more than 600 patient advocacy organizations.[75,76] In addition to advocating for RD, these organizations can also collaborate with developers and physicians to raise awareness for AI-based diagnosis and strategies to apply AI powers to use the limited amount of available data to better treat RDs.

Rare Diseases Data Meta-Repositories

The ability of AI technologies to integrate and analyze data from different structured and unstructured sources (eg, radiomics, patient registries, anecdotal evidence, genetic variation, and molecular profiling)[77,78] can be used to overcome RD data challenges (eg, low diagnostic rates, limited number of patients in each RD category, geographic dispersion, and heterogenous clinical presentation). Nevertheless, there is a lack of central RD data repositories for AI training.[23] Although there are specialized repositories in existence, such as The Cancer Imaging Archive (TCIA),[79] it is vital to further expand the availability of similar datasets for RD and link different types of data together for each patient.

Sharing of anonymized health data sets enables a deeper and broader understanding of the nature of RD and affected patient populations.[80] The move toward "Big Data" provides substantial evidence for advancing model training and tuning, shortening the TTD, clinical outcomes, as well as the development of treatments for RDs.[81] Patients are often supportive of safe and transparent sharing of their anonymized electronic health records (EHR) for research.[82] Consenting to PHI sharing, as Figueiredo states, may also be a method of repaying society's investment in science through public-funded research or charity.[83] To this end, it is a *social responsibility* of public institutions, private centers, schools, hospitals, etc. to share their high-quality, exquisitely curated, privacy-preserved diverse health and consumer data on patients with RDs for curating a central RD and CD data repository for AI training and testing. Professional societies (e.g. Society of Nuclear Medicine and Molecular Imaging (SNMMI), Society of Imaging Informatics in Medicine (SIIM), Radiological Society of North America (RSNA), and American Medical Informatics Association (AMIA), among others) can help address institutional *barriers to data sharing* and act as a liaison between stakeholders and associated organizations.

The National Institutes of Health (*NIH*) are also committed to providing long and short-term support to the RD community and to promoting AI research in areas whereby there may otherwise be insufficient attention or action.[84] To achieve this goal, *NORD* and the Rare Disease Clinical Research Network (RDCRN)[85] at the National Center for Advancing Translational Sciences (NCATS) have curated RD registries that are available for patients, researchers, and clinicians.[86] Such registries not only facilitate communication between health care professionals, patients, and the multidisciplinary team but also highlight critical aspects of data quality, governance, and access.[77]

Rare Diseases Awareness at Artificial Intelligence Conceptualization/Development Stage

It is of utmost importance for RDs to be considered in all stages of model and decision support system development. Specifically, RD awareness at the design stage relates to the inclusion of RDs alongside CDs in datasets used for model training, validation, and testing of performance. The model should be able to categorize each disease pattern into a certain identified rare or CD pattern. For example, the AI-based imaging device should be able to perform a classification task related to RD and CD identification with reasonable accuracy and precision. For an AI-based imaging device, RD categories must be included in image recognition, annotation of radiomics, disease ranking, diagnosis, and prediction. To accomplish this, the diversity of RD and CD patterns must be included in the derivation and validation of AI models. This conceptualization minimizes chances that a rare event or incidence triggers either an *aberrant error*, is misplaced into a CD category based on resemblance, or is identified as an unknown pattern.

Class imbalance

Inductive approaches are employed in computational phenotyping algorithms to find correlations or patterns within datasets. The diagnostic accuracy and informative value of the resulting phenotyping tools are determined by the amount, variety, and accuracy of data used in model training and testing.[87] As a result, creating a representative database for algorithm training is critical to the effectiveness of computational phenotyping in RDs.[88] However, inherent to RDs, available sample sizes for the training of algorithms are often limited. This leads to class imbalance issues. Through multi-institutional collaborations (direct sharing of data and/or use of federated learning), physicians and scientists should make efforts to address this limitation. In any case, even with much needed concerted efforts, class imbalance problems are likely to persist.

To tackle this, first, we note that poor performances in class imbalance problems can be hidden if limited metrics are used for assessment; for example, for an AI algorithm that performs poorly at detecting a rare minority class, overall area-under-the-receiver-operator-characteristic-curve (AUC ROC), accuracy or specificity used as metrics may still show excellent performances ("the accuracy paradox"), due to the dominance of the majority class (e.g. healthy patients or CD). As such, a range of evaluation metrics especially those de-emphasizing true negatives (i.e. correctly classified majority class) should be reported such as recall, precision, F1 score, false-discovery rate, and the area-under-the-precision-recall-curve (AUC PR)[89] to better reveal poor performances of AI algorithms in class imbalanced datasets.

To tackle poor performances in class-imbalanced problems, computational methods including majority class undersampling and/or minority class oversampling/data augmentation can be invoked (e.g. SMOTE,[90] ADASYN[91]). In particular, data augmentation can be performed on the training data to increase the size of datasets and limit overfitting. Conventional techniques of image transformations can be used such as rotating, cropping, and zooming.[92] Additionally, AI itself might be capable of providing solutions to this matter; for example, using Generative Adversarial Networks (GANs) as used in many disciplines to generate new, synthetic instances of data that can pass for real data[93] and used for data augmentation purposes.[94] Use of AI-based Style Transfer[95] for data augmentation can also be further explored.

Instead of augmenting/manipulating the datasets directly, it is also possible to use other techniques that enhance the overall model architecture, making it more suited for a class-imbalanced problem. Some of these include using weighted loss functions such as the focal loss[96] that gives different weights for calculating the loss values related to the majority and the minority classes or using penalized models such as cost-sensitive support vector machine (SVM)[97] with inbuilt hyperparameters that can be weighted as per the importance of each class (with the minority class getting more weight). Certain other techniques such as anomaly detection[98] attempt to solve this issue by redefining the class-imbalance problem (i.e. with a majority and a minority class) into a problem of outlier/novelty detection (with the minority class being the outlier/novelty) in a normal (majority class) dataset.

To this end, while training an AI algorithm, the prevalence and/or importance of RD can be further enhanced (as discussed above), enabling the derivation of AI models that are effective in detecting common conditions as well as uncommon diseases. This approach is similar to the expectation that exists in medical education, including board certification examinations, to train physicians that are capable of diagnosing and treating patients with CDs as well as RDs. Therefore, it is critical to recognize this challenge and to make active efforts to provide technical best practice recommendations and guidelines.

Oversight and Regulation

Appropriate development and deployment of AI-based medical tools necessitate continuous ethics, safety, and performance assessment by objective oversight and evaluation frameworks that are inclusive of RDs. At this exciting transitional stage, whereby AI is increasingly used in health care across the world, there are numerous opportunities compounded with AI governance difficulties.[99] The federal and local policies are often not able to keep up with the exponential growth of AI technology in health care. For this reason, a regulatory agency or public organization can ensure the proper implementation of AI-aware policies for RD diagnosis and treatment. The creation of legislation may potentially follow an industrial and political complex path[100] and must address the collective needs of patients with RDs. In regard to the US, the regulation of drugs, biologics, and devices are predominantly overseen by the FDA.[44]

One aspect of regulation for RD-aware AI entails inclusivity monitoring, which can be conducted either by the FDA or an independent professional credentialing organization similar to the certification and recertification of medical professionals. The regulatory body should ensure the generalizability of the AI to all patients suffering from a particular condition regardless of extraneous personal characteristics. Individuals who are underrepresented or suffer from RDs should not be excluded from the creation, assessment, and deployment stages of AI systems. Appropriate validation testing on standardized sets that include a diverse patient population, including rare or unusual presentation of disease, is critical to assess for the presence of bias in results.[37,48] More specifically, the oversight must include the assessment of performance that is, equitable, diverse, and includes relevant CDs and RDs. To achieve this goal, oversight can enforce and monitor the safety, security, ethics of SaMDs at every stage of conceptualization, development, and deployment.[88,99]

Another highly important regulatory aspect pertains to information security and the nondiscriminatory use of AI for RD diagnosis and management. If AI-based medical imaging systems improve the diagnostic capabilities for RDs, the knowledge of this RD cannot be used by third parties to pose potential health, financial, or societal harm (stigmatization) toward the individual. Thus, the implementation of AI systems in health care will require a recalibration of confidentiality and other core tenets of professional ethics. As discussed previously, gathering more complex medical information on patients with RDs require legal protection against unintended harm (i.e. available informed consent forms). Due to the novelty of AI in medicine, there have not been many legal cases against AI, however, predictably, potential unintended discrimination and stigmatization can happen as the result of widespread AI use in medicine. Patients with RDs are even more prone to discrimination and have been previously neglected care and treatment due to their illnesses or survival rates. Medical programs and health institutions should rethink their strategy, ensuring individualized evaluations and preventing the exclusion of patients based on their RD group membership.[35] Additionally, AI-based diagnosis of a RD and associated data should not be used to discriminate against this group or deny or delay care. We need to create legal protections for vulnerable populations including those with diagnosed RDs. Acknowledgment and adoption of policies similar to the Genetic Information Nondiscrimination Act (GINA)[101] that prohibits discrimination by health insurance and employers for information for medical AI may be imperative if we are to prevent harm before the deployment of AI for the management and diagnosis of RDs.

EMERGING APPLICATIONS OF ARTIFICIAL INTELLIGENCE IN MOLECULAR IMAGING OF RARE DISEASES
Synergism of Artificial Intelligence and Positron Emission Tomography to Accelerate Orphan Drug Development

Less is different
Orphan drug development is not merely drug development on a smaller scale. The challenges are not just the limited market.[102] Here, *less is different*. Considering the limited number of affected individuals eligible for clinical trials, translation of preclinical targets to clinical phase studies requires extra care (*precise translation*).[103] Drug development, in general, benefits from AI for more successful target selection[104] as less than 9% of investigational drugs entering phase 1 clinical trials reach the FDA approval.[105] For CDs, this is an improvement but for RDs, it is essential: population-based data for physiologically based pharmacokinetic modeling might be insufficient and the limited number of eligible candidates makes the pharmacokinetic estimations more prone to error due to smaller sample size and sparse data. AI-based PET kinetic modelings have the potential to produce valuable data regarding the pharmacokinetics of the investigational drugs with a limited number of subjects by the implementation of TB-PET dynamic imaging (**Figs. 2 and 3**).[106] The depth of such information in addition to AI-augmented pharmacochemistry provides a platform for nuanced structural fine-tuning of the selected target.[107] In summary, advanced computational techniques in systems biology and multi-scale modeling in addition to the novel technology of dynamic TB-PET imaging and AI-empowered complex systems modeling can aid in the creation of virtual replicates of patients, also known as digital twins.[78,108]

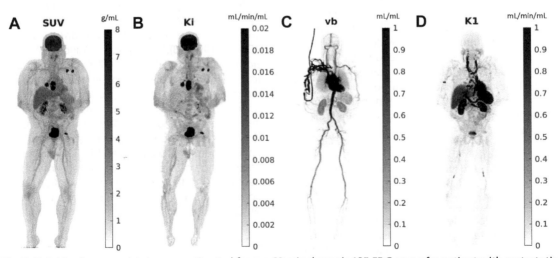

Fig. 2. Total-body parametric images estimated from a 60-min dynamic 18F-FDG scan of a patient with metastatic cancer on the uEXPLORER: (*A*) SUV, (*B*) FDG net influx rate Ki, (*C*) fractional blood volume vb, and (*D*) FDG delivery rate K1. (*From* Wang Y, Li E, Cherry SR, Wang G. Total-Body PET Kinetic Modeling and Potential Opportunities Using Deep Learning. PET Clinics. 2021;16(4):613 to 625.: with permission.)

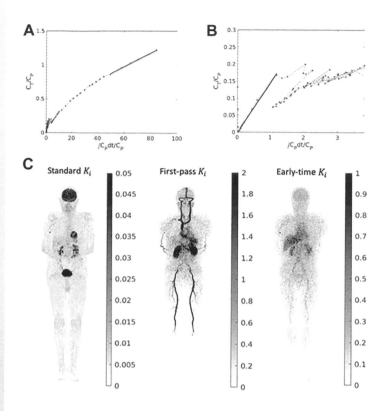

Fig. 3. High-temporal resolution Patlak plot and parametric imaging.30 (*A*) Patlak plot of 1-h dynamic FDG data; (*B*) zoom-in of the first 2- min data; (*C*) parametric images of the slope at 3 different phases—standard Ki (30–60 minutes), first-pass Ki (20–30 s), and early-time Ki (1–2 minutes). Shown are the MIP images. The unit of Ki is mL/min/mL. (*From* Wang Y, Li E, Cherry SR, Wang G. Total-Body PET Kinetic Modeling and Potential Opportunities Using Deep Learning. PET Clinics. 2021;16(4):613 to 625.: with permission.)

Diagnosis of Rare Diseases with Artificial Intelligence and Molecular Imaging- Can We Shorten the Diagnostic Odyssey?

The multi-regional nature of routine PET images (from the base of skull and neck, through chest, abdomen, and pelvis to the upper aspect of thighs) provides comprehensive coverage to combine various imaging findings in many organs and assemble a multi-regional multi-organ pathology profile. Such information is invaluable for image-based phenotyping (radiophenomics). A simple suggestion by the AI software can remind the nuclear medicine physician of a possibility of a RD pattern and this may trigger a further investigation if deemed appropriate based on other clinical findings.

Artificial Intelligence-Based Positron Emission Tomography Solutions for Management of Patients with Rare Diseases

It is crucial to develop RD-specific AI algorithms that understand the *pre-test probability* of screening and diagnosis in patients with RDs. For instance, as a medical imaging physician is reviewing an imaging study of a patient with MEN2A syndrome, abnormal adrenal gland findings could be more for an adrenal malignancy. AI algorithms should be developed to use radiomics information to incorporate such clinical information pertinent to the management of patients with RDs.[109] Both the accuracy of the probability scale (i.e. 70% chance of MEN2A) and the optimal threshold that is applied to the image may vary based on the pretest probability.

PET is an important imaging modality in management of patients with RDs,[110–112] such as multiple endocrine neoplasia syndromes (MEN1, MEN2A, MEN2B),[113] tumoral calcinosis,[114] Von-Hippel Lindau (VHL),[115] familial carcinoid syndrome,[116] metastatic pheochromocytoma, and paraganglioma,[117] hemangioendothelioma, and other hereditary cancer syndromes.[118] Appropriately employing the capabilities of AI in conjunction with PET could improve monitoring and management of RDs. AI-based PET models have already shown to be capable of performing segmentation, detection, and classification tasks more objectively and efficiently than expert clinicians.[119,120,121]

SUMMARY

If applied properly, AI-based Positron Emission Tomography (PET) has enormous potential to revolutionize the detection and management of RDs, particularly considering the richness of data in emerging TB-PET.[122,123] However, the RDs community and stakeholders must be recognized and present at the table of AI stakeholders. A national archive of RD data is a necessary precondition for a just AI environment. AI medical systems should provide a clear notice stating that any differential diagnostic support system may miss some RDs, if not appropriately trained and validated. There should be technical guidelines on data augmentation for AI training, including a greater proportion of RD data in training sets than is currently the case. The RD community should be safeguarded against any exploitation or abuse of AI systems that result in discrimination toward those living with these conditions. This could be accomplished in a variety of ways, including teaching medical/scientific communities' ethical leaders about the critical nature of RD inclusion, as well as through regulatory mandates.

CLINICS CARE POINTS

- Medicine is the art of compassionate care using scientific wisdom and the best available tools. AI medical devices (AIMDs) are among those tools. It is the responsibility of physicians and healthcare system to understand the beneficial uses and dangerous misuses of this new technology, particularly in relation to the rare disease community.

- If the performance of AIMDs is not evaluated in rare diseases carefully, there might be an ethical obligation to disclose the potential harms (for example, the device could have a clear disclaimer stating that some RDs may be missed in the differential diagnosis support system).

- The rare disease community should be recognized as a stakeholder in the lifecycle of AIMDs and they should be involved in all phases of development, deployment, and oversight.

- AI solutions for RD patients could be actualized through sustainable cooperation among all stakeholders (from creation of data metarepositories, to social awareness at all phases of development and implementation).

ACKNOWLEDGMENTS AND DISCLOSURES

This research was supported in part by the Intramural Research Program of the NIH, Clinical Center. The opinions expressed in this publication are the author's own and do not reflect the view of the National Institutes of Health, the Department of Health and Human Services, or the United States government.

The authors acknowledge valuable feedback by Shadab Ahamed on the class imbalance problem. The authors acknowledge and thank Dr. David Magnus for his contributions.

REFERENCES

1. Kwok ESH, Calder LA, Barlow-Krelina E, et al. Implementation of a structured hospital-wide morbidity and mortality rounds model. BMJ Qual Saf 2017;26(6):439–48.

2. Sharma N, Aggarwal LM. Automated medical image segmentation techniques. J Med Phys 2010; 35(1):3–14.

3. Act C. Orphan drug act of 1983. Public L 1983;97: 414. Available at: https://www.fda.gov/media/99546/download.

4. Office of the Commissioner. Rare diseases at FDA. Available at: https://www.fda.gov/patients/rare-diseases-fda. Accessed July 6, 2021.

5. Ekins S. Industrializing rare disease therapy discovery and development. Nat Biotechnol 2017; 35(2):117–8.

6. RARE facts. Available at: https://globalgenes.org/rare-facts/. Accessed July 6, 2021.

7. Burden of Rare Disease Study - EveryLife Foundation for Rare Diseases. Available at: https://everylifefoundation.org/burden-study/. Accessed September 18, 2021.

8. Navarrete-Opazo AA, Singh M, Tisdale A, et al. Can you hear us now? The impact of health-care utilization by rare disease patients in the United States. Genet Med 2021. https://doi.org/10.1038/s41436-021-01241-7.

9. FAQs about rare diseases. Available at: https://rarediseases.info.nih.gov/diseases/pages/31/faqs-about-rare-diseases. Accessed September 18, 2021.

10. Multiple endocrine neoplasia type 1 - NORD (national organization for rare disorders). 2015. Available at: https://rarediseases.org/rare-diseases/multiple-endocrine-neoplasia-type-1/. Accessed July 21, 2021.

11. Von Hippel-Lindau Disease - NORD (National Organization for Rare Disorders). 2015. Available at: https://rarediseases.org/rare-diseases/von-hippel-lindau-disease/. Accessed July 21, 2021.

12. Pheochromocytoma - NORD (National Organization for Rare Disorders). 2015. Available at: https://rarediseases.org/rare-diseases/pheochromocytoma/. Accessed July 21, 2021.

13. Carcinoid syndrome - NORD (national organization for rare disorders). 2015. Available at: https://

rarediseases.org/rare-diseases/carcinoid-syndrome/
. Accessed July 21, 2021.

14. Erdheim Chester Disease - NORD (National Organization for Rare Disorders). 2015. Available at: https://rarediseases.org/rare-diseases/erdheim-chester-disease/. Accessed July 22, 2021.

15. Duchenne muscular dystrophy - NORD (national organization for rare disorders). 2015. Available at: https://rarediseases.org/rare-diseases/duchenne-muscular-dystrophy/. Accessed July 21, 2021.

16. Black N, Martineau F, Manacorda T. Diagnostic odyssey for rare diseases: exploration of potential indicators. Available at: https://piru.ac.uk/assets/files/Rare%20diseases%20Final%20report.pdf. Accessed July 7, 2021.

17. Contributer G. The rare disease diagnostic odyssey: a medical student's perspective. Available at: https://www.findacure.org.uk/2018/07/06/the-rare-disease-diagnostic-odyssey-a-medical-students-perspective/. Accessed July 6, 2021.

18. The Lancet Diabetes Endocrinology. Spotlight on rare diseases. Lancet Diabetes Endocrinol 2019; 7(2):75.

19. Vandeborne L, van Overbeeke E, Dooms M, et al. Information needs of physicians regarding the diagnosis of rare diseases: a questionnaire-based study in Belgium. Orphanet J Rare Dis 2019;14(1).99.

20. Hempel H. Accurate diagnosis of rare diseases remains difficult despite strong physician interest. 2014. Available at: https://globalgenes.org/2014/03/06/accurate-diagnosis-of-rare-diseases-remains-difficult-despite-strong-physician-interest/. Accessed July 22, 2021.

21. Alves R, Piñol M, Vilaplana J, et al. Computer-assisted initial diagnosis of rare diseases. PeerJ 2016;4: e2211. https://doi.org/10.7717/peerj.2211.

22. Hirsch MC, Ronicke S, Krusche M, et al. Rare diseases 2030: how augmented AI will support diagnosis and treatment of rare diseases in the future. Ann Rheum Dis 2020;79(6):740–3.

23. Brasil S, Pascoal C, Francisco R, et al. Artificial intelligence (AI) in rare diseases: is the future Brighter? Genes 2019;10(12). https://doi.org/10.3390/genes10120978.

24. Schaefer J, Lehne M, Schepers J, et al. The use of machine learning in rare diseases: a scoping review. Orphanet J Rare Dis 2020;15(1):145.

25. Becker AS, Marcon M, Ghafoor S, et al. Deep learning in mammography: diagnostic accuracy of a multipurpose image analysis software in the detection of breast cancer. Invest Radiol 2017;52(7):434–40.

26. Comelli A, Stefano A, Russo G, et al. A smart and operator independent system to delineate tumours in positron emission tomography scans. Comput Biol Med 2018;102:1–15.

27. Kijowski R, Liu F, Caliva F, et al. Deep learning for lesion detection, progression, and prediction of musculoskeletal disease. J Magn Reson Imaging 2020;52(6):1607–19.

28. Cortes C, Jackel LD. Limits on learning machine accuracy imposed by data quality. Available at: https://www.aaai.org/Papers/KDD/1995/KDD95-007.pdf. Accessed July 19, 2021.

29. Shinozaki A. Electronic medical records and machine learning in approaches to drug development. In: Cassidy JW, Taylor B, editors. Artificial intelligence in Oncology drug discovery and development. IntechOpen; 2020. https://doi.org/10.5772/intechopen.92613.

30. Sachdeva S, Bhalla S. Semantic interoperability in standardized electronic health record databases. J Data Inf Qual 2012;3(1):1–37.

31. Martinez-Martin N, Magnus D. Privacy and ethical challenges in next-generation sequencing. Expert Rev Precis Med Drug Dev 2019;4(2):95–104.

32. Char DS, Lázaro-Muñoz G, Barnes A, et al. Genomic contraindications for heart transplantation. Pediatrics 2017;139(4). https://doi.org/10.1542/peds.2016-3471.

33. A guide to disability rights laws. Available at: https://www.ada.gov/cguide.htm. Accessed July 24, 2021.

34. Genetic discrimination. Available at: https://www.genome.gov/about-genomics/policy-issues/Genetic-Discrimination. Accessed September 18, 2021.

35. Wall A, Lee GH, Maldonado J, et al. Genetic disease and intellectual disability as contraindications to transplant listing in the United States: a survey of heart, kidney, liver, and lung transplant programs. Pediatr Transpl 2020;24(7):e13837.

36. Lee SS-J, Fullerton SM, Saperstein A, et al. Ethics of inclusion: cultivate trust in precision medicine. Science 2019;364(6444):941–2.

37. Kuhlman C, Jackson L, Chunara R. No computation without representation: avoiding data and algorithm biases through diversity. Available at: http://arxiv.org/abs/2002.11836. Accessed September 10, 2021.

38. Burke W, Edwards KA, Goering S, et al. Achieving justice in genomic translation: re-thinking the pathway to benefit. Oxford University Press; 2011. Available at: https://play.google.com/store/books/details?id=KA5pAgAAQBAJ.

39. Lewis ACF. Where bioethics meets machine ethics. Am J Bioeth 2020;20(11):22–4.

40. Burgart AM, Magnus D, Tabor HK, et al. Ethical challenges confronted when providing nusinersen treatment for spinal muscular atrophy. JAMA Pediatr 2018;172(2):188–92.

41. Chiruvella V, Guddati AK. Ethical issues in patient data ownership. Interact J Med Res 2021;10(2): e22269.

42. Milner LC, Garrison NA, Cho MK, et al. Genomics in the clinic: ethical and policy challenges in clinical next-

generation sequencing programs at early adopter USA institutions. Per Med 2015;12(3):269–82.

43. Cutillo CM, Sharma KR, Foschini L, et al. Machine intelligence in healthcare-perspectives on trustworthiness, explainability, usability, and transparency. NPJ Digit Med 2020;3:47.

44. Pesapane F, Volonté C, Codari M, et al. Artificial intelligence as a medical device in radiology: ethical and regulatory issues in Europe and the United States. Insights Imaging 2018;9(5):745–53.

45. Institute of Medicine. Board on health sciences policy, committee on Accelerating rare diseases research and orphan Product development. Rare diseases and orphan Products: Accelerating research and development. National Academies Press; 2011. Available at: https://play.google.com/store/books/details?id=HnYyeNIY3WwC.

46. Groft SC, Posada M, Taruscio D. Progress, challenges and global approaches to rare diseases. Acta Paediatr 2021;9. https://doi.org/10.1111/apa.15974.

47. Valdez R, Ouyang L, Bolen J. Public health and rare diseases: Oxymoron No more. Prev Chronic Dis 2016;13:E05.

48. Allen B, Dreyer K. The role of the ACR data science Institute in advancing health equity in radiology. J Am Coll Radiol 2019;16(4 Pt B):644–8.

49. Zou J, Schiebinger L. Ensuring that biomedical AI benefits diverse populations. EBioMedicine 2021; 67:103358.

50. Fletcher RR, Nakeshimana A, Olubeko O. Addressing fairness, bias, and appropriate use of artificial intelligence and machine learning in global health. Front Artif Intell 2020;3:561802.

51. Hurvitz N, Azmanov H, Kesler A, et al. Establishing a second-generation artificial intelligence-based system for improving diagnosis, treatment, and monitoring of patients with rare diseases. Eur J Hum Genet 2021; 19. https://doi.org/10.1038/s41431-021-00928-4.

52. Juth N. For the Sake of Justice: should We prioritize rare diseases? Health Care Anal 2017;25(1):1–20.

53. Scherman D. The dynamic and urgent path of rare disease and orphan drug research. Rare Dis Orphan Drugs J. Published online 2021. doi: 10.20517/rdodj.2021.01

54. Morris MA, Saboury B, Burkett B, et al. Reinventing radiology: big data and the future of medical imaging. J Thorac Imaging 2018;33(1):4–16.

55. Hosny A, Parmar C, Quackenbush J, et al. Artificial intelligence in radiology. Nat Rev Cancer 2018; 18(8):500–10.

56. Pirasteh A, Riedl C, Mayerhoefer ME, et al. PET/MRI for neuroendocrine tumors: a match made in heaven or just another hype? Clin Transl Imaging 2019;7(6):405–13.

57. Blumenrath SH, Lee BY, Low L, et al. Tackling rare diseases: clinical trials on chips. Exp Biol Med 2020;245(13):1155–62.

58. de Mello CPP, Rumsey J, Slaughter V, et al. A human-on-a-chip approach to tackling rare diseases. Drug Discov Today 2019;24(11):2139–51.

59. Paul A, Shen TC, Lee S, et al. Generalized Zero-shot Chest X-ray Diagnosis through Trait-Guided Multi-view Semantic Embedding with Self-training. IEEE Transactions on Medical Imaging. 2021.

60. Paul A, Tang YX, Shen TC,et al. Discriminative ensemble learning for few-shot chest x-ray diagnosis. Medical Image Analysis. 2021 Feb 1;68: 101911.

61. Paul A, Tang YX, Summers RM. Fast few-shot transfer learning for disease identification from chest x-ray images using autoencoder ensemble. In Medical Imaging 2020: Computer-Aided Diagnosis 2020 Mar 16 (Vol. 11314, p. 1131407). International Society for Optics and Photonics.

62. Piñol M, Alves R, Teixidó I, et al. Rare disease discovery: an optimized disease ranking system. IEEE Trans Ind Inf 2017;13(3):1184–92.

63. Gurovich Y, Hanani Y, Bar O, et al. Identifying facial phenotypes of genetic disorders using deep learning. Nat Med 2019;25(1):60–4.

64. Ekins S, Puhl AC, Zorn KM, et al. Exploiting machine learning for end-to-end drug discovery and development. Nat Mater 2019;18(5):435–41.

65. Li Q, Zhao K, Bustamante CD, et al. Xrare: a machine learning method jointly modeling phenotypes and genetic evidence for rare disease diagnosis. Genet Med 2019;21(9):2126–34.

66. Progress in fighting rare diseases. Available at: https://www.phrma.org/en/Media/Progress-in-Fighting-Rare-Diseases. Accessed July 19, 2021.

67. Gough A, Soto-Gutierrez A, Vernetti L, et al. Human biomimetic liver microphysiology systems in drug development and precision medicine. Nat Rev Gastroenterol Hepatol 2021;18(4):252–68.

68. Hargrove-Grimes P, Low LA, Tagle DA. Microphysiological systems: what it takes for community adoption. Exp Biol Med 2021. https://doi.org/10.1177/15353702211008872.

69. Akobeng AK. Understanding diagnostic tests 2: likelihood ratios, pre- and post-test probabilities and their use in clinical practice. Acta Paediatr 2007;96(4):487–91.

70. Bond RR, Novotny T, Andrsova I, et al. Automation bias in medicine: the influence of automated diagnoses on interpreter accuracy and uncertainty when reading electrocardiograms. J Electrocardiol 2018; 51(6S):S6–11.

71. Rare disease advocacy - NORD's rare action NetworkTM - NORD (national organization for rare disorders). 2014. Available at: https://rarediseases.org/for-patient-organizations/ways-partner/advocacy/. Accessed July 18, 2021.

72. CME - NORD (National Organization for Rare Disorders). Available at: https://rarediseases.org/for-

clinicians-and-researchers/resources/cme/. Accessed July 18, 2021.

73. Chan Zuckerberg. Initiative. Available at: https://chanzuckerberg.com/. Accessed September 19, 2021.

74. Advocacy, Education & Empowerment. Available at: http://www.geneticalliance.org/. Accessed July 21, 2021.

75. Schieppati A, Henter J-I, Daina E, et al. Why rare diseases are an important medical and social issue. Lancet 2008;371(9629):2039–41.

76. Genetic and Rare Diseases Information Center (GARD). Available at: https://ncats.nih.gov/gard. Accessed July 6, 2021.

77. Ali SR, Bryce J, Tan LE, et al. The EuRRECa Project as a model for data access and governance policies for rare disease registries that Collect clinical outcomes. Int J Environ Res Public Health 2020; 17(23). https://doi.org/10.3390/ijerph17238743.

78. Saboury B, Morris MA, Farhadi F, et al. Reinventing molecular imaging with total-body PET, Part I: technical revolution in Evolution. PET Clin 2020;15(4):427–38.

79. Prior F, Smith K, Sharma A, et al. The public cancer radiology imaging collections of the Cancer Imaging Archive. Sci Data 2017;4:170124.

80. El Emam K, Rodgers S, Malin B. Anonymising and sharing individual patient data. BMJ 2015;350: h1139. https://doi.org/10.1136/bmj.h1139.

81. Courbier S, Dimond R, Bros-Facer V. Share and protect our health data: an evidence based approach to rare disease patients' perspectives on data sharing and data protection - quantitative survey and recommendations. Orphanet J Rare Dis 2019;14(1):175.

82. Spencer K, Sanders C, Whitley EA, et al. Patient perspectives on sharing anonymized personal health data using a digital system for dynamic consent and research feedback: a Qualitative study. J Med Internet Res 2016;18(4):e66.

83. Figueiredo AS. Data sharing: convert challenges into opportunities. Front Public Health 2017;5:327.

84. Rare diseases. Available at: https://www.nih.gov/about-nih/what-we-do/nih-turning-discovery-into-health/rare-diseases. Accessed July 19, 2021.

85. Find Diseases We Study. Available at: https://www.rarediseasesnetwork.org/diseases. Accessed September 19, 2021.

86. Genetic Alliance - NORD (national organization for rare disorders). 2015. Available at: https://rarediseases.org/organizations/genetic-alliance/. Accessed July 6, 2021.

87. Ghosh P (guha). The impact of data quality in the machine learning era - DATAVERSITY. Available at: https://www.dataversity.net/impact-data-quality-machine-learning-era/. Accessed July 17, 2021.

88. Hallowell N, Parker M, Nellåker C. Big data phenotyping in rare diseases: some ethical issues. Genet Med 2019;21(2):272–4.

89. Yousefirizi F, Jha AK, Brosch-Lenz J, et al. Toward high-Throughput artificial intelligence-based segmentation in oncological PET imaging. PET Clin 2021;16(4):577–96.

90. Arslan M, Guzel M, Demirci M, et al. SMOTE and gaussian noise based sensor data augmentation. In: 2019 4th International Conference on computer science and Engineering (UBMK):Samsun, Turkey; 11-15 Sept. 2019:1-5. doi:10.1109/UBMK.2019.8907003.

91. dos Santos Tanaka FHK, Aranha C. Data augmentation using GANs. Available at: http://arxiv.org/abs/1904.09135.

92. Mikołajczyk A, Grochowski M. Data augmentation for improving deep learning in image classification problem. In: 2018 International Interdisciplinary PhD Workshop (IIPhDW):Cie, Poland. ieeexplore.ieee.org; 9-12 May 2018:117-122. doi:10.1109/IIPHDW.2018.8388338

93. Frid-Adar M, Diamant I, Klang E, et al. GAN-based synthetic medical image augmentation for increased CNN performance in liver lesion classification. Neurocomputing 2018;321:321–31.

94. Frid-Adar M, Klang E, Amitai M, Goldberger J, Greenspan H. Synthetic data augmentation using GAN for improved liver lesion classification. In: 2018 IEEE 15th International Symposium on Biomedical Imaging:Washington, DC (ISBI 2018). ; 4-7 April 2018:289-293. doi:10.1109/ISBI.2018.8363576

95. Zheng X, Chalasani T, Ghosal K, Lutz S, Smolic A. STaDA: Style Transfer as Data Augmentation. In: Proceedings of the 14th International Joint Conference on Computer Vision, Imaging and Computer Graphics Theory and Applications:Prague, Czech Republic. SCITEPRESS - Science and Technology Publications; 25-27, 2019. doi: 10.5220/0007353401070114

96. Qin R, Qiao K, Wang L, Zeng L, Chen J, Yan B. Weighted Focal Loss: An Effective Loss Function to Overcome Unbalance Problem of Chest X-ray14. IOP Conference Series: Materials Science and Engineering:Chengdu, China. 19-22 July 2018;428:012022. doi:10.1088/1757-899x/428/1/012022

97. Zhi-huan ZE-HP. Cost sensitive support vector machines. Control Decis. 2006. Available at: https://en.cnki.com.cn/article_en/cjfdtotal-kzyc200604024.htm. Accessed September 10, 2021.

98. Wei Q, Ren Y, Hou R, et al. Anomaly detection for medical images based on a one-class classification. Medical imaging 2018: Computer-Aided diagnosis, 10575. SPIE; 2018. p. 375–80. https://doi.org/10.1117/12.2293408.

99. Ganapathy K. Artificial intelligence and healthcare regulatory and legal concerns. TMT 2021. https://doi.org/10.30953/tmt.v6.252.

100. Khosla N, Valdez R. A compilation of national plans, policies and government actions for rare diseases in 23 countries. Intractable Rare Dis Res 2018;7(4):213–22.

101. Hudson KL, Holohan MK, Collins FS. Keeping pace with the times–the genetic information Nondiscrimination act of 2008. N Engl J Med 2008;358(25): 2661–3.

102. Melnikova I. Rare diseases and orphan drugs. Nat Rev Drug Discov 2012;11(4):267–8.

103. Heemstra HE, van Weely S, Büller HA, et al. Translation of rare disease research into orphan drug development: disease matters. Drug Discov Today 2009;14(23–24):1166–73.

104. Liu B, He H, Luo H, et al. Artificial intelligence and big data facilitated targeted drug discovery. Stroke Vasc Neurol 2019;4(4):206–13.

105. New study shows the rate of drug approvals lower than previously reported. Available at: https://archive.bio.org/media/press-release/new-study-shows-rate-drug-approvals-lower-previously-reported. Accessed September 20, 2021.

106. Wang Y, Li E, Cherry SR, et al. Total-body PET kinetic modeling and potential opportunities using deep learning. PET Clin 2021;16(4):613–25.

107. Ataeinia B, Heidari P. Artificial intelligence and the future of diagnostic and therapeutic radiopharmaceutical development. PET Clin 2021;16(4):513–23.

108. Saboury B, Morris MA, Nikpanah M, et al. Reinventing molecular imaging with total-body PET, Part II. PET Clin 2020;15(4):463–75.

109. Morgenstern J. Why pretest probability is absolutely essential. First10EM blog. Published online 2019. doi:10.51684/firs.9601.

110. Nikpanah M, Saboury B, Farhadi F, et al. Pictorial review of the 18F-FDG PET/CT Manifestations of Erdheim-Chester disease. J Nucl Med 2019; 60(supplement 1):1141. Available at: https://jnm.snmjournals.org/content/60/supplement_1/1141.short. Accessed September 18, 2021.

111. Cuthbertson DJ, Barriuso J, Lamarca A, et al. The impact of 68Gallium DOTA PET/CT in managing patients with sporadic and familial pancreatic neuroendocrine tumours. Front Endocrinol 2021;12:654975. https://doi.org/10.3389/fendo.2021.654975.

112. Boér A, Szakáll S Jr, Klein I, et al. FDG PET imaging in hereditary thyroid cancer. Eur J Surg Oncol 2003;29(10):922–8.

113. July M, Santhanam P, Giovanella L, et al. Role of positron emission tomography imaging in Multiple Endocrine Neoplasia syndromes. Clin Physiol Funct Imaging 2018;38(1):4–9.

114. Duryea DM, Walker ER, Brian PL. Two foci of FDG-avid secondary tumoral calcinosis incidentally noted in a patient with small-cell lung carcinoma after PET/CT. Radiol Case Rep 2014;9(4):998.

115. Oh J-R, Kulkarni H, Carreras C, et al. Ga-68 Somatostatin Receptor PET/CT in von Hippel-Lindau disease. Nucl Med Mol Imaging 2012;46(2): 129–33.

116. Hughes MS, Azoury SC, Assadipour Y, et al. Prospective evaluation and treatment of familial carcinoid small intestine neuroendocrine tumors (SI-NETs). Surgery 2016;159(1):350–6.

117. Čtvrtlík F, Koranda P, Schovánek J, et al. Current diagnostic imaging of pheochromocytomas and implications for therapeutic strategy. Exp Ther Med 2018;15(4):3151–60.

118. Anand SS, Singh H, Dash AK. Clinical applications of PET and PET-CT. Armed Forces Med J India 2009;65(4):353–8.

119. Weisman AJ, Kim J, Lee I, et al. Automated quantification of baseline imaging PET metrics on FDG PET/CT images of pediatric Hodgkin lymphoma patients. EJNMMI Phys 2020;7(1):76.

120. Yang R, Yu Y. Artificial Convolutional neural Network in Object detection and semantic segmentation for medical imaging Analysis. Front Oncol 2021;11:638182. https://doi.org/10.3389/fonc.2021.638182.

121. Lee Y-S, Krishnan A, Oughtred R, et al. A Computational Framework for Genome-wide Characterization of the Human Disease Landscape. Cell Syst. 2019;8(2):152-162.e6.

122. Saboury B, Morris MA, Nikpanah M, et al. Reinventing Molecular Imaging with Total-Body PET, Part II: Clinical Applications [published correction appears in PET Clin. 2021 Jan;16(1):xv]. PET Clin 2021;15(4):463–75. https://doi.org/10.1016/j.cpet.2020.06.013.

123. Saboury B, Morris MA, Farhadi F, et al. Reinventing Molecular Imaging with Total-Body PET, Part I: Technical Revolution in Evolution. PET Clin 2020 Oct;15(4):427–38. https://doi.org/10.1016/j.cpet.2020.06.012.

Artificial Intelligence and Positron Emission Tomography Imaging Workflow:
Technologists' Perspective

Cheryl Beegle, JD, CRA, R.T. (R)(N) ARRT, CNMT[a,1], Navid Hasani, BS[a,b,1],
Roberto Maass-Moreno, PhD, DABR[a],
Babak Saboury, MD, MPH, DABR, DABNM[a,c,d,*], Eliot Siegel, MD, FSIIM, FACR[e,*]

KEYWORDS

• Artificial intelligence • Medical imaging • Nuclear medicine technologists • Imaging workflow

KEY POINTS

• Artificial intelligence (AI) can reduce burdens and redundancies associated with clinical documentation while increasing image acquisition and processing quality and efficiency.
• By automating mundane tasks, AI enables future nuclear medicine (NM) technologists to reimagine their role, ensuring improved communication with patients and guaranteeing an exceptional patient experience.
• Stakeholder committees, including NM technologists, should develop frameworks laying out the actions that must be taken to advance and implement the use of AI systems.
• More than simplifying the tasks of technologists, AI will redirect their intellectual and technical resources to more challenging and satisfying tasks.
• Strong imaging leadership is required to encourage, strengthen, and develop a patient-focused AI-empowered workflow and ensure delivery of high-quality care.

INTRODUCTION

In the era of AI-enabled medical imaging, AI applications extend well beyond voxel-based algorithms, auto-segmentation of lesions of interest, or analysis of images and reports.[1] Although AI-enabled image acquisition and processing have been a stepping stone, the nuclear medicine (NM) practice of tomorrow will be largely structured around acknowledging the ethos of personalized health care. With the patient at the center, NM technologists will continue to serve as a critical part of the medical team working in conjunction with patients and radiologists to optimize each patient's imaging experience and oversee the performance of integrated artificial intelligence (AI) applications.

[a] Department of Radiology and Imaging Sciences, Clinical Center, National Institutes of Health, 9000 Rockville Pike, Building 10, Room 1C455, Bethesda, MD 20892, USA; [b] University of Queensland Faculty of Medicine, Ochsner Clinical School, New Orleans, LA 70121, USA; [c] Department of Computer Science and Electrical Engineering, University of Maryland, Baltimore Country, Baltimore, MD, USA; [d] Department of Radiology, Hospital of the University of Pennsylvania, Philadelphia, PA, USA; [e] Department of Radiology and Nuclear Medicine, University of Maryland Medical Center, 655 W. Baltimore Street, Baltimore, MD 21201, USA
[1] Co-first authors: contributed equally to this paper.
* Corresponding authors. Department of Radiology and Nuclear Medicine, University of Maryland Medical Center, 655 W. Baltimore Street, Baltimore, MD 21201, USA (E.S); Department of Radiology and Imaging Sciences, Clinical Center, National Institutes of Health, 9000 Rockville Pike, Building 10, Room 1C455, Bethesda, MD 20892, USA (B.S).
E-mail addresses: babak.saboury@nih.gov (B.S.); Esiegel@umaryland.edu (E.S.)

PET Clin 17 (2022) 31–39
https://doi.org/10.1016/j.cpet.2021.09.008

The process of patient care begins well before patients present at the imaging center. When the patient arrives, the process begins with the accurate collection of critical demographic and clinical information, the identification of their potential needs, the verification of the type/purpose of imaging study requested, scheduling needs, and so on. The patient's experience at an imaging center may also depend on the information that is provided, for instance, regarding what needs to be conducted during the study and after their appointment.[2] AI can help NM technologists to facilitate such tasks at every stage of imaging workflow and improve the quality of care before and after imaging. AI, when incorporated properly, can enable future NM technologists to focus on the human interaction aspect of patient care. The experience of the patient after image acquisition is also highly dependent on this human interaction.

Although some studies have been conducted to better understand the perspectives and readiness of technologists in the integration of AI in imaging workflow,[3–5] to the best of our knowledge, there is limited literature on the current and anticipated future integration of AI into the NM imaging workflow from the perspective of the technologist.

NUCLEAR MEDICINE TECHNOLOGISTS OF TOMORROW

Although the imaging workflow might vary among different settings (ie, inpatient and outpatient), a substantial portion of NM technologists' current workflow involves explaining the procedures to patients, preparing and administering radiotracers under the supervision of a physician, operating NM scanners for image acquisition, and working with postprocessing applications for advanced image quantifications.[6] Technologists are also responsible for patients' physical and psychological well-being before, during, and after imaging procedures.

From a global perspective, there is a growing medical imaging workload, shortage of providers and tachnologists, and suboptimal infrastructure often causing slowed down workflow and backlogs of unreported imaging studies, particularly in underfunded health care systems.[7,8] Even more evident with the COVID-19 pandemic, overcrowding stresses the ability and reduces the performance of our hospitals including imaging departments. With so much at stake, this is bound to trigger considerable interest in seeking opportunities to incorporate AI systems for medical imaging workflow tracking and automation. The overall goal is then to free

radiologists and technologists to support better informed decision making, personalized care, and better attention to emerging conditions.

Thus, the transition from the current state of medical imaging to a future of AI-enabled imaging departments seems inevitable. In such an environment, AI will significantly reduce the mundane tasks which only aim at "transmission of data" (such as obtaining the insurance records, updating the contact information, patient check-in and processing, and acquisition-set up and post-processing). The technologists, as the primary dedicated and responsive persons to the care of the individual patient, will oversee, but not perform, these time-consuming and attention-grabbing routine tasks.

As we transition into this 4th industrial revolution in medicine, we must reimagine the role of NM technologists to best enable patient-centered care. They will be first in line to identify failures and will become better translators of such events into innovative quality assurance and control requirements or new technology needs. Better still, because AI adapts as it learns, technologists will be in a privileged position to perceive subtle changes in the prevalence and patterns of diseases or changes in patient behavior. In other words, technologists will be more closely connected to medical care itself.

As a profession, diagnostic imaging has undergone numerous important advances through disruptive technologies in the past; notably, the creation and deployment of the picture archiving and communication system (PACS) environment and computer-aided diagnosis (CADs), which were once thought to be the end of the profession.[6,9,10,11] Those did not affect the growth of the discipline in a negative manner and possibly enhanced the prosperous progression of the field on multiple fronts. Imaging informatics did enhance the patient experience, as well as the delivery of services, and as a result, promoted the growth of the radiology community.[12] Similarly, AI technology will change the mode of clinical practice in NM positively and NM technologists' incorporation of AI systems will improve service quality and expand the growth of this profession. However, to perform appropriate supervision for AI systems the technologists must develop a good understanding of how AI systems work, their power, and their limits. Like any other medical subsystem, AI will require monitoring and its own quality assurance and control. Again, they will interact with both humans and machines but at a completely different level; hopefully, less with machines and more with the patient and their curative evolution.

Nuclear Medicine Advanced Technologist (n.)

/'nukliər 'mɛdəsən əd'vænst tek'nɑlədʒɪst/

Skillful and certified nuclear medicine technologist who has achieved additional qualifications through education and clinical training that enables them to be a valuable contribution to nuclear medicine physician-led teams in the artificial intelligence era.

ANTICIPATED ROLE OF ARTIFICIAL INTELLIGENCE IN TECHNOLOGISTS WORKFLOW

Before the COVID-19 pandemic, what was just an irritation for patients, such as waiting in a crowded waiting room before an imaging study, in the COVID-19 and post–COVID-19 era may prompt significant distress. Patient perceptions of what makes them "vulnerable" have shifted, and patients expect the medical staff to assist them in reducing those vulnerable times. To accommodate this expectation and pursue patient-centered care, NM technologists and health systems should strive to leverage AI technologies and achieve an automated workflow system that is, not only more efficient but also improves the quality of care. As such, in this section, we will explore ways to improve the current NM imaging workflow (**Fig. 1**) by embracing AI technologies at various stages of the workflow.

Scheduling and Triage

AI incorporated into scheduling and triage algorithms can significantly streamline appointments, self-scheduling, rescheduling, and prioritizing certain visits.[13] In an outpatient setting, the AI has the potential to enable patients to determine a location and time that works best for them. Additionally, an AI algorithm can help personalize information regarding the optimal match for a particular patient depending on their individual study and needs. Many elements, including a type of customer review system similar to modern web-based trends in accountability and customer feedback used by restaurants, hotels, and so forth, can be used by AI to determine the appropriate imaging centers for a certain patient with a specific study. Many web-based electronic health record (EHR) systems and practice websites already collect and publish customer review information for providers privately within the system or for patients publicly (ie, Kareo).[14] In the in-patient setting, an AI algorithm incorporated into the imaging triage system can automatically prioritize certain examinations with the goal of optimizing patient care.[15]

Quality Control

NM technologists perform scanner quality control (QC) daily to ensure a properly functioning nuclear imaging system.[16,17] No patient should ever ingest or be injected with a radiotracer compound without first establishing the imaging equipment's ability to acquire the study effectively. QC can also be undertaken on a weekly, monthly, or quarterly basis. It is critical to understand whether each scanner is operational each day. These duties are critical in part because without daily QC testing, there is no method of determining when a scanner ceased to work optimally.[8] Daily QC permits timely service calls to be placed, ensuring operational integrity, and quality imaging.

Over many years, equipment vendors have tried to automate the daily QC processes with mixed reviews. Pontoriero and colleagues have demonstrated the feasibility of automatic QC of

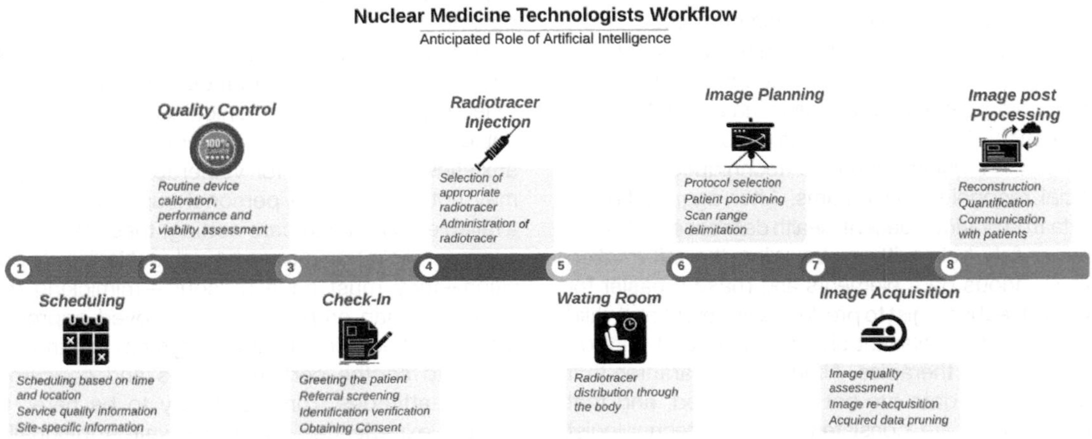

Nuclear Medicine Technologists Workflow
Anticipated Role of Artificial Intelligence

Fig. 1. Nuclear medicine imaging and technologists workflow.

18F-FDOPA PET imaging using deep learning.[18] Similar methods have the potential to be applied to various PET tracers in both brain and nonbrain applications. Current day scanner systems can unload the detector collimators and bring a source into the field of view (FOV) of the detector array. The scanner acquires the QC data during off-hours and stores the information in the acquisition terminal awaiting review and acceptance by the technologist. Since QC is performed before the scanner being used, QC is a task that decreases the amount of time that technologists are available to interact with and scan patients. This results in inefficiencies in the scheduling of scanners and reduces the number of patients and imaging sequences that can be acquired in a single day.

Often, depending on the number of scanners in an NM/PET imaging suite, QC downtime can make multiple systems unavailable for patient scanning. QC can take as little as 30 minutes or as long as three or more hours. This time can require roughly 25% of a technologist's eight-hour workday, that is, not spent performing direct patient care or imaging tasks. Often, multiple technologists are involved in QC activities. Therefore, AI-based QC systems can significantly improve the efficiency of NM technologists and departments.

Check-in

The check-in process for imaging patients has 2 critical parts (1) obtaining identification information from the patient and confirming appropriate imaging procedure (2) an interpersonal interaction; creating eye contact with the patient, greeting, and warmly welcoming them into the imaging center. AI systems have shown to be able to perform the automatic mundane parts of patient check-in allowing the technologist to focus on comforting the patient and properly greeting them, easing anxieties associated with the procedure, and ensuring better patient cooperation with the examination protocol.

AI systems for check-in can help with automatic screening of referrals and prescriptions as well as confirming patient identification via interaction with the EHR.[19] AI systems can also enable identification verification using biometric techniques such as facial recognition algorithms. After aggregation of data from various patient-health databases, AI could immensely help with synthesizing the information from various data elements and make it easier for the NM technologist to produce a coherent and valid compilation of relevant clinical history and prior diagnoses and therapies. Although to guarantee that patient EHR data are not compromised, and that AI decisions are consistent, the NM technologist oversight remains necessary.

Radiotracer Injection

The future of AI-enabled imaging workflow should verify the person at each stage of the imaging study and automatically select the specific tracer and a "smart" syringe[20] that can track the dose and the patient receiving the tracer. By automating the selection of the radiotracer and subsequently AI-verified injection, we can significantly reduce the chances of human errors. For instance, a framework such as the human factors analysis and classification system (HFACS)[21] integrated into AI medical systems can enable the identification of human errors based on historical recurring accidents and system breakdowns, thereby reducing the percentage of accidents and improving patient safety.[22] AI systems will allow redundant methods for cross-verify procedure appropriateness to significantly decrease or eliminate the preventable mistakes of today's NM routine workflows (ie, erroneous data entry at the point-of-care, including patient identifiers, relevant biologic data such as weight and height, specific study instance, and the proper type and amount of radiotracer administered).

Waiting Room

Many PET and NM studies require patients to wait in a secluded waiting environment for a certain period while the radioactive tracer distributes throughout their bodies. During this waiting period, the patient is radioactive and may not be in contact with family members or technologists. In some instances, certain movements may impact tracer uptake and are to be avoided. AI can be used in this setting to support patient compliance and appropriate tracer distribution during the waiting period. For instance, emotionally intelligent AI-based devices can be uniquely beneficial to provide care and support compliance tailored appropriately based on the study obtained by the patient.

Additionally, deploying 'AI-based companions' such as smart chatbots that use machine learning to learn about and communicate with the patients could also be beneficial in this environment to ease anxieties, particularly for vulnerable patients who may not have strong personal support networks available. In a health care setting, these 'AI-based companions' should have a kind and loving disposition—they must have a "soul"—mimicking the best of human empathy.[23] If deployed appropriately, an AI emotional support system has the potential to soothe certain feelings and concerns, altering attitudes from "unhappy to be here" to positive experiences during the wait. Additionally, devices such as smartwatches or sensors that contain accelerometers can help to detect undesirable patient motion or activity and provide feedback to the patients and technologists to help enhance the quality of a study.

Image Planning ("Protocolling")

NM technologists are required to choose the correct scanning protocol depending on the prescribed diagnostic test protocoled by senior technologists and confirmed with the NM physician. AI and deep learning algorithms have already been integrated into PACS for protocol selection.[24] AI algorithms can improve workflow efficiency by suggesting appropriate protocols for a specific patient using available pertinent clinical information in the EHR.[25] Intelligent systems might also be used to optimize contrast volume and injection rates based on patient characteristics.[26,27] In addition, prior imaging findings could guide the current field-of-view selection; for example, if a lesion was previously present in the calf on prior PET examination or even of another modality such as MRI, the AI can alert the technologist to ensure that this area is acquired in the present examination's field of view or excluded by educated decision making rather than excluded by uninformed decision making.

Technologists often perform patient positioning tasks using their expertise and judgment. This process as well as the determination of the appropriate field of view, both currently conducted by PET technologists, can become less subjective and more accurate using AI-enabled automatic positioning. This has been previously demonstrated in CT studies[28] and can be similarly implemented into the PET workflow. For example, an AI-based 2 or 3-dimentional camera system mounted on the ceiling can be used to automatically measure distances between two points inside its field of vision. In this case, as the AI or technologist select the appropriate study protocol, an automatic patient positioning mechanism will use anatomic references and range information to determine important landmarks as well as the start and stop positions of the scanner.[29]

The desired range of scanning should be marked on topogram (range delimitation) of AI-based PET/CT imaging can be a promising avenue whereby scan-framing (range delimitation) can be precisely and objectively defined, reducing the potential for human error. Demircioğlu and colleagues demonstrated that in chest CT, software-based, fully automatic scan range delimitation is possible with great accuracy and robustness (**Fig. 2**).[30] Similar algorithms can be incorporated into the NM imaging workflow to further improve the accuracy of scan range delimitation in PET/CT.

Image Acquisition

During the image acquisition and scanning stage, it is also vital to investigate how digital equipment might be used to increase imaging quality and efficiency.[31,32] AI's applications for accelerating scanning time and for dosage reduction[31] are also promising avenues that can be applied to NM and other imaging modalities. In the future, real-time medical image quality assessment evaluation may become a critical component of patient quality and safety data, as well as accreditation institutions. Through this methodology, technologists will be notified of potential examination quality issues, which would be corrected either by *reacquisition* or *post-acquisition data error correction*. This approach will decrease the need

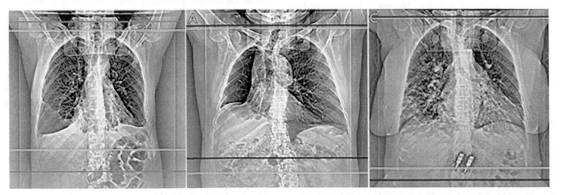

Fig. 2. Demircioglu and colleagues[30] demonstrate the feasibility of AI-based automated delimitation that is comparable with radiologists' and technologists' delimitation. Part A Illustration of a radiologist's (*in green*) and radiographer's scan range limitation (*in orange*). Part B shows delimitations of the scan ranges for the two expert radiologists (*green*) and the generative adversarial neural (GAN) network (*in blue*). Correlation analysis performed between the AI-generated and radiologists' scan range delimitations evaluated a Dice score of 0.99 in 1149 patients and all subgroups. (*From* Demircioğlu A, Kim M-S, Stein MC, Guberina N, Umutlu L, Nassenstein K. Automatic Scan Range Delimitation in Chest CT Using Deep Learning. *Radiol Artif Intell*. 2021;3(3):e200211.)

for patient recall for another imaging sequence and help avoid having to deal with significant image degradation. The process of recall in NM has significant financial and radiation costs and real-time identification of suboptimal image acquisition could reduce the impact, by simple remedies such as limited field-of-view *image reacquisition*- or *acquired data pruning*, of corrupted data.

Moreover, AI systems could also alert the patient in real-time during the scan if they have unintended movements or help them to adjust their position (such as the prevention of "upward creep" of the heart). Additionally, wearable AI health devices such as smart watches or smart rings can be optimized to engage the patient under the scanner, helping lower the anxiety or stress that some patients feel while in the scanner.

Image Postprocessing

Quantification is one of the hallmarks of NM imaging. The rich history of quantitative measures in this field makes the incorporation of AI into the workflow easier. Innovative approaches could dramatically help with labor-intensive tasks such as image registration, region-of-interest (ROI) drawing, and quantification workflow navigation.[33,34]

One of the most significant advantages of AI applications for image processing is that it will save time for technologists, increase reproducibility, and decrease redundancy in the work, allowing them to focus more on developing interpersonal ties with patients and answering patient questions.

AI can act as a personal assistant or scribe for the documentation of imaging studies. This can allow auto-suggestions that facilitate technologists' documentation of study results into the reporting system (similar to web search auto-completion). Such approaches could automatically fill the report with the relevant information and allow the technologist to accept or reject the suggested results and input their findings.[35] This accelerates the workflow from registration, documentation, and processing to billing, and into the EHR system, therefore, enabling the NM technologists to dedicate more time explaining procedures to the patient, answering any question or concerns the patient has after the study is over. This would release technologists from noncritical roles to reinforce the focus of professional roles based on the patient, enabling technologists to better serve as caregivers with imaging and therapy expertise. There are many tedious and redundant tasks that the technologist does that are not related to quality assurance, many of which can be delegated to AI.

IMPORTANT FUTURE DIRECTIONS
Need for Frameworks and Roadmaps

Comprehensive policy frameworks and roadmaps for AI implementation in medical imaging should be based on inclusive and extensive dialogue between all stakeholders and are needed to address ethical and practical challenges. On-the-job AI training programs and implementation roadmaps for a transition from conventional ways of practice to AI-enabled workflow are needed in the field of NM.[5] A future with AI assisting in the active engagement of technologists will be necessary to successfully implement these advanced technologies in medical imaging. Medical imaging professional societies and colleges should be in charge of designing and implementing frameworks and guideline for the profession. These recommendations must include a set of standards for use and validation of specific AI system. These task forces and committees may then assist local and federal policymakers in drafting legislations and establishing regulations for the safe use of AI.[36]

In this process NM technologists should aim to embrace, adopt, and adapt to the technology, ensuring that practice is based on the ethos of patient-centered care. To improve patient care, radiology and NM technologists should become active stakeholders in building the framework for ethical, practical, patient safety, and clinical aspects of AI. The machine and human relationship should be viewed as a symbiotic relationship whereby the machines will assist technologists and optimize patient outcomes, whereas in return technologists help to control, create and design the AI-based systems.

Smooth translation and integration of AI into medical imaging requires the technologists support and engagement as they are often the interface between patients and AI-enabled imaging workflow. Technologists should be a part of the design of AI and enhance their knowledge of its potential especially as they understand the workflow and NM systems the best. NM technologists must act as active participants in forming the future of NM imaging in order to contribute their valuable viewpoints regarding the technology's implementation and related policies.

Integration of Artificial Intelligence-Related Content into Technologist Training Curriculum and Accreditation

The technologists of tomorrow must be managers and supervisors of multiple AI systems that are integrated within the workflow of imaging.[3,6] As a result of this significant change in job skills and responsibilities, there is a critical need for an adaptation of training curriculum and accreditation standards accordingly.[37] The technologists should be able to understand how algorithms arrive at decisions and the potential for inevitable errors within these systems to enable effective communication of findings to patients. To do so, it is imperative to prioritize the integration of AI content into technologists' professional education. Curriculums should include learning about AI health data curation and quality,[38] integration,[39] and governance, as well as working with EHRs, AI basics, and AI ethical and legal problems.[39] Coursework in AI rigorous appraisal and statistical interpretation is equally vital.[40] Accreditation organizations and hospitals should also shift their standards and expectations to advocate for more AI-awareness and AI-enabled medical services in medical imaging.

Currently, there is no registry for technologists that address the competencies and skills required for AI-rich workflows by either the American Registry of Radiologic Technology (ARRT) or the Nuclear Medicine Technology Certification Board (NMTCB). The registry for Medical Dosimetry, offered by the Medical Dosimetrist Certification Board (MDCB),[41] has a focus on external beam dosimetry for radiation oncology. The Nuclear Medicine Technology Certification Board (NMTCB) offers the Nuclear Medicine Advanced Associate Registry (NMAA)[42] that functions as a physician extender in a similar fashion as a Physician Assistant (PA) and the ARRT physician extender. NMAAs facilitate the care and management of patients while in the NM department. With the growing role of AI in health care and the importance of molecular imaging biomarker labs and precision dosimetry for radiopharmaceutical therapy, it is more than ever vital to train NM advanced technologists (NMAT). This link between NM imaging and AI is critical to the development of precision dosimetry that informs radiopharmaceutical therapeutic treatment.[43,44] Without such a background, the dosimetry/theranostics technologist of the future will fall short of the needed basic understanding of the field that defines the basis for advanced therapeutic treatment planning. As NMTCB is currently responsible for NMT accreditation, they should be the ones who certify future NMAT as well.

As AI application grows and integrates itself within NM imaging, the ability of algorithms to provide more precise direction in identifying significant patient tumor burden also grows[45] [see Hasani and colleagues' article, "Artificial Intelligence in Lymphoma PET Imaging: A Scoping Review (Current Trends and Future Directions)," in this issue]. To achieve the full potential of AI we must aspire toward a trustworthy AI ecosystem whereby all stakeholders, including NMAT, have an active role in all stages of the AI lifecycle [see Hasani and colleagues' article, "Trustworthy AI in Medical Imaging," in this issue].

This active participation, however, is not achievable unless NM technologists are trained and accredited in the clinical implantation of these technologies.

SUMMARY

At first glance, AI seems to threaten the role of the NM technologist, however, there are numerous opportunities for greater professional autonomy, improved personal connection with patients, and extension of the roles of technologists. Additionally, NM technologists will take on the role of AI supervisors, overseeing many aspects of imaging such as QC in conjunction with AI systems. These opportunities can only come to fruition if technologists are active stakeholders in the development and deployment process. They must take the steps to best define how they wish to envision their professional evolution to successfully prepare for, and adapt to, the work in an AI-enabled environment. The future demands inevitable changes in roles and culture. By embracing change, we can assure and prepare all medical imaging technologists with the abilities needed to connect with tomorrow's.

CLINICS CARE POINTS

- AI will enable imaging technologists to shift their focus from simply performing tasks to engaging with their patients, discussing their concerns and listening to their expressed needs, promoting patient well-being, and helping to form relationships that will provide for more effective care.

- Strong imaging leadership is required to encourage and strengthen the development of this patient-focused AI-driven workflow and ensure the continued delivery of high-quality care.

- Nuclear Medicine Advanced Technologist (NMAT) provide opportunities for expanded professional growth will develop in tandem with the implementation of all types of AI, ML, and DL paradigms not just in imaging but throughout the new and more comprehensive approach to health care delivery worldwide.

ACKNOWLEDGMENTS AND DISCLOSURES

This research was supported in part by the Intramural Research Program of the NIH, Clinical Center. The opinions expressed in this publication are the author's own and do not reflect the view of the National Institutes of Health, the Department of

Health and Human Services, or the United States government.

REFERENCES

1. Lakhani P, Prater AB, Hutson RK, et al. Machine learning in radiology: applications beyond image interpretation. J Am Coll Radiol 2018;15(2):350–9.
2. Kyono T, Gilbert FJ, van der Schaar M. Improving workflow efficiency for mammography using machine learning. J Am Coll Radiol 2020;17(1 Pt A):56–63.
3. Botwe BO, Antwi WK, Arkoh S, et al. Radiographers' perspectives on the emerging integration of artificial intelligence into diagnostic imaging: The Ghana study. J Med Radiat Sci 2021;14. https://doi.org/10.1002/jmrs.460.
4. Antwi WK, Akudjedu TN, Botwe BO. Artificial intelligence in medical imaging practice in Africa: a qualitative content analysis study of radiographers' perspectives. Insights Imaging 2021;12:80.
5. Botwe BO, Akudjedu TN, Antwi WK, et al. The integration of artificial intelligence in medical imaging practice: Perspectives of African radiographers. Radiography 2021;27(3):861–6.
6. Hardy M, Harvey H. Artificial intelligence in diagnostic imaging: impact on the radiography profession. Br J Radiol 2020;93(1108):20190840.
7. Smith-Bindman R, Kwan ML, Marlow EC, et al. Trends in use of medical imaging in US Health care systems and in Ontario, Canada, 2000-2016. JAMA 2019;322(9):843–56.
8. Smith-Bindman R, Miglioretti DL, Larson EB. Rising use of diagnostic medical imaging in a large integrated health system. Health Aff 2008;27(6):1491–502.
9. Dinesh Peter J, Fernandes SL, Thomaz CE, et al. Computer aided Intervention and diagnostics in clinical and medical images. NY, USA: Springer; 2019.
10. Richardson ML, Garwood ER, Lee Y, et al. Noninterpretive uses of artificial intelligence in radiology. Acad Radiol 2021;28(9):1225–35.
11. Langlotz CP. Will artificial intelligence replace radiologists? Radiol Artif Intelligence 2019;1(3):e190058.
12. Reardon S. Rise of Robot Radiologists. Nature 2019;576(7787):S54–8.
13. Srinivas S, Ravindran AR. Optimizing outpatient appointment system using machine learning algorithms and scheduling rules: A prescriptive analytics framework. Expert Syst Appl 2018;102:245–61.
14. Kareo EHR Patient Portal. Available at: https://www.kareo.com/kareo-ehr-patient-portal. Accessed September 20, 2021.
15. Weisberg EM, Chu LC, Fishman EK. The first use of artificial intelligence (AI) in the ER: triage not diagnosis. Emerg Radiol 2020;27(4):361–6.
16. Zanzonico P. Routine quality control of clinical nuclear medicine instrumentation: a brief review. J Nucl Med 2008;49(7):1114–31.
17. Santos JC, Wong JHD, Pallath V, et al. The perceptions of medical physicists towards relevance and impact of artificial intelligence. Australas Phys Eng Sci Med 2021;44(3):833–41.
18. Pontoriero AD, Nordio G, Easmin R, et al. Automated data quality control in FDOPA brain PET imaging using deep learning. Comput Methods Programs Biomed 2021;208:106239.
19. No matter how you slice it, this AI tech is changing MR neuro imaging. Available at: https://www.gehealthcare.com/article/no-matter-how-you-slice-it-this-ai-tech-is-changing-mr-neuro-imaging/. Accessed August 9, 2021.
20. Market Growth Insight. Smart syringe market to witness an outstanding growth during 2020 – 2025 – Welltok, Intel, Nvidia, Google. Available at: https://www.medgadget.com/2021/02/smart-syringe-market-to-witness-an-outstanding-growth-during-2020-2025-welltok-intel-nvidia-google.html. Accessed August 22, 2021.
21. HFACS, Inc.. Available at: https://hfacs.com/hfacs-framework.html. Accessed September 19, 2021.
22. Asan O, Choudhury A. Research trends in artificial intelligence applications in human factors health care: mapping review. JMIR Hum Factors 2021;8(2):e28236.
23. Griffin A. Improving the patient waiting room experience: chatbots could be the prescription we need – Tech 2025. Available at: https://www.tech2025.com/2017/05/18/improving-the-patient-waiting-room-experience-chatbots-could-be-the-prescription-we-need/. Accessed August 10, 2021.
24. Brown AD, Marotta TR. Using machine learning for sequence-level automated MRI protocol selection in neuroradiology. J Am Med Inform Assoc 2018;25(5):568–71.
25. Häggström I, Schmidtlein CR, Campanella G, et al. DeepPET: A deep encoder-decoder network for directly solving the PET image reconstruction inverse problem. Med Image Anal 2019;54:253–62.
26. Santini G, Zumbo LM, Martini N, et al. Synthetic contrast enhancement in cardiac CT with Deep Learning. Available at: http://arxiv.org/abs/1807.01779.
27. Feng S-T, Zhu H, Peng Z, et al. An individually optimized protocol of contrast medium injection in enhanced CT scan for liver imaging. Contrast Media Mol Imaging 2017;2017.7350429.
28. FAST Integrated Workflow. Available at: https://www.siemens-healthineers.com/computed-tomography/technologies-and-innovations/fast-integrated-workflow. Accessed August 20, 2021.
29. Gang Y, Chen X, Li H, et al. A comparison between manual and artificial intelligence-based automatic positioning in CT imaging for COVID-19 patients. Eur Radiol 2021;31(8):6049–58.

30. Demircioğlu A, Kim M-S, Stein MC, et al. Automatic scan range delimitation in chest CT using deep learning. Radiol Artif Intell 2021;3(3):e200211.

31. Qi J, Matej S, Wang G, et al. 3D/4D reconstruction and quantitative total body imaging. PET Clin 2021;16(1):41–54.

32. Liu J, Malekzadeh M, Mirian N, et al. Artificial intelligence-based image enhancement in PET imaging: noise reduction and resolution Enhancement. Available at: http://arxiv.org/abs/2107.13595.

33. Ledig C, Theis L, Huszar F, et al. Photo-Realistic Single Image Super-Resolution Using a Generative Adversarial Network. arXiv [csCV]. 2016. Available at: http://arxiv.org/abs/1609.04802.

34. Tong N, Gou S, Yang S, et al. Fully automatic multi-organ segmentation for head and neck cancer radiotherapy using shape representation model constrained fully convolutional neural networks. Med Phys 2018;45(10):4558–67.

35. Adam Bohr KM. The rise of artificial intelligence in healthcare applications. Artif Intelligence Healthc 2020;25.

36. Liew C. The future of radiology augmented with Artificial Intelligence: A strategy for success. Eur J Radiol 2018;102:152–6.

37. Paranjape K, Schinkel M, Nannan Panday R, et al. Introducing artificial intelligence training in medical education. JMIR Med Educ 2019;5(2):e16048.

38. Ranschaert ER, Morozov S, Algra PR. In: Ranschaert ER, Morozov S, Algra PR, editors. Artificial intelligence in medical imaging: opportunities, applications and risks. Cham: Springer; 2019.

39. Prasser F, Kohlbacher O, Mansmann U, et al. Data integration for future medicine (DIFUTURE). Methods Inf Med 2018;57(S 01):e57–65.

40. The Topol Review — NHS Health Education England. Available at: https://topol.hee.nhs.uk/. Accessed August 22, 2021.

41. About MDCB. Available at: https://www.mdcb.org/about-mdcb. Accessed September 19, 2021.

42. Nuclear Medicine Advanced Associate (NMAA) Exam. Available at: https://www.nmtcb.org/exams/nmaa. Accessed September 19, 2021.

43. Owen MA, Sinotte KN, Bolus N, et al. Nuclear medicine advanced associates: physician extenders in nuclear medicine—now is the time. J Nucl Med Technol 2020;48(3):241–5.

44. Lindqwister AL, Hassanpour S, Lewis PJ, et al. AI-RADS: An artificial intelligence curriculum for residents. Acad Radiol. Published online October 15, 2020. doi:10.1016/j.acra.2020.09.017

45. Esses SJ, Lu X, Zhao T, et al. Automated image quality evaluation of T2-weighted liver MRI utilizing deep learning architecture. J Magn Reson Imaging 2018;47(3):723–8.

Demystifying Medico-legal Challenges of Artificial Intelligence Applications in Molecular Imaging and Therapy

Jonathan Lee Mezrich, MD, JD, MBA, LLM*

KEYWORDS

- Artificial intelligence • Machine learning • Deep learning • Medico-legal • Standard of care
- Malpractice • Negligence • Liability

KEY POINTS

- Artificial intelligence (AI) is rapidly becoming incorporated into imaging practice, and it is likely that some of the biggest hurdles to AI going forward will not be technological but legal.
- Although the laws applicable to AI are as yet poorly delineated, potential causes of action that may be implicated in cases of medical error in the AI setting include medical malpractice, vicarious liability, and products liability.
- Legislation and practice guidelines covering AI use would be beneficial to delineate standard-of-care benchmarks, and physician advocacy for such legislative/professional rules is recommended.

INTRODUCTION -

For well over the past decade, it has been a popular mantra to suggest that artificial intelligence/deep learning (AI) will soon replace physicians working in diagnostic radiology and nuclear medicine.[1] It seems only logical: computers are relatively cost effective, they never tire, can work 24/7, and offer a degree of consistency and precision that few humans can. Imaging specialties, with their dependence on technology, emphasis on search patterns and pattern recognition, and relatively limited need to interface with patients seem to be ripe for automation. Many physicians chose these fields precisely because of the ability to combine medicine with interests in technological innovation.

AI has been rapidly embraced by the imaging fields, featured in countless articles, and the featured topic of many national meetings. Many practices have begun to incorporate aspects of AI into practice, ranging from relatively limited computer detection software tools to more sophisticated deep learning algorithms/neural networks. Computer-aided detection (CAD), an early form of AI, has been in use in breast imaging for decades. More recent uses of AI as an adjunct to radiology practice include identification of pulmonary embolisms, pneumothoraces, intracranial hemorrhage, cervical and rib fractures, and the like. CAD performs a specific task based on predefined criteria, whereas more advanced forms of AI (machine learning/deep learning/neural networks) go a step beyond and incorporate an ability to learn from previously seen data.

Nuclear medicine offers ample opportunities for use of AI, not only in terms of lesion detection by highlighting potential areas of concern on imaging based on standardized uptake value calculations/counts and interval change, but also in terms of image quality, such as reconstruction/attenuation correction,[2,3] which in turn may offer opportunities for lower dose scanning and shorter scan times.[4]

Department of Radiology and Biomedical Imaging, Emergency Radiology, Yale School of Medicine, 333 Cedar Street, New Haven, CT 06510, USA
* 2111 Jennifers Drive, Guilford, CT 06437.
E-mail address: Jonathan.Mezrich@yale.edu

PET Clin 17 (2022) 41–49
https://doi.org/10.1016/j.cpet.2021.08.002
1556-8598/22/© 2021 Elsevier Inc. All rights reserved.

AI ultimately may be incorporated in image interpretation of findings and reporting of results. There also may be opportunity to use AI in the design of the radiotracers themselves.

Although the incorporation of AI into radiology/nuclear medicine practice has been slower than some pundits originally predicted, in part because of oversimplistic notions of imagers as mere pattern recognition experts, it is likely that this technology will persevere, and that AI will continue to make significant inroads into our specialty. As such, the biggest hurdles to AI will likely not be technological, but legal.

DISCUSSION
Mistakes, Malpractice, and Liability

AI will enable physicians to handle greater volumes of patient imaging. With great volumes, errors are inevitable, and at some point AI will make a mistake, and the law will seek to make the injured patient, an innocent victim, whole, by means of a lawsuit or settlement. Tort law is the branch of civil liability in which an individual damaged by the wrongful act or mistake of another may seek damages.[5] Types of tort claims that may come into play in the health care setting include medical malpractice, vicarious liability, and products liability.[5]

Elements of a Medical Malpractice Claim

Before we consider the issue of potential liability for AI, an overview of the potentially applicable tort laws is helpful. When a physician makes a mistake, the injured patient might opt to pursue damages by bringing a civil lawsuit against the physician for medical malpractice. To successfully establish a medical malpractice cause of action, the injured patient, as "plaintiff," must prove 4 key elements against the physician as "defendant": (1) that the physician owed a legal duty of care to the patient, (2) that there was a breach of that duty, (3) causation, and (4) resultant harm/damages.[6] We look at each of these elements in turn.

First, for there to be a duty, a physician-patient relationship must be established. When a physician-patient relationship is established, a physician will owe a legal duty to practice within the accepted standards of care for that specialty.[7,8] Although imagers may not always meet or speak with a patient directly, a physician-patient relationship will generally be established as soon as the patient arrives at the imaging department for a study.[7,8]

A breach of duty occurs when the treating physician does not meet the accepted "standard of care." The standard of care is the degree of care that a reasonably prudent physician of that specialty would be expected to exercise under the same or similar circumstances.[9] Not meeting this standard of care is strong indicia of malpractice.[10] Essentially, to show he or she has breached a standard of care, the imager must be shown to have either done something he or she should not have done, or failed to do something he or she should have done. The question of liability comes down to a benchmark of reasonableness: "what would the reasonably prudent imager have done in this situation?" To a large extent, this standard of care will be determined in the courtroom setting based on expert testimony, whereby other members of the specialty will be engaged to testify as to what, in their professional opinion, would be a reasonable action in this situation.[11] The standard of care may also derive from clinical practical guidelines, regulations, or an institution's rules, which may be admitted in litigation either as the basis of an expert's opinion or to assist the court or jury as a "learned treatise" or other exception under the Federal Rules of Evidence.[12] Practice guidelines enacted by the specialty are not the standard of care, but can be used in litigation as evidence of the standard.

To prove causation, a plaintiff will need to prove that a physician's negligence was the cause of his or her damages, that is, the harm would not have occurred if the standard of care was met.[13] For example, a patient who suffered harm in the setting of a negligent review of an imaging study would need to show that there was a substantial likelihood that he or she would have been unharmed (or at least better off) had the evaluation been performed without deviation from the standard of care.

Finally, the plaintiff needs to show damages. A patient must show he or she was actually harmed as a result of the imager's actions.[13]

The injured patient has the burden of proof, and must present enough evidence to support the claim by a preponderance of the evidence.[10(p43)] Preponderance of the evidence means more likely than not.[14] For the patient to prevail the scale needs to be tipped to "more likely." The patient loses if he or she is unable to prove any of the preceding 4 elements (duty, beach, causation, damages).

Vicarious liability
Vicarious liability (in Latin, *respondeat superior*, "let the master answer") is a legal doctrine of imputed negligence whereby an agent of an individual creates liability for that individual notwithstanding that the individual him or herself is free

of personal fault.[15] As such, the negligence of the agent/servant becomes the negligence of the otherwise innocent defendant. For instance, if a physician asked a technologist to scan a patient, and the technologist negligently injured the patient, that negligence could be imputed to the physician. An AI algorithm, acting autonomously in diagnosing patients in a nuclear medicine department could theoretically be regarded as functionally analogous to an agent/employee of that department, with the result that its negligence might be imputed to the supervising radiologist or institution. As algorithms become more autonomous, this may become a favored approach by courts, as the department or radiologist has more or less fictitious "control" of the AI, has set it in motion, and profits from it. Courts may favor this approach as a matter of policy, as it serves to make an injured patient whole, and ascribes liability to a party better able to absorb the costs.

Products liability
Products liability is the area of law involving liability of those supplying goods and products with respect to customers (and bystanders).[16] Product liability law may be implicated when a patient is injured by a product that is not reasonably safe due to defect in design, manufacture, or warning.[5(p162),17] There are several hurdles with respect to applying products liability law to AI. First, AI tends not to be a tangible product, but rather a software algorithm, and the law has been loath to apply products liability law to software[18]; the case may be different where that software is incorporated into an actual tangible product, as in the case of an autonomous ("self-driving") car. Second, the goal of machine learning is that the algorithm will learn and evolve based on experience, such that the original algorithm a vendor develops and sells may not be exactly the same as the one that ultimately causes an injury at a later date.

Learned intermediary exception
In addition, an exception to products liability that could come into play here would be the "learned intermediary" exception. To the extent an imager (the "learned intermediary") had an opportunity to review findings before a report was issued and a patient was injured, that physician would bear the brunt of the liability: a physician would not be permitted to act as a passive messenger of negligent AI findings.[18(p9)] The physician's intervening failure to catch the mistake essentially absolves the AI algorithm developer's downstream negligence.[18(p9)] This is most obvious in the use of CAD, where the AI is to be used more as a second set of eyes and the physician clearly chooses to accept or reject the AI findings, but may become more convoluted to the extent the AI software directly interfaces with patients.

Who Bears the Responsibility for Harmful Errors?
Once harm occurs in conjunction with AI, the question becomes: who is responsible for these mistakes? That question will depend on the role of AI in practice, and physicians need to be cognizant of these risks.

Because AI is such new technology, the tort law that applies to AI is not yet well developed. Not every bad outcome will have legal significance; as mentioned, a suit for malpractice requires a breach of duty and a deviation from the standard of care. Such negligence in the context of AI could reflect a failure of programming, supervision/evaluation, actions of the physician, or of the algorithm itself. It may also stem from training of the algorithm that precedes the injured patient encounter. "Medical AI may be trained in inappropriate environments, using imperfect techniques, or on incomplete data."[19]

Simplest analysis: artificial intelligence as a second set of eyes, for example, computer-aided detection
If AI is merely used as a tool to make the radiologist more efficient: to "bird dog" findings for the physician's review, much like CAD is currently used in mammography, or to put acute things higher on the worklist, review medical records, and help populate the report, but the imaging physician essentially makes all final determinations and signs the report, the physician will clearly be the party at risk for liability, with medical malpractice laws potentially applicable. The physician will be negligent or not based on his or her own independent determinations, with the AI simply making sure the physician did not overlook anything, or give him or her regions to double check. Tort law creates a significant incentive to limit AI to this function, as unless and until widespread use of AI becomes the standard of care, "the 'safest' way to use medical AI from a liability perspective is as a confirmatory tool to support existing decision-making processes, rather than as a source to improve care."[19] Malpractice law involving physician error is well established and predictable, but laws governing AI are not, and so there is a legal bias toward keeping AI categorized as a physician tool rather than an independent decision-making member of the health care team.

Using limited AI such as CAD as a "second set of eyes" should increase diagnostic accuracy and prevent negative outcomes, decreasing risk of liability.[20] But even relegating AI use merely to CAD functions is not without liability risk: use of CAD can result in "reviewer bias" where an imager is more likely to consider a finding positive when flagged by CAD, which could lead to unnecessary treatment and ultimately lead to a lawsuit.[20] On the flip side, a negative finding by CAD could provide false reassurance and a missed finding, which also could subject an imager to liability.[20] Use of CAD may also create an obligation for the physician to address AI findings in the report and explain his or her reasons for disregarding such findings, which could create additional work for the imager; it would not do for a physician to disregard a positive, ultimately validated CAD finding not mentioned in the report and then have to explain this omission in front of a jury. In the CAD setting, the computer becomes the built-in expert witness against the defendant physician.[11]

Artificial intelligence as a true, independent "assistant"

As AI functions become more widely adopted and AI starts to fill a role of an assistant/employee/servant of the radiologist, at times acting independently but under regular or periodic supervision, essentially acting as the "agent" of the physician, doctrines of vicarious liability would likely come into play, and the physician (and the physician's employers) would still be liable.[5(p162),17(p67)] The physician/employer is the party with control over the AI, and who profits from this AI "subordinate's" actions and so under the law would be liable for the negligence of his or her subordinate. This doctrine may be an imperfect fit with respect to automation, but liability of health care providers for negligently failing to exercise due care in supervising or maintaining the AI may also be applicable.[5(p162)] In this respect, the negligence would essentially be that of negligent supervision in allowing the error to occur, rather than causing the error itself.

Artificial intelligence as a replacement for the imaging physician

Because many advocates of AI see this technology as having a role in actually supplanting/replacing imaging physicians,[1] rather than merely making them more efficient, that opens another whole can of worms. If a physician is neither making a final decision on findings nor supervising or controlling the AI algorithm in any meaningful way before it independently issues its report, the analysis becomes more difficult. Questions then depend on whether the algorithm is a "product" such that the tort laws of products liability come into play. As mentioned, software is generally not in and of itself a product for products liability purposes,[17(p71),18(p7)] although products that incorporate software/algorithms might be, and as such, the manufacturer/vendor may have some legal exposure. If developed by an outside vendor as an "off-the-shelf"–type product, then it may subject the software developers themselves to liability, with the caveat that if the physician's role was intended to intervene between the manufacturer and end user/patient (eg, the physician used AI as decision support rather than let AI make the decisions) or the physician did not provide adequate disclosure of risks to the patient, the physician would bear the brunt of liability (the learned intermediary exception described previously).[5(p162),17(p71),18(p9)] If developed or customized in-house, concepts of "enterprise liability" will come into play and the developing/customizing hospital will also potentially bear liability.[21] Although AI software developers may be relatively small start-ups as compared with the relatively "deep pocket" of a large hospital and its insurance carrier, a lawsuit would likely name both of these entities as defendants and let the courts apportion the liability.

Artificial intelligence as a "medical device"?

Another wrinkle will be if the Food and Drug Administration (FDA) treats AI-containing products, or the algorithms themselves, as medical devices, in which case some have argued that the doctrine of "preemption" should come into play. Preemption, in simple terms, is a doctrine that clarifies that in cases in which state law obligations differ from federal law obligations, the federal laws will preempt those of the state. So once the FDA, a federal agency acting pursuant to federal regulations, has approved a medical product for certain types of usage with certain delineated risks, and if a hospital/physician appropriately uses it as such, and the patient is made aware of these risks, state malpractice law will be "preempted" by these federal regulations and the use of the product in the way delineated and approved by the FDA may not be deemed negligent, notwithstanding bad outcomes.[21,22] However, preemption has been somewhat inconsistently applied by the courts.[21] The problem with this analysis may be confounded by the fact that algorithms are not static products: deep learning algorithms/neural networks are designed to evolve and learn; the algorithm itself changes based on increased experience, such that the algorithm approved by the FDA originally may not bear an exact likeness to that which caused the error months or years later.[21] Some have suggested that to obtain FDA approval an algorithm may need to employ "locking," whereby an algorithm's capacity is frozen once it has been sufficiently trained, but this approach is unsatisfying as it ultimately limits the benefit and utility of AI and would serve as a ceiling for AI evolution.[23]

Novel suggestion for addressing artificial intelligence liability: artificial intelligence personhood

Several authors have suggested a possible solution to AI liability: confer the AI algorithm "personhood," make it required to carry its own insurance and be available to be sued directly, the same as any other physician.[5(p164)] It has also been suggested in the literature that recent examples of AI, such as IBM's Watson, are functionally analogous to a medical student, with a role in patient care, not constantly supervised in all functions, but without the autonomy or decision-making authority of the attending physician[17(p69)]; it is suggested that the AI should "be able to be held liable in its student-like capacity," with the physician also directly or vicariously liable for failing to properly consider the AI's recommendations.[17(p70)] "What we are arguing is that Watson should be classified as a legal person for the purposes of apportioning liability so that Watson's activities can be insured at a level that rises to that of a medical student."[17(p73)] Although the implications of bestowing "personhood" on inanimate objects may have unforeseen implications down the road, it should be noted that use of this legal fiction is not without precedent; corporate entities have been bestowed a multitude of rights of "personhood" under US tax and other laws.

Artificial Intelligence Litigation and Lack of Precedent

The law of AI is still in its infancy and it remains to be seen how courts will allocate liability for AI mishaps. Most of these issues will play themselves out in court, and the mistakes that occur will impact the development of liability for AI. Although the function and risks are somewhat different, the legal history of autonomous vehicles (so-called "self-driving cars") will be instructive. Some states, anticipating legal issues with autonomous vehicles, have preempted the issue by passing laws explicitly placing liability on the vehicle's human operator.[24] Even without such explicit statutory obligations, tort law principles in these cases will turn on the element of control: the operator is liable to the extent they reasonably could have prevented the accident. The question will then be,

would complete reliance on technology in operating a vehicle ever be considered reasonable? And if the answer is no in the case of a self-driving car, why should it be any different in the case of a self-driving physician?[24] If a jury would be troubled by a person going to sleep and letting his or her car navigate a school zone unattended, would the analysis be different where a physician takes a nap and lets a computer diagnose a tumor? It should be noted that autonomous vehicle manufacturers tend to be deep pocket defendants (major automobile manufacturers), whereas medical algorithm software developers may be small start-ups, and there is the fact that self-driving algorithms will be integrated into a discrete tangible product (a car) to a greater extent than a medical algorithm, so approaches by a plaintiff's attorneys in terms of which party is sued and whether a products liability versus negligence route is pursued may be different. The early lawsuits in the area of autonomous vehicles have ended in settlement, and a court's determination of liability in such cases remains a mystery.[24–26]

Robots Make Bad Defendants

It should be intuitive that a medically harmed patient, or family of an injured or deceased patient tends to make a very sympathetic witness, and an AI algorithm that erred will make for a very unsympathetic defendant. Defense attorneys will have the opportunity to paint a picture of technology running amok, with impassionate robots making decisions, imagery that will play at the heartstrings of jurors predisposed to the dangers of technology both because they do not understand it and because of decades of exposure to science fiction dystopias. The notion that a hospital would replace a compassionate physician for a more cost-efficient, faster machine in order to maximize profits will also not sit well with a juror.

Will Artificial Intelligence Become the Standard of Care

As AI use becomes more ubiquitous, there will be a point in which using AI will become the expected standard of care.[11,21] As such, a radiologist/hospital not using AI would be hard-pressed to defend against a claim of negligence in any case in which AI would have picked up a lesion or made the salient finding. A somewhat perplexing corollary was demonstrated in a study by Tobia and colleagues,[27] where mock jurors showed a significant bias toward deeming reasonable a physician's acceptance of not only a standard-of-care recommendation from AI but also nonstandard recommendations, meaning that "if physicians receive a nonstandard AI recommendation, they do not necessarily make themselves safer from liability by rejecting it,"[27(p19)] and that "[g]iven that physicians who receive nonstandard advice are worse off in terms of liability than physicians who accept standard of advice, health-care institutions might consider whether to make AI systems available to physicians."[27(p19)] In other words, once AI is adopted, this study suggests jurors will expect physicians to follow AI recommendations, even if nonstandard, and to ignore it at one's own peril (see also Ref.[19(p1766)]).

In the current early AI environment, to the extent a physician intends to ignore an AI finding, he or she should make an effort to explain away these findings in his or her report, as simply ignoring an AI finding could be regarded as negligent. In this respect, AI may sometimes result in more work for the physician, although hopefully with an increase in accuracy.

Security and Privacy Risks with Artificial Intelligence

Letting a machine "learn" on thousands of cases means thousands of opportunities to breach privacy. Although somewhat beyond the scope of this analysis, AI requires access to a large library/database of patient imaging and data from which to train. Such extensive access may create additional risks of these data to hackers, Health Insurance Portability and Accountability Act violations, and the like. Although these issues are not insurmountable, the risks need to be acknowledged and addressed.[28]

What Can be Done Legislatively to Address Artificial Intelligence Issues?

Avoid the courts
There is an often paraphrased adage "hard cases make bad law." Letting the courts address errors in AI could result in a delineating of liability in ways counterproductive to AI development, and may have the effect of snuffing out this technology in its relative infancy. When a court makes law, its impact is less instructional and more remedial. Given the underlying risk inherent in health care, when faced with significant lawsuits, the risks of liability may be too great for smaller start-up AI development companies.

Legislative action
Legislators would be better positioned than the courts to issue legislation that does not stifle AI in its infancy while still protecting the public from potential dangers when AI judgment replaces that of humans. Many states have already enacted

legislation in the area of autonomous vehicles in order to foster growth and testing.[24(pp7–9)] To allow for robust AI development in the medical area, advocates have suggested a variety of legislative actions/regulations, with some emphasis on the need for standardization. Having a set of regulations to adhere to would allow health care interests to demonstrate that they were abiding by the standard of care. Although of less impact than legislation, clinical practice guidelines issued by professional organizations also may be useful in delineating a standard of care for use in AI.

Some investigators have advocated an approach pioneered decades ago to protect the vaccine industry.[23(p22),24(p6)] In the 1980s there was an onslaught of litigation filed against manufacturers and developers of childhood vaccines, and there was national concern that vaccine companies would determine the risk of lawsuits too great and withdraw from the industry. To bolster this sector, the US government created a federally administered fund based on taxes on vaccines, and uses this fund to award judgments for injuries from certain delineated reactions to certain childhood vaccines under the National Vaccine Injury Compensation Program.[29] This federal legislation proved beneficial both because it allowed vaccine manufacturers to continue producing vaccines without the constant threat of massive lawsuits, but also because a specialized adjunct court within the US Court of Federal Claims, with expertise on vaccines and reactions was hearing these cases rather than a jury, and the awards tended to be less variable and emotionally charged and more needs driven/less punitive.[29] A similar opportunity could be available with AI, as there are certainly national benefits to incorporating AI into health care, AI use carries with it significant litigation risk, AI's use will presumably become a technical fee in billing that could easily be "taxed" to compose a fund, and specialized judges rather than jurors simply would make more sense to oversee AI cases given the complexity of the technology involved.

REGULATION OF AI

The extent to which AI software may be regulated will turn on whether it is treated as a medical device, and the classification assigned to it by the FDA. The FDA categorizes medical devices into one of three classes (Class I, II and III, respectively) based on risks and the necessary regulatory controls to assure safety and effectiveness.[31]Class I are devices used in medical care which present minimal potential for harm, Class II are intermediate risk devices, and Class III are high risk devices that are very important to health or sustaining life.[32] The treatment of CADe and CADx respectively is illustrative. The FDA initially distinguished the type of software application CADe, Computer Aided Detection, "intended to identify, mark, highlight or otherwise direct attention to portions of an image" from what we term CADx, Computer Aided Diagnosis, "intended to provide information beyond identifying… abnormalities, such as an assessment of disease".[33] As such, software that flags findings for an imager to consider are categorized as CADe, while software that provides a more comprehensive diagnostic assessment, such as tumor grading, would be considered CADx. Federal regulations address radiological computer assisted diagnostic software (including CADx), and describes that it is a device that characterizes lesions based on features or information extracted from the images and provides information about the lesion(s) to the user…" noting that "[d]iagnostic and patient management decisions are made by the clinical user".[34] The functions of CADe are covered by another provision, addressing software that is intended to incorporate pattern recognition and flag findings on previously acquired images for an imager to consider.[35] Under current legislation, both of these functions now fall under Class II.[33,36–38]

As mentioned above, the FDA has historically sidestepped the issue of addressing learning/evolving algorithms, and cleared a number of AI based medical devices using "locked algorithms".[39] While it remains to be seen how a more autonomous continuous learning AI algorithm would be addressed and categorized by the FDA, the FDA has indicated that they may require a "predetermined change control plan" involving a greater degree of transparency in premarket submissions and real world monitoring and updates in conjunction with FDA oversight and monitoring of AI/Machine Learning devices.[40] It remains to be seen how this may impact the development and applications of this fledgling technology going forward.

SUMMARY: FINAL THOUGHTS AND RECOMMENDATIONS

AI is rapidly becoming incorporated into nuclear medicine and other health care fields and offers significant upside in terms of diagnostic accuracy, cost-effectiveness, and potentially even scan time/dose reduction. However, the legal ramifications of AI are as yet poorly delineated, and imagers would be wise to stay abreast of legal developments with respect to this new technology. Specifically, imaging physicians working in practices that are incorporating AI should[19(p1766),30(p121)] do the following:

- Educate themselves on their AI software: learn better how to use and interpret AI algorithms, and thoroughly train those employees involved in the use of AI.
- Advocate for professional organization guidelines, governmental regulations. These will provide a standard-of-care benchmark to adhere to when using AI.
- Make sure AI products are adequately vetted before use; FDA approved where possible.
- Monitor the results of AI systems and make sure they are making medically appropriate recommendations: some form of regular, continuous auditing process is suggested.
- Confirm with malpractice carrier to what extent you are covered for AI use/reliance.
- Obtain informed consent of patients before incorporating AI use into their care. Disclaimers are unlikely to be enforceable in cases of medical negligence, but patients should be made aware of the extent of reliance on AI in their care.
- When using CAD applications, acknowledge the CAD findings in your report, and explain your reasoning when disagreeing with a CAD finding.
- Maintain robust cybersecurity and privacy controls.

CLINICS CARE POINTS

- In order to establish a medical malpractice case, a plaintiff must establish that a physician had a duty of care, that there was a breach of that duty, prove causation and demonstrate damages.
- It remains unclear whether negligence in the setting of AI will result in liability to the treating physician, likely via a doctrine of vicarious liability or as a learned intermediary, or whether the AI manufacturer will bear liability under products liability law.
- Whether the law ultimately treats AI as a mere physician enhancement tool versus an autonomous "person", as well as evolving FDA regulation of AI as a medical device, will have profound impact on the future development of this industry.
- Clinicians utilizing AI should educate themselves on the AI software they use, monitor/audit results and advocate for sensible organizational guidelines and legislative regulations to establish a standard of care for use of AI in the field.

DISCLOSURE

The author has nothing to disclose.

REFERENCES

1. Walter M. If you think AI will never replace radiologists – you may want to think again. Radiology Business; 2018. Available at: https://www.radiologybusiness.com/topics/artificial-intelligence/if-you-think-ai-will-never-replace-radiologists-you-may-want-think. Accessed March 6, 2021.
2. Froelich JW, Salavati A. Artificial intelligence in PET/CT is about to make whole-body tumor burden measurements a clinical reality. Radiology 2020;2094:453–4.
3. Sibille L, Seifert R, Avramovic N, et al. 18F-FDG PET/CT uptake classification in lymphoma and lung cancer by using deep convolutional neural networks. Radiology 2020;294:445–52.
4. Wang T, Lei Y, Fu Y, et al. Machine learning in quantitative PET: a review of attenuation correction and low-count image reconstruction methods. Phys Med 2020;76:294–306.
5. Sullivan HR, Schweikart SJ. Are current tort liability doctrines adequate for addressing injury caused by AI? AMA J Ethics 2019;21(2):E160–6. at 161. Available at: https://journalofethics.ama-assn.org/article/are-current-tort-liability-doctrines-adequate-addressing-injury-caused-ai/2019-02. Accessed September 25, 2021.
6. Achar S, Wu W. How to reduce malpractice risk; family practice management. 2012. Available at: www.aafp.org/fpm.
7. Berlin L. Malpractice issues in radiology: curbstone consultations. AJR Am J Roentgenol 2002;178(6):1353–9.
8. Francis A. Is this a real doctor-patient relationship? Medscape; 2012. Available at: https://www.medscape.com/viewarticle/759163. Accessed March 6, 2021.
9. Black HC. Black's law dictionary. 5th edition. St Paul: West Publishing Co; 1979.
10. Eisenberg RL. Radiology and the law: malpractice and other issues. New York: Springer-Verlag; 2004.
11. Mezrich JL, Siegel EL. Legal ramifications of computer-aided detection in mammography. J Am Coll Radiol 2015;12(6):572–4.
12. Federal rules of evidence, rule 803 (18). Available at: https://www.law.cornell.edu/rules/fre/rule_803. Accessed March 6, 2021.
13. Mezrich J. Hiding in the hedges: tips to minimize your malpractice risks as a radiologist. Am J Roentgen 2019;213:1037–41. at 1038.
14. Crisler RS. The burden of proof in medical liability cases: a preponderance of the evidence. American Academy of Orthopaedic Surgeons Bulletin; 2006. Available at: http://www2.aaos.org/bulletin/feb06/rskman2.asp. Accessed Match 6, 2021.
15. Keeton WP, editor. Prosser and Keeton on the law of torts. 5th edition. St. Paul, MN: West Publishing; 1984. p. 499. ch. 12.
16. Prosser, supra, chapter 17. pp. 677.
17. Chung J, Zink A, Watson Hey. Can I sue you for malpractice? Examining the liability of artificial intelligence in medicine. Asia Pac J Health L Ethics 2018;11(2):51–80. at 68.
18. Harned Z, Lungren MP, Rajpurkar P. Machine vision, medical AI, and malpractice. Harv J Law Technol 2019. at 7. Available at: https://jolt.law.harvard.edu/digest/machine-vision-medical-ai-and-malpractice. Accessed March 6, 2021.
19. Price WN, Gerke S, Cohen IG. Potential liability for physicians using artificial intelligence. J Am Med Assoc 2019;322(18):1765–6. at 1765.
20. Keris MP. Artificial intelligence in medicine creates real risk management and litigation issues. J Healthc Risk Manag 2020;40(2):21–6. at 2.
21. Jha S. Can you sue an algorithm for malpractice? It depends. STAT; 2020. Available at: https://www.statnews.com/2020/03/09/can-you-sue-artificial-intelligence-algorithm-for-malpractice/. Accessed March 6, 2021.
22. Riegel V. Medtronic, Inc, 552 U.S. 312 (2008).
23. Jorstad KT. Intersection of artificial intelligence and medicine: tort liability in the technological age. J Med Artif Intellig 2020;3(17):1–28. at 7. Available at: https://jmai.amegroups.com/article/view/5938. Accessed September 25, 2021.
24. Silverman C, Goldberg P, Wilson J, et al. Torts of the future: autonomous vehicles. Addressing the liability and regulatory implications of emerging technologies. U.S. Chamber Institute for Legal Reform; 2018. at 4.
25. Shepardson D. GM settles lawsuit with motorcyclist hit by self-driving car, Reuters. 2018. Available at: https://www.reuters.com/article/us-gm-selfdriving/gm-settles-lawsuit-with-motorcyclist-hit-by-self-driving-car-idUSKCN1IX604. Accessed March 6, 21.
26. Siddiqui F. Uber reaches settlement with family of victim killed after being struck by self driving vehicles. Chicago Tribune; 2018 (While Uber settled this civil suit, the driver was subsequently charged criminally for negligent homicide). Available at: https://www.chicagotribune.com/business/ct-biz-uber-self-driving-car-settlement-20180330-story.html. Accessed March 6, 2021.
27. Tobia K, Nielsen A, Stremitzer A. When does physician use of AI increase liability? J Nucl Med 2021;62:17–21.
28. Klenske N. Protecting patient privacy in the era of artificial intelligence. RSNA News; 2021. Available at: https://www.rsna.org/news/2021/february/protecting-patient-privacy. Accessed March 6, 2021.

29. Mezrich J, Proving a claim under the national vaccine injury compensation program, 23 American Jurisprudence, Proof of facts 3d. 71 (1993).
30. Giuffrida I, Treece T. Keeping AI under observation: anticipated impacts on physician's standard of care. Faculty Publications; 2020. Available at: https://scholarship.law.wm.edu/facpubs/2002. Accessed March 6, 2021.
31. Overview of Medical Device Classification and Reclassification. Available at. www.fda.gov.
32. Jin J, FDA Authorization of Medical Devices, JAMA, 2014;311(4): 435. Available at www.jamanetwork.com.
33. Van Leeuwen F, A 101f guide to the FDA regulatory process for AI radiology software, Quantib, Nov. 20, 2019. Available at. www.quantib.com.
34. 21 C.F.R. 892.2060 (a).
35. 21.C.F.R. 892.2070 (a).
36. Ridley, EL, FDA finalizes easier rules for CADe software, Auntminnie.com, Jan.21, 2020. Available at. www.auntminnie.com.
37. 21 C.F.R. 892.2070 (b).
38. 21 C.F.R. 892.2060 (b).
39. Benjamens S, Dhunnoo P, Mesko B, The state of artificial intelligence-based FDA-approved medical devices and algorithms: an online database, npj Digitial Medicine 3:118 (2020).
40. Artificial Intelligence/Machine Learning (AI/ML)-Based Software as a Medical Device (SaMD) Action Plan, US Food and Drug Administration, January 2021. Available at. www.fda.gov.

Evidence-Based Artificial Intelligence in Medical Imaging

David L. Streiner, PhD, CPsych[a,b,c], Babak Saboury, MD, MPH, DABR, DABNM[d,e,f], Katherine A. Zukotynski, MD, PhD, FRCPC, PEng[g,h,i],*

KEYWORDS

• Evidence-based • Medical imaging • Artificial intelligence

KEY POINTS

- It is imperative that articles discussing artificial intelligence (AI) in medical imaging be evaluated critically using an evidence-based approach, as has been proposed for other types of research.
- In the field of AI in medical imaging, 5 questions can be applied to determine if the model being suggested is applicable to the situation at hand.
- These questions are: (1) Who was in the training sample?, (2) How was the model trained?, (3) How reliable is the algorithm?, (4) How was the model evaluated?, and (5) How useable is the algorithm?.

THE 5-STEP EVIDENCE-BASED APPROACH TO ARTIFICIAL INTELLIGENCE IN MEDICAL IMAGING

In medical imaging, images are typically acquired to answer a specific clinical question. Artificial intelligence (AI) relies on the use of algorithms to accomplish a given task. To gather insight into the algorithm best suited for a task, and the cost needed to achieve the desired output, it has been recommended that a checklist be included for reporting the algorithm in the context of the task performed. **Table 1** provides our top 5 points to include, for the purposes of clarity.[1]

However, while answering the questions above helps to describe an algorithm and its performance for completing a specific task, in such a way that results can be more easily reproduced and compared, it does not answer the ultimate question of how applicable an algorithm is to answer a given clinical question.

Similar to the evidence-based approach that we are already familiar with throughout the field of medicine, adopting an evidence-based approach to AI in medical imaging entails asking the following questions and analyzing the answers. Specifically: (1) Who was in the training sample?, (2) How was the model trained?, (3) How reliable is the algorithm?, (4) How was the model validated?, and (5) How useable is the algorithm? (**Box 1**). We provide additional details regarding these questions later in discussion.

[a] Department of Psychiatry and Behavioural Neurosciences, McMaster University; [b] Department of Psychiatry, University of Toronto; [c] St. Joseph's Healthcare, West 5th Campus, 100 West 5th Street, Hamilton, Ontario L8N 3K7, Canada; [d] Department of Radiology and Imaging Sciences, Clinical Center, National Institutes of Health, Bethesda, MD, USA; [e] Department of Computer Science and Electrical Engineering, University of Maryland, Baltimore County, Baltimore, MD, USA; [f] Department of Radiology, Hospital of the University of Pennsylvania, Philadelphia, PA, USA; [g] Departments of Radiology and Medicine, McMaster University, 1200 Main St. W., Hamilton, ON L8N 3Z5, Canada; [h] School of Biomedical Engineering, McMaster University, 1280 Main St. W., Hamilton, ON L8S 4K1, Canada; [i] Edward S. Rogers Sr. Department of Electrical and Computer Engineering, University of Toronto, 10 King's College Rd., Toronto, ON M5S 3G8, Canada
* Corresponding author. Department of Medicine, McMaster University, 1200 Main Street West, Hamilton, Ontario L8N 3Z5, Canada.
E-mail address: katherine.zukotynski@utoronto.ca

PET Clin 17 (2022) 51–55
https://doi.org/10.1016/j.cpet.2021.09.005
1556-8598/22/© 2021 Elsevier Inc. All rights reserved.

Table 1
Suggested checklist to include for algorithm reporting

Question	Possible Metric	Comment
1. Algorithm used?	Family of algorithms	that is, Convolutional neural network (CNN), random forest...
2. Architecture details?	Dependent on algorithm	that is, for a CNN report number of layers, kernel size, strides, and show a complete block diagram with sufficient detail that the model could be independently reconstructed.
3. Computational cost?	Number of parameters	that is, while consulting a computing expert, similar to consulting a statistician for clinical trials, is suggested, authors may generate this themselves.
4. Data?	Training, validation, testing	that is, data type, number of validation/testing cases, use of cross-validation, data source (algorithms trained with data from a single institution might not perform well using data from another institution).
5. Figure of merit?	Classification accuracy, dose reduction...	that is, key numerical performance results should be given such as classification accuracy... ultimately this should be standardized for a given application.

Box 1
Checklist for appraising an article

1. Who was in the training sample?
   a. Was the sample adequately described in terms of demographic information?
   b. Did this article indicate any inclusion/exclusion criteria?
   c. Was the setting described?
   d. Was there a full spectrum of diseases, including normals?
   e. Were any diagnoses overrepresented?
   f. Were the data transformed in any way, and if so, how?

2. How was the model trained?
   a. How was the criterion diagnosis established?
   b. If there were 2 or more raters, was their reliability reported?
   c. How were cases whereby there was no agreement handled?
   d. How many images were in the training set?

3. How reliable are the results?
   a. Was reliability checked by using the algorithm twice on the same data?
   b. How high was the reliability?
   c. Was the estimate of reliability determined in a sample of patients similar to yours?

4. How was the model validated?
   a. How large was the internal validation set?
   b. How large was the external validation set?
   c. Were the judgments of the clinicians made without knowledge of the model diagnosis?
   d. How were the results reported?

5. How useable is the algorithm?
   a. Does it diagnose the conditions in which you are interested?
   b. Is it designed for research or clinical purposes?
   c. Can the end-user modify or adapt it?
   d. Does the vendor provide periodic updates?
   e. Can it be integrated into the clinical workflow?

Who Was in the Training Sample?

AI algorithms used in medical imaging may be supervised or unsupervised. In the case of a supervised algorithm, training requires access to a database of existing images. Thus, the accuracy of the output, for example, a diagnosis based on new images depends on the degree to which those new images (presumably the images seen in clinical practice) are similar to those images in the training set. This can be determined only if there is a complete description of the cases in the training set. For example, details on the training data such as image acquisition technique, equipment used, patient age, disease diagnoses, and how the patient cohort was selected (eg, all cases; only those that met certain criteria, etc.), among other details, are needed. Also, the training sample should include the full spectrum of pathology that can be diagnosed from the images, including normal cases, and the distribution of disease should be similar to what is encountered in clinical practice. Over or underrepresentation of one disease subtype can bias the results.[2] Finally, there should be a description of how the data were transformed before being entered into the database.

How Was the Algorithm Trained?

Most commonly, a supervised algorithm is trained using a label or diagnosis attached to each of the images in the dataset, also called using tagged data. Of course, the accuracy of the algorithm depends heavily on the accuracy of the labels. These may be based on the clinical notes, the judgment of clinicians, or a combination of the 2. Under ideal circumstances, 2 or more judges would independently come to a decision, using whatever information is available, and this raises 2 points. First, the agreement between or among the judges should be reported, using either Cohen's kappa[3] or an extension of it for 3 or more raters, such as the intraclass correlation coefficient (ICC[4]). Second, there may be some cases whereby the judges disagree. If so, how were these cases handled? Were they deleted from the training set or were they kept in, and, in the latter case, which, if any, diagnosis was assigned?

A more difficult question is whether there were enough cases in the dataset to fully reflect the data that might be encountered in clinical practice. There are many heuristics that can be considered, such as X cases for each output class, or Y times the number of input features, or Z times the number of model parameters. The problem is that no one knows the right values for X, Y, or Z. What is known (or at least strongly suspected) is that these

values are high, such as 500 to 1000 cases for each output class. If there are too few cases, there is a very real danger of overfitting the model, meaning that there are too many parameters or features given the sample size.[5,6] This will result in an algorithm that fits the training data very well, but will have very little predictive power when applied to new data.

How Reliable Is the Algorithm?

Reliability can be defined as "the extent to which measurements of individuals obtained under different circumstances yield similar results".[7] Although there are several different ways of establishing reliability, the most important for a diagnostic test is referred to as *test–retest reliability*. That is, if the same scan is analyzed by the algorithm on 2 separate occasions, do they yield the same result? If the outcome is dichotomous (eg, disease present or absent), one would analyze the results using Cohen's kappa (κ), which is a measure of agreement corrected for chance agreement[3]; whereas for categorical results (eg, present/absent/indeterminate), one would use weighted kappa (κ_W[8]) or the ICC.[4,9] If the output will be used solely for research purposes, values between 0.70 and 0.90 are acceptable. However, when used for clinical purposes, the reliability should be at least 0.95.[10]

It is important to bear in mind that reliability is not a fixed property of a tool, but is highly dependent on the sample in which it is assessed.[11] Another way of defining reliability is a tool's ability to differentiate among people. If the sample is heterogeneous, reliability tends to be high. However, the same instrument used with a more homogeneous sample will have lower reliability. Thus, you should trust the reported reliability only if it was determined in a sample of patients with characteristics similar to your own.

How Was the Algorithm Validated?

In most cases, the data set is divided into 3 groups: the training set, a validation set, and a testing set. The validation set, which is usually smaller than the training set, allows the model parameters to be fine-tuned. The final model should then be tested.[2] It is mandatory that no cases in this testing set be in the training or validation sets. Otherwise, there will be "criterion contamination",[7] in which the algorithm is being correlated in part with itself.

Although this is a necessary step, it is not sufficient because the testing data is drawn from the same pool of cases as the training and validation data. Thus, whatever biases exist in the latter, with respect to diagnostic mix, ethnicity, age,

Table 2
Reporting the results of validity studies

		Gold Standard		Total
		Present	Absent	
Model Result	Present	A True Positive	B False Positive	A + B
	Absent	C False Negative	D True Negative	C + D
	Total	A + C	B + D	N

and so on, will also exist in the training set. A true test of the validity of the algorithms would be an external testing data set, ideally drawn from a different setting. Regardless, it is imperative that the judgment of the clinician be made without knowledge of the diagnosis from the algorithms. Again, violation of this would result in criterion contamination.

There are several ways to report the accuracy of the algorithm. Perhaps the easiest to understand is with a 2 × 2 table, as illustrated in **Table 2**, whereby the columns reflect the "gold standard" (eg, the consensus diagnosis of 2 or more clinicians, made without knowing the results of the algorithm) and the rows are the output from the model. Cell A represents the number of cases whereby both the gold standard and the algorithm agree a disease is present (ie, true positives), Cell B whereby the gold standard indicates that a disease is not present but the algorithm says it is (false positives), and so forth (**Table 2**).

The *sensitivity* of the algorithm is defined as A/(A + C); that is, the proportion of true cases detected by the algorithm. Similarly, the *specificity* is D/(B+ D); the proportion of noncases labeled by the algorithm as noncases. Although these are important properties of any diagnostic tool, they do not tell the whole story. Once the algorithm is used routinely, the gold standard will not be available to the clinicians. All they will have are several cases deemed to have the disease by the algorithm (ie, Cells A + B) and a number labeled as disease-free (Cells C + D). The important questions are then: Of all cases called positive by the program, what proportion are actually from people who have the disease; that is, A/(A + B)? This is called the *positive predictive value* (PPV) of the algorithm. In the same way, the second question is what proportion of cases deemed disease-free by the algorithm are actually from people who do not have the disease; the *negative predictive value* (NPV), defined as D/(C + D)?

It is assumed that if the patients seen in one's clinical practice are similar to the ones in the training set, then the sensitivity and specificity should remain constant. However, the PPV and NPV are very dependent on the prevalence of the disease in one's caseload. When the prevalence is low, the PPV tends to be poor, resulting in many false-positive cases; whereas the NPV is high, meaning that the algorithm is good for ruling out the disorder. Conversely, when the prevalence is high, the PPV is high but the NPV is low. These are universal laws that hold for all diagnostic tests. For more on interpreting the results of diagnostic tests, see Streiner.[12,13]

How Useable Is the Algorithm?

No matter how accurate the algorithm is, it is of little use unless it can be integrated into clinical practice. Omoumi and colleagues[14] list several factors that must be considered in evaluating an AI system. First, is it designed to identify the medical conditions that you are interested in? Second, was it designed to be used for clinical or research purposes, or both? Third, can the end-user modify or adapt the algorithm in light of experience or the characteristics of the clinical population being seen? Fourth, does the vendor provide periodic updates? And finally, can it be easily integrated into the clinical workflow? The article also discusses several other possible considerations and should be read by anyone contemplating using such a system.

SUMMARY

At the end of the day, one must have a clear understanding of the clinical task, patient population, data for training including the process by which imaging was acquired and data extracted, algorithm training and reliability, the validation method used, and the applicability of the algorithm into clinical practice. Armed with this, one has the ability to apply a generalizable evidence-based approach to AI in medical imaging!

DISCLOSURE

Please note that Dr D. Streiner, Dr K.A. Zukotynski, and Dr B. Saboury have nothing to disclose.

REFERENCES

1. Zukotynski K, Gaudet V, Uribe CF, et al. Machine learning in nuclear medicine: Part 2—neural networks and clinical aspects. J Nucl Med 2021; 62(1):22–9.
2. Faes L, Liu X, Wagner SK, et al. A clinician's guide to artificial intelligence: how to critically appraise machine learning studies. Transl Vis Sci Technol 2020; 9(2):7.
3. Cohen J. A coefficient of agreement for nominal scales. Educ Psychol Meas 1960;20(1):37–46.
4. Shrout PE, Fleiss JL. Intraclass correlations: uses in assessing rater reliability. Psychol Bull 1979;86(2): 420–8.
5. Collins GS, Moons KGM. Reporting of artificial intelligence prediction models. Lancet 2019;393(10181): 1577–9.
6. Norgeot B, Quer G, Beaulieu-Jones BK, et al. Minimum information about clinical artificial intelligence modeling: the MI-CLAIM checklist. Nat Med 2020; 26(9):1320–4.
7. Streiner DL, Norman GR, Cairney J. Health measurement scales: a practical guide to their development and use. 5th edition. Oxford (England): Oxford University Press; 2015.
8. Cohen J. Weighted kappa: nominal scale agreement provision for scaled disagreement or partial credit. Psychol Bull 1968;70(4):213–20.
9. Fleiss JL, Cohen J. The equivalence of weighted kappa and the intraclass correlation coefficient as measures of reliability. Educ Psychol Meas 1973; 33(3):613–9.
10. Nunnally J, Bernstein I. Psychometric theory. 3rd edition. New York: McGraw-Hill; 1994.
11. Streiner DL. Reliability. J Clin Psychopharmacol 2016;36(4):305–7.
12. Streiner DL. Diagnosing tests: using and misusing diagnostic and screening tests. J Pers Assess 2003;81(3):209–19.
13. Streiner DL. Using diagnostic tests; or the search for universal truths. J Clin Psychopharmacol 2017; 37(4):391–3.
14. Omoumi P, Ducarouge A, Tournier A, et al. To buy or not to buy—evaluating commercial AI solutions in radiology (the ECLAIR guidelines). Eur Radiol 2021;31(6):3786–96.

Clinical

Artificial Intelligence for Brain Molecular Imaging

Donna J. Cross, PhD[a,*], Seisaku Komori[b], Satoshi Minoshima, MD, PhD[a]

KEYWORDS

• Artificial intelligence • Deep learning • Brain molecular imaging • PET

KEY POINTS

- "Artificial Intelligence" or "AI" was initially developed in the mid-twentieth century. In the past decade, the field of AI has seen explosive growth due to increases in computational resources, availability of "big data," and investment by industry and academia.
- A neural network includes an input training dataset, which is propagated through hidden layers for the feature extraction and determination of the weights. The resultant output is compared with the curated training output through an iterative process. The trained algorithm analyzes a new input dataset and predicts output.
- "Deep Learning" algorithms can be distinguished from simple multilayer machine learning models in that they use more complex, nested, and/or hierarchical information combined with algorithms, which can both extract features and optimize the assignment of the weights to achieve accurate diagnostic classification.
- We propose a "Tier" concept to classify AI health care applications: Tier 1, AI-based imaging applications can be considered "Operations" including ones that facilitate workflow and image generation. Tier 2-type applications are focused on cognitive skills/decision-making, such as diagnosis and/or evaluating prognosis. Tier 3 includes AI algorithms, which are "superhuman," and can achieve outcomes that are not possible by human experts.
- Even with the growing level of sophistication, these advanced AI networks will still require expert human supervision for appropriate application and accurate interpretation in medical imaging practice at this time.

INTRODUCTION

The concept of "Artificial Intelligence" or "AI" was developed in the mid-twentieth Century whereby terms such as "Neural Nets,"[1] artificial neural networks (ANNs), or "Perceptrons,"[2] and "backpropagation"[3] were coined. However, limitations in computational power resulted in slow research progress for such concepts during the mid to late 1970s. In the early 1980s, with the algorithmic advancement of "Convolutional Neural Networks" or "CNN," AI development resumed, including applications to more complex imaging datasets.[4,5]

Still, development in the field of AI was limited by computational hardware in the early 1990s. The modern era of AI development and more widespread application began in the late 1990s and was facilitated by technical advancements in data processing, storage, and transmission capabilities as well as the accumulation of large datasets for algorithmic training. Within the past decade, the field of AI has seen explosive growth, mostly due to the above-mentioned increases in computational resources and "big data." In addition, a growing awareness of its transformative potential, as well as substantial academic and

[a] Department of Radiology and Imaging Sciences, University of Utah, 30 North 1900 East #1A71, Salt Lake City, UT 84132-2140, USA; [b] Future Design Lab, New Concept Design, Global Strategic Challenge Center, Hamamatsu Photonics K.K. 5000, Hirakuchi, Hamakita-ku, Hamamatsu-City, 434-8601 Japan
* Corresponding author. Department of Radiology and Imaging Sciences, University of Utah, 30 North 1900 East #1A71, Salt Lake City, UT 84132-2140.
E-mail address: d.cross@utah.edu

PET Clin 17 (2022) 57–64
https://doi.org/10.1016/j.cpet.2021.08.001
1556-8598/22/© 2021 Elsevier Inc. All rights reserved.

industry investment has led to readily available software platforms, which can be easily implemented. Such open-source platforms include U-Net, OpenNN, TensorFlow, and many others.

EVOLUTION OF ARTIFICIAL INTELLIGENCE DEVELOPMENT FOR MEDICAL IMAGING
Artificial Neural Networks

Despite the development of increasingly sophisticated algorithms for AI applications, most modern methods implement basic processes that have been established over years. These concepts, including neural networks with multilayer perceptrons (MLPs), deep learning, machine learning, and convolutional neural networks are the foundation of the software platforms, which are used for image-based AI applications.

The basic versions of AI are neural networks such as MLPs. Within this framework, the initial training dataset is fed into the "Input Layer," processed via backpropagation throughout the hidden layers and the resultant information becomes the "Output Layer," which is compared with the training output. Most importantly, the training dataset is curated, particularly the output data, which represents the ground truth or "gold standard," and is the objective of the AI algorithmic outcome. During the training phase, with sufficient training input and curated output data, backpropagation throughout the hidden layers results in the estimation of weights for various features, which produce a match of the resultant output layer with the curated training output (Fig. 1A). Once the neural network is trained, including an estimation of the weights, a new input dataset, the validation data, is fed into the trained network, and the resultant product is the new output (Fig. 1B).

These most basic neural networks have been applied to imaging data. In fact, the application to brain molecular imaging is one of the first clinical applications of AI in the field of Radiology. As early as 1992, a study by Kippenhan and colleagues used a region of interest (ROI)-based approach combined with a backpropagation neural network to discriminate normal versus abnormal on ^{18}F-fluorodeoxyglucose positron emission tomography (FDG-PET) from probable patients with Alzheimer's disease (AD) versus age-matched controls.[6] On the ROC curve evaluation, they found that the discriminatory performance of the neural net was better than the statistical "discriminant analysis" method, but not quite as good as that of a trained expert reader. In another study published in 2000, Lee and colleagues used a relatively simple MLP neural network applied to FDG-PET images of patients with temporal lobe epilepsy to identify the epileptogenic foci.[7] The ANN performed better than traditional discriminatory analysis but also was slightly improved from the expert diagnosis. Even over this relatively short time, these fairly simple ANNs were able to meet or exceed the diagnostic performance of expert readers. Another application of an ANN distinguished Parkinson's disease from normal controls on [99mTc]TRODAT-1 SPECT imaging, and achieved 91.4%, 97.5%, and 94.4% for the sensitivity, specificity, and accuracy, respectively.[8] These values were greatly improved from "best observer" numbers of 88.3%, 87.7%, and 88.0%. Also, Bose and colleagues used an ANN model to classify schizophrenic patients from normal controls based on 6-[18]F- fluoro-L-DOPA PET images.[9] Using the ^{18}F-FDOPA rate constants in the anterior–posterior subdivisions of the striatum, they found that the ANN model correctly discriminated controls from patients, with a sensitivity of 89% and a specificity of 94%. These examples illustrate that even relatively simple AI models such as neural networks can achieve levels of diagnostic classification for brain molecular imaging, which equals or exceeds the performance of medical experts.

Deep Learning

Early studies of AI imaging applications were mostly based on the initial extraction of ROIs or region-extracted features, which required user supervision to reach optimal discriminatory capabilities and served to reduce the total amount of data input to the network. As the technology evolved to permit greater computational power, the feature extraction step could be integrated into the AI algorithms to permit user-independent models. These "Deep Learning" algorithms can be distinguished from simple multilayer machine learning models in that they use more complex, nested, and/or hierarchical information combined with algorithms, which can both extract features and optimize the assignment of the weights to achieve accurate diagnostic classification. These more sophisticated models use a greater number of hidden processing layers with more complex connectivity. The drawback of deep learning AI is that the algorithms are computationally expensive, but also they require extremely large datasets for training because there are more parameters to be estimated. This can be a significant obstacle with brain molecular imaging applications because the acquisition of large curated imaging datasets can be a challenge to obtain and also very expensive cost-wise. However, deep learning has been

A

Neural Network: Multilayer Perceptrons (MLP)

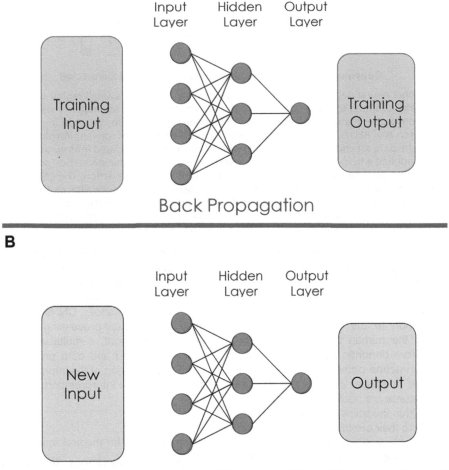

Fig. 1. Neural network architecture incorporating multilayer perceptrons. (*A*) Represents the curated training data for a neural network including the input dataset, which is propagated throughout the hidden layers for the feature extraction and determination of the weights. The resultant output is compared with the curated training output, preferably representing a "gold standard" or ground truth, through this iterative process. (*B*) Once the algorithm is trained, it can analyze the new input to predict the output.

readily applied to various fields for which large datasets exist, such as language processing and speech recognition, image recognition and restoration, drug discovery, bioinformatics, management operations, finance, the gaming industry, and marketing.

Several types of deep learning algorithms have been developed, which are more specific to medical imaging applications. These include convolutional neural networks (CNNs), recurrent neural networks (eg, LSTM), and recursive neural networks. CNNs are the most widely applied for image analysis. With CNN processing, the input image undergoes feature extraction within the hidden layers of the algorithm whereby the steps involve the application of convolution filters plus rectified linear units (RELUs), then pooling, followed by more iterations of convolution plus RELUs, then pooling, to compress the data set and assign the weights within the spatially associated information (**Fig. 2**). The convolution filters, which are applied within the hidden layers, are diverse and can discriminate vertical and horizontal direction, gradients, different colors, and so forth, for the purpose of feature detection and extraction. The concept of convolution filters is

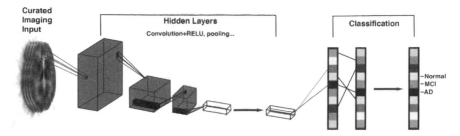

Convolutional Layer -> Pooling Layer -> -> -> Fully Connected

Fig. 2. Convolutional neural networks (CNNs) for image analysis. In a CNN, a small region of the input layer, a local receptive field, connects to the hidden layers, and is translated across an image to create a feature map. The input image undergoes feature extraction within the hidden layers whereby the steps involve the application of convolution filters plus RELUs, then pooling, followed by more iterations of convolution plus RELUs, then pooling, to compress the data set and assign the weights within the spatially associated information. The convolution filters, which are applied within the hidden layers are diverse and can discriminate vertical and horizontal direction, gradients, different colors, and so forth, for the purpose of feature extraction. The CNN model learns the weights during the training process. The pooling step reduces the dimensionality of the feature map by condensing the output. This simplifies the subsequent layers and reduces the number of parameters. The resultant spatially interconnected and compressed imaging data are then "flattened" into a fully connected layer for the classification output which is subsequently compared with the curated output in the training phase.

familiar to nuclear medicine and molecular imaging specialists because similar approaches have been applied to image reconstruction and processing. The RELUs are activation functions, which serve as the decision tool to sum the weights, in relation to the convolutional filters. The analogy to the human brain would be the ramp function from dendritic input which results in the firing of an action potential in the neuronal axon. Within the multilayer construct, data with these similar features are pooled through many iterations. Also within the training process, the data are weighted as to their contribution to the correct outcome, which ultimately shrinks the overall size of the dataset as well as eliminates image noise. The resultant spatially interconnected and compressed imaging data are then "flattened" into a fully connected layer for the classification output which is subsequently than the curated output in the training phase.

To further relate the CNN algorithmic process to actual brain function, it can be compared with how the human brain processes visual information (Fig. 3). The cells within the retina receive information related to the original image, and transmit feature-specific data via neuronal firing to the next layer within the lateral geniculate nucleus (LGN).[10] From there, the information is further "expanded" as it is processed in the primary (V1) and secondary (V2) visual cortices. The original visual input is further processed through this visual hierarchy, which identifies and encodes information such as edge detection, orientation, color, motion, and so forth, similar to the convolution filters, RELUs, and pooling layers of a CNN. Finally,

within the visual association cortex including the lateral occipital cortex (LOC), the information is consolidated and certain specific cells respond to more abstract categorizations such as "face" or "cat." In this manner, CNNs were designed to mimic human visual processing in that there is an original visual input, a multilayer approach with feature extraction and data processing followed by the consolidation of the information for classification and image interpretation.

AI applications for medical imaging

- *Tier 1* – Operations (image formation, workflow)
- *Tier 2* – Decision making (diagnosis, prediction)
- *Tier 3* – Superhuman (better than human experts)

APPLICATIONS OF ARTIFICIAL INTELLIGENCE TO BRAIN MOLECULAR IMAGING

We propose that artificial intelligence (AI) for brain molecular imaging applications be broadly divided into 3 categories. Many imaging applications are "Operations" including ones that facilitate image generation and workflow, which may be considered first level or "Tier 1." Second level or "Tier 2" type applications are focused on decision-making and applications mimicking human cognitive functions, such as diagnosis and/or disease

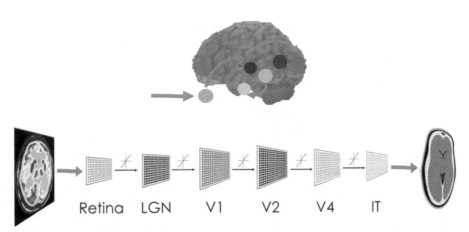

Retina LGN V1 V2 V4 IT

Fig. 3. Human brain versus CNN: the visual system. The retina receives information related to the original image and transmits feature-specific data via neuronal firing to the next layer within the LGN. The original visual input is "expanded" as it is processed in the primary (V1) and secondary (V2) visual cortices. This visual hierarchy identifies and encodes information such as edge detection, orientation, color, motion, and so forth, similar to the convolution filters, RELUs, and pooling layers of a CNN. Finally, within the visual association cortex including the LOC and the inferior temporal cortex (IT), the information is consolidated and certain specific cells respond to more general categorizations such as "cat" or "brain." In this manner, CNNs were designed to mimic human visual processing in that there is an original visual input, a multilayer approach with feature extraction and data processing. The process continues and becomes more and more abstract within each layer. The deeper layers extract high-order features such as shapes or specific objects. The last layers of the network integrate all of those complex features and product classifications.

prognostic prediction. The last level, "Tier 3" would be AI algorithms which are "superhuman," that is, they can achieve outcomes that are not possible by human experts. Most often applications of this level become critical when using multimodal information including imaging and other clinical outcomes to derive new information about health and disease.

Operations: Workflow and Image Generation

Tier 1 image reconstruction and attenuation correction-focused studies have been developed for various brain molecular imaging modalities. In one such study, Hwang and colleagues reported a method for brain PET attenuation correction using only the emission scan from ^{18}F-florinated-N-3-fluoropropyl-2-β-carboxymethoxy3-β-(4-iodo-phenyl)nortropane [^{18}F-FP-CIT] PET with specific binding to the striatum.[11] They applied 3 different CNN architectures, U-NET, a convolutional autoencoder (CAE), and a hybrid CAE, which were trained and compared with actual acquired computed tomography (CT) using imaging datasets from 40 patients with suspected Parkinson's disease. The resultant outputs from the 3 CNNs were compared with the maximum-likelihood reconstruction of activity and attenuation (MLAA) correction. They found that the CNNs generated less noisy and more uniform attenuation maps than the MLAA. In a similar study, the investigators used a deep learning CAE network to generate

pseudo–CT attenuation correction maps for PET images from magnetic resonance images (MRIs) acquired on a PET/MR scanner.[12] The deep MR imaging-based attenuation correction (MRAC) method compared the pseudo–CT scans generated from 30 T1-weighted MR scans to the acquired CT scans during the training and then validated the algorithm in an additional 10 subjects. In the final step, the trained algorithm was applied prospectively to PET/MR images from 5 subjects. They found that the deep MRAC produced accurate pseudo–CT scans with Dice coefficients of 0.971, 0,936, and 0,803 for air, soft tissue, and bone, respectively. In addition, when compared with Dixon-based soft tissue and air segmentation and anatomic CT-based template registration, the deep MRAC resulted in significantly lower PET reconstruction errors.

Another molecular imaging AI application with very important clinical implications is the generation of high-quality images from those acquired with very low radiotracer doses. A recent study by Zaharchuk and colleagues applied CNNs to [^{18}F]–florbetaben amyloid PET images from 39 patients, which were acquired on a PET/MR scanner.[13] The authors trained the CNN using one-hundredth of the raw list-mode PET data to simulate "low dose" and evaluated both "PET-only" and "PET plus MR" for the input data. The output was compared with the actual "full dose" amyloid PET images. As would be expected, they found that the synthesized images were markedly improved over the "low-dose" images, and in particular, the PET plus MR trained output was very similar to the actual full-dose images.

The same group also applied a deep CNN to MR Imaging-based arterial spin labeling (ASL) plus structural MR images to predict ^{15}O-water PET of cerebral blood flow (CBF) images,[14] as ^{15}O-water PET is considered to be a current gold standard. The trained output from healthy controls and patients with cerebrovascular disease was compared with ^{15}O-water PET images simultaneously acquired by PET/MR. The trained algorithm resulted in CBF images with improved estimation error in both controls and patients, that were better correlated with the PET images. This example illustrates the potential for trained algorithms to synthesize brain PET image information from only MR Imaging input.

Our group recently developed an image-based deep-learning technique to generate amyloid PET images using only the first 0 to 20 min of radiotracer uptake.[15] Currently, ^{11}C-Pittsburgh Compound-B (PiB) accumulation requires more than 50 minutes after injection to obtain sufficient image quality for an accurate diagnosis. A U-net CNN was used with a conditional generative adversarial network (C-GAN) for data augmentation. Using only early-phase amyloid PET, we generated corresponding delayed images using the trained network. The actual delayed images and predicted delayed images were interpreted by imaging expert readers for amyloid positivity. The concordance of amyloid positivity between the actual versus predicted images was 79%($\kappa = 0.60$) for the 2 radiologists. The statistical comparison of the actual versus the predicted delayed images resulted in a peak signal-to-noise ratio (PSNR) of 21.8 dB, and a structural similarity index (SSIM) of 0.45, which indicated good agreement.

These different examples can all be considered Tier 1 type applications in that the desired outcomes ranged from image reconstruction and attenuation correction, to noise filtering, and compensation for low tracer doses, as well as the generation of actual images from other imaging modalities or datasets. Numerous studies of such applications can be found in the literature and the benefits of AI to these types of tasks for brain molecular imaging are very well-established.

Decision Making: Diagnosis and Prediction

The next level of sophistication in the application of AI to brain molecular imaging can be considered "decision-making" or classification. The purpose of the network training is to diagnose or differentiate disease conditions or make predictions regarding future disease progression. These Tier 2 level studies may use more complex deep learning architectures and often use multimodal imaging datasets to accomplish training for the desired outcomes.

Diagnosis and prediction of neurodegenerative conditions such as AD have been a focus of such research efforts. Recent developments in potential AD therapeutics have underscored the importance of early diagnosis/detection for optimal treatment outcomes. AI and deep learning methods can greatly advance the use of imaging to support these efforts. A study by Katako and colleagues compared different classification strategies applied to FDG-PET images to predict the future development of AD from mild cognitive impairment (MCI), and found that a support vector machine with an iterative single data algorithm resulted in a sensitivity of 0.84 and specificity of 0.95.[16] Choi and colleagues used multi-modal imaging including FDG and amyloid PET images from 139 AD, 171 MCI, and 182 normal subjects to train the deep learning CNN.[17] Notably, the images were minimally processed and not spatially normalized before the training. The accuracy of prediction for the conversion of MCI to AD was 84.2%, which was better than conventional feature-based quantification approaches and the performance using the multimodal dataset was better than either amyloid or FDG PET alone. Another study applied a deep neural network with a multimodal training dataset, which included AV-45 amyloid PET, MR Imaging, and clinical data to differentiate early and late MCI and AD from controls.[18] The trained network was able to classify early MCI and AD from normal controls with an accuracy of 84.0% and 96.8%, respectively. The above studies all used the AD neuroimaging initiative database (ADNI: http://adni.loni.usc.edu/) for the research. The development of this imaging resource began in 2004, and it is the largest multimodal imaging database for AD. The composite imaging data from thousands of subjects can be accessed by researchers worldwide. The implementation of such large data repositories is critical to the further development of AI-based methods for brain molecular imaging.

Superhuman Artificial Intelligence

The advanced level of AI for brain molecular imaging can be considered "superhuman" in which deep learning algorithms can generate outputs that are not readily possible by human experts. In general, this process may involve multidimensional data including imaging and can make predictions beyond what human brains can achieve. An example that approaches this "Tier 3" type level of AI is a study by Papp and colleagues, which used supervised machine learning with ^{11}C-methionine PET, clinical symptoms, and ex vivo histopathologic characteristics to predict survival in patients with treatment naïve glioma.[19] The machine-learning architecture identified the relevant in vivo, ex vivo, and patient features along with the relative weights, and these were used to establish 3 predictive models for 36-month survival. One model used a combination of in vivo, ex vivo, and clinical patient information. The second model used in vivo and patient information only. The third one used only the in vivo information. The models were validated by a Monte Carlo cross-validation scheme. The investigators found that the most prominent machine-learning weighted features were patient and ex vivo derived, followed by the in vivo features. This study also illustrates the point that the human brain has more difficulty incorporating such multidimensional information, which may be better managed by a trained AI.

IS ARTIFICIAL INTELLIGENCE GOING TO REPLACE RADIOLOGISTS?

With these rapid advancements, imaging specialists including radiologists and nuclear medicine physicians as well as medical students may wonder "will AI take my job"? Although no one can confidently predict what the future holds, we can reassure ourselves by looking to other examples in medicine whereby technological advancements seemed to threaten physician job security. One such situation occurred in the 1970s when automatic electrocardiograms (ECGs) were invented. At the time, many people had concerns such as, "can it be trusted," "will ECG improve efficiency," "is it cost-effective," and, most importantly, "will this replace cardiologists"? In fact, the automatic ECG readout can be useful in certain clinical settings to screen for major abnormalities when cardiac specialists are unavailable. Also, has turned out to be cost-effective because software can be added to the machine to enhance performance. However, after a half-century of automatic ECG recordings, the technology is used primarily to supplement the diagnosis and care provided by cardiologists and health care workers. The more important aspect of using technologies such as AI for medical imaging practice is to establish who will decide how to use such tools in a clinical setting to improve patient care quality. Even with advanced "superhuman" type applications, the role of the AI will be to facilitate and supplement medical care by the physician and staff, and not replace them, at least for now.

PRACTICAL CONSIDERATIONS

Despite considerable progress in the development of AI-based tools for brain molecular imaging, there remain some challenges to be addressed before these methods can be implemented in routine clinical practice. There is considerable uncertainty as to how the various architectures derive weights and produce the resultant trained output, and the term "black box" is often applied to describe such cryptic processes. Another concern is that methods for the quality assurance and verification of the accuracy of the output are somewhat limited. As mentioned previously, AI training depends on large, curated datasets, which can be difficult and costly to obtain for brain molecular imaging, in particular. Within the medical field in general, regulatory approval is required for clinical implementation. This has been obtained for certain software platforms and particular applications; however, the way in which AI methods for brain imaging are regulated and approved needs to be further clarified. Also, to a certain extent, computational resources still need to improve, including networks and data transfer speeds, to facilitate cloud-based analytical approaches.

SUMMARY

AI has been developed and applied to brain molecular imaging for over 30 years. The past 2 decades, in particular, have seen explosive progress in the field with no indications of a decline. AI applications span from operations-type processes such as attenuation correction and image generation to disease diagnosis and/or prediction. As the level of sophistication in AI software platforms increases and the availability of large imaging data repositories become common, future studies will incorporate more multidimensional datasets and information that may truly reach "superhuman" levels in the field of brain molecular imaging. However, even with the growing level of capability and sophistication, these advanced networks will still require human supervision for appropriate application and accurate interpretation in medical imaging practice.

ACKNOWLEDGEMENTS

Some support was provided by Hamamatsu Photonics K.K. and Hitachi, Ltd.

REFERENCES

1. McCulloch WS, Pitts W. A logical calculus of the ideas immanent in nervous activity. Bull Math Biophys 1943;5:115–33.
2. Rosenblatt F. The perceptron: a probabilistic model for information storage and organization in the brain. Psychol Rev 1958;65:386–408.
3. Kelley HJ. Gradient theory of optimal flight paths. ARS 1960;30:947–54.
4. Fukushima K. Neocognitron: a self organizing neural network model for a mechanism of pattern recognition unaffected by shift in position. Biol Cybern 1980;36:193–202.
5. Zhang W, Hasegawa A, Itoh K, et al. Image processing of human corneal endothelium based on a learning network. Appl Opt 1991;30:4211–7.
6. Kippenhan JS, Barker WW, Pascal S, et al. Evaluation of a neural-network classifier for PET scans of normal and Alzheimer's disease subjects. J Nucl Med 1992;33:1459–67.
7. Lee JS, Lee DS, Kim S-K, et al. Localization of epileptogenic zones in F-18 FDG brain PET of patients with temporal lobe epilepsy using artificial neural network. IEEE Trans Med Imaging 2000;19:347–55.
8. Acton PD, Newberg A. Artificial neural network classifier for the diagnosis of Parkinson's disease using [99m Tc]TRODAT-1 and SPECT. Phys Med Biol 2006;51:3057–66.
9. Bose SK, Turkheimer FE, Howes OD, et al. Classification of schizophrenic patients and healthy controls using [18F] fluorodopa PET imaging. Schizophr Res 2008;106:148–55.
10. Grill-Spector K, Malach R. The human visual cortex. Annu Rev Neurosci 2004;27:649–77.
11. Hwang D, Kim KY, Kang SK, et al. Improving the accuracy of simultaneously reconstructed activity and attenuation maps using deep learning. J Nucl Med 2018;59:1624–9.
12. Liu F, Jang H, Kijowski R, et al. Deep learning MR imaging-based attenuation correction for PET/MR imaging. Radiology 2018;286:676–84.
13. Chen KT, Gong E, Macruz FBdC, et al. Ultra–low-dose 18 F-florbetaben amyloid PET imaging using deep learning with multi-contrast MRI inputs. Radiology 2019;290:649–56.
14. Guo J, Gong E, Fan AP, et al. Predicting 15O-Water PET cerebral blood flow maps from multi-contrast MRI using a deep convolutional neural network with evaluation of training cohort bias. J Cereb Blood Flow Metab 2019;40:2240–53.
15. Komori S, Kimura Y, Hatano K, et al. Image-based deep-learning prediction of future FDG PET patterns in aging and dementia. J Nucl Med 2019;60:1211.
16. Katako A, Shelton P, Goertzen AL, et al. Machine learning identified an Alzheimer's disease-related FDG-PET pattern which is also expressed in Lewy body dementia and Parkinson's disease dementia. Sci Rep 2018;8:13236.
17. Choi H, Jin KH, Alzheimer's Disease Neuroimaging I. Predicting cognitive decline with deep learning of brain metabolism and amyloid imaging. Behav Brain Res 2018;344:103–9.
18. Forouzannezhad P, Abbaspour A, Li C, et al (2018). A deep neural network approach for early diagnosis of mild cognitive impairment using multiple features. Orlando FL:Dec 17-20, 2018;17th IEEE international conference on machine learning and applications (ICMLA),1341-1346.
19. Papp L, Pötsch N, Grahovac M, et al. Glioma survival prediction with combined analysis of in vivo 11C-MET PET features, ex vivo features, and patient features by supervised machine learning. J Nucl Med 2018;59:892–9.

Clinical Application of Artificial Intelligence in PET Imaging of Head and Neck Cancer

Seyed Mohammad H. Gharavi, MD*, Armaghan Faghihimehr, MD

KEYWORDS

• PET • Deep learning • Neural network • Artificial intelligence • Head and neck cancer

KEY POINTS

- Machine learning models using PET imaging can be used in prognostication, prediction of response to treatment, and prediction of tumor markers in head and neck cancers.
- Machine learning models using PET imaging can be used for gross tumor and lymph node volume segmentation to enhance radiation therapy simulation.
- Different challenges need to be overcome before artificial intelligence models can be deployed in head and neck cancer imaging.

INTRODUCTION

Most of the head and neck cancers are squamous cell carcinomas (HNSCC) arising from the upper aerodigestive tract's mucosal lining.[1] The incidence of squamous cell carcinoma, particularly among young individuals, has shown an incremental trend in the last 3 decades, despite decreased smoking rates.[1,2]

The American Joint Committee on Cancer (AJCC) TNM staging of HNSCC is based on multiple components, including the size of the primary tumor, size, number, and laterality of involved locoregional lymph nodes and the presence or absence of distant metastasis. In the latest revision of AJCC, HPV status has been incorporated into the staging of oropharyngeal cancers.[3] Depending on tumor stage, typical treatment options for HNSCC include radiation therapy with or without chemotherapy and surgical resection with lymph node dissection.

In conjunction with physical examination and endoscopy, medical imaging plays a crucial role in the diagnosis, staging, and management of HNSCC. PET with fludeoxyglucose (FDG-PET)/computed tomography (CT), contrast-enhanced CT, and MR imaging are among the most frequently used modalities in imaging of head and neck tumors. FDG-PET has a key advantage in primary tumor localization among patients with cervical lymphadenopathy and unknown primary cancer sites. PET increases the accuracy of the initial staging of the primary tumor, offers sensitive detection of possible second primaries, and can provide semiquantitative estimates of treatment response.[4] FDG-PET/CT has direct application in the Neck Imaging Reporting and Data System, the standardized radiological posttreatment surveillance staging system used for predicting the risk of treatment failure in HNSCC.[5,6]

The head and neck's complex anatomy, high concentration of vital structures, and treatment-related distortion of the normal anatomy render diagnostic imaging of head and neck cancer challenging even among experienced radiologists. In the era of increasing demand for precision

---

a Virginia Commonwealth University, VCU School of Medicine, Department of Radiology, West Hospital, 1200 East Broad Street, North Wing, Room 2-013, Box 980470, Richmond, VA 23298-0470, USA
* Corresponding author.
E-mail address: Seyedmohammad.gharavi@vcuhealth.org

PET Clin 17 (2022) 65–76
https://doi.org/10.1016/j.cpet.2021.09.004
1556-8598/22/© 2021 Elsevier Inc. All rights reserved.

medicine and the promise of rapidly progressing artificial intelligence (AI), diagnosticians and clinicians alike are encouraged to embrace the union of advanced oncologic imaging and machine learning to enhance both personalized health care and population health as a whole.

Artificial Intelligence

The term "artificial intelligence" (AI), a concept of computerized synthetic human cognitive function, was first introduced in 1956 at Dartmouth University.[7] Since its inception, and especially in recent years, there has been an exponential expansion of AI with widespread application among various industries including automotive engineering, gaming, and health care.

In the past 10 years, with emerging massive amounts of digital information known as "big data" and significant computer processing power progression, AI and its application in different aspects of human life are becoming more practical.

"Machine learning" is a subfield of AI that refers to computer algorithms that analyze data input and infer a function to predict the output of unseen observations. Machine learning can be used for both "supervised" and "unsupervised" learning applications. In supervised training, data are labeled as empirical data—or "ground truth"—and the model learns to predict the output on the test data. On the other hand, unsupervised training does not provide this empirical data, and the model identifies the patterns and clusters in a dataset autonomously.

Machine learning approaches include more traditional mathematic models such as linear regression, support-vector machines, random forest, and decision tree, as well as novel deep learning methods using neural networks, which is an emulation of complex human neuronal interconnections. A neural network can be as simple as a single computational unit—or "node"—between the input and a binary output, called "logistic regression," or a more sophisticated network with multinodal layers, each connecting to the immediate earlier and deeper layers. Input to each layer will be multiplied by the nodes' weights in that layer and then transferred to the deeper layer.

Readily accessible archives of enormous digital data in medical imaging have made radiology a leader in exploring medical applications of AI. Although the initial hype of AI in radiology was a perceived threat to the profession,[8] current attitudes have largely deviated toward augmenting radiology and improving the health care quality.

In particular, quantitative oncologic imaging with PET has great potential to leverage AI technology in the pursuit of precision medicine. In this article, the authors aim to review current AI applications in PET imaging of head and neck cancers, beginning with radiomics and followed by deep learning in each section.

Radiomics

The term "radiomics" was first introduced in the literature in 2012, referring to extraction and analysis of large amounts of advanced quantitative imaging features obtained with CT, PET, or MR imaging.[9] The main objective of radiomics is to convert radiologic images to higher-order dimensional data for subsequent data mining and improved decision support. The initial process consists of image acquisition, region of interest or volume of interest identification, and total or subtotal tumor segmentation. These data are extracted as *semantic* (commonly used in the radiologic lexicon, ie, shape or size) and *agnostic* (mathematical formulaic) features to populate a searchable database for mining as an independent subset or in combination with other clinical, demographic, or genomic data to develop an outcome-predicting model.[10]

The image analysis and feature extraction process in the radiomic approach does not need AI. It can be performed by computerized image analysis software or what is called the "hand-crafted method." Machine learning models may then be implemented to construct a predictive model using radiomic features as input data. Therefore, radiomic pipelines are a combination of a non-AI and AI processes.[11]

Deep learning

Deep learning is the subset of machine learning referring to more sophisticated neural networks with multiple hidden layers, usually more than 20.[7,11] Convolutional neural network (CNN) is a deep learning method that has been increasingly implemented in computer vision tasks such as image classification, segmentation, and object detection.[12–15] Complex CNNs such as AlexNet, VGGNet, GoogLeNet, and ResNet have shown remarkable performance in image classification.[16–18] The convolutional layers act to extract features, the pooling layers to reduce the size, and the fully connected layers to predict the model. CNN can handle the entire process of feature extraction, selection, and prediction in an end-to-end fashion, therefore obviating the hand-crafted feature extraction with radiomics.[11]

APPLICATION OF ARTIFICIAL INTELLIGENCE IN HEAD AND NECK CANCER
Prognosis, Recurrence Rate, and Treatment Outcome Prediction

Recognizing the potential high-risk patients with head and neck cancer is critical in tailoring the individual therapy for this group of patients. CT and magnetic resonance radiomics have accurately predicted the prognostic measures in head and neck cancers such as overall survival,[19] risk of distant metastasis,[20] and recurrence patterns after radiotherapy.[21] Combining PET with CT radiomic features can lead to an even more accurate prediction of such measures.

Vallières and colleagues[22] extracted 1615 radiomic features from the pretreatment FDG-PET/CT (CT-only, PET-only, and PET/CT) of 300 patients with head and neck cancer and predicted the chance of locoregional recurrence, distant metastasis, and overall survival by applying random forest model on the extracted features. The highest performance was achieved by using PET/CT radiomics combined with clinical variables for locoregional recurrence (area under the curve [AUC] of 0.69) and combined PET radiomics and clinical variables for overall survival (AUC of 0.74).

In a study on 190 patients with oropharyngeal squamous cell carcinoma (OPSCC), Haider and colleagues[23] extracted PET and CT radiomic features from 190 primary tumors and 266 metastatic lymph nodes and used a random forest model to predict the risk of locoregional progression after curative treatment. The optimized model achieved an interquartile range C-index of 0.76 for combined PET/CT radiomics. In another study on 311 patients with OPSCC, they designed a model based on radiomic features that outperformed those based on AJCC variables in predicting the progression-free survival[24] (**Fig. 1**).

Folkert and colleagues,[25] proposed a machine learning–based model to predict the local failure, distant metastasis, and all-cause mortality based on the extracted radiomics from PET/CT of 174

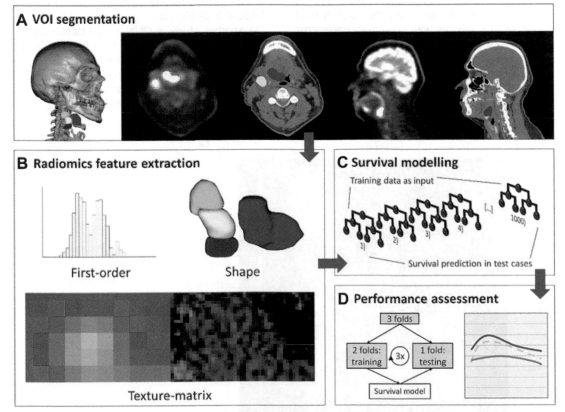

Fig. 1. Segmentation, radiomics feature extraction, and survival modeling pipeline. (*A*) manual segmentation of the primary tumor and individual metastatic cervical lymph nodes on PET and CT. (*B*) Extraction of first-order, shape, and texture matrix features. (*C*) Random forest machine-learning models with 1000 decision trees were applied for survival prediction and risk stratification. (*D*) Model performance was assessed in 3-fold cross-validation (*left*). Model performance was visualized in performance curves (*right*). (*From* Haider SP, Zeevi T, Baumeister P, et al. Potential added value of PET/CT radiomics for survival prognostication beyond AJCC 8th edition staging in oropharyngeal squamous cell carcinoma. *Cancers.* 2020;12(7):1-16.)

patients with high-stage OPSCC. They yielded statistically significant performance after 5-fold cross-validation for all 3 endpoints (AUC = 0.65, 0.73, and 0.66 for all-cause mortality, local failure, and distant metastasis, respectively).

A combination of hand-crafted and CNN-extracted PET/CT radiomic features were used by Peng and colleagues[26] to predict the disease-free survival in patients with advanced nasopharyngeal carcinoma. They were able to identify the high-risk patients who could benefit from induction chemotherapy before radiation treatment.

Despite certain advantages of the radiomics approach in feature extraction, the hand-crafted radiomics approach can be complicated and time-consuming. The end-to-end CNN approach can be a more efficient method and therefore enhances the performance by detecting patterns that hand-crafted techniques cannot discover.[27] However, only a few studies have implemented CNNs in predicting the prognostic measures in head and neck cancers. Fujima and colleagues[28] proposed a CNN model that predicted the disease-free survival based on the FDG-PET/CT images of 113 patients with oral cavity carcinoma and yielded a diagnostic accuracy, sensitivity, and specificity of 0.8, 0.8, and 0.8, respectively.

In another study, Wang and colleagues[29] proposed a CNN model that predicted the PET image of the tumor after radiation therapy based on the pretherapy FDG-PET and planned dose distribution. They trained the model with 61 and tested it with 5 patients with OPSCC. Their model accurately predicted the SUV$_{mean}$ values of the gross tumor volume (GTV) and clinical target volume (**Fig. 2**).

Applications in Radiotherapy

Accurate tumor delineation in head and neck cancers is a crucial step in radiation simulation, which often is a challenging task for radiation oncologists due to the complexity of the anatomy and potential artifacts in the region. Lately, the application of AI in GTV delineation has been the focus of several types of research.

Huang and colleagues[30] proposed a CNN model to predict GTV from PET/CT images of patients with HNC. Their dataset consisted of 22 patients with 1034 CT and PET slices. They used GTV manually segmented by a radiation oncologist and subsequently verified by a radiologist as their gold standard. Their model predicted the GTV with a median Dice similarity coefficient (DSC) of 0.785 (0.482–0.863) (**Fig. 3**).

In another study, a CNN model based on PET/CT images of 197 patients with head and neck cancers identified 86% of the true GTV structures, whereas models built solely on CT images identified only 55% of the true structures. The mean Dice scores were 55%, 69%, and 71% for the

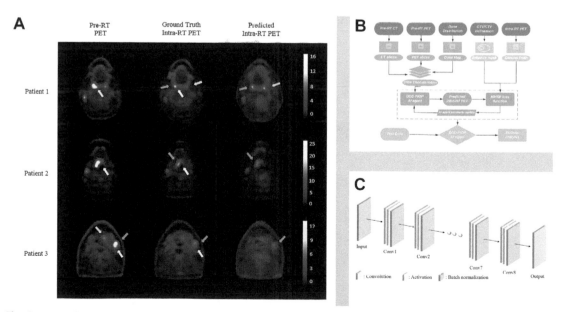

Fig. 2. Postradiation interim outcome prediction model. (*A*) Results of 3 test patients. Left column: pre-RT PET; middle column: ground truth intra-RT PET; right column: predicted intra-RT PET. Yellow arrows: SUV reduction after 20 Gy as treatment response; blue and white arrows: model predictions–captured ground-truth results. (*B*) Model workflow. (*C*) Model CNN architecture. RT, radiation therapy. (*From* Wang C, Liu C, Chang Y, et al. Dose-Distribution-Driven PET Image-Based Outcome Prediction (DDD-PIOP): A Deep Learning Study for Oropharyngeal Cancer IMRT Application. *Front Oncol.* 2020; 10:1592.)

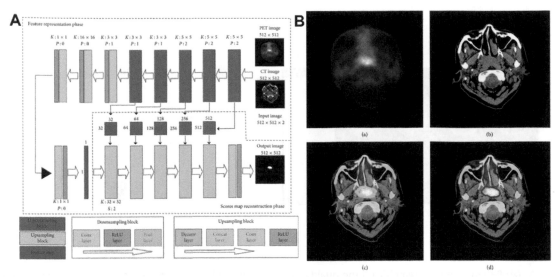

Fig. 3. (*A*) Architecture of the proposed CNN model for GTV prediction in HNC. The proposed network includes 2 phases: the feature representation phase and scores map reconstruction phase. (*B*) An example of HNC tumor segmentation with high accuracy. Automatic segmentation result presented on the fused PET-CT image (*green line*). The gold standard of gross tumor volume drawn on the combined PET-CT image (*red line*). (*From* Huang B, Chen Z, Wu P-M, et al. Fully Automated Delineation of Gross Tumor Volume for Head and Neck Cancer on PET-CT Using Deep Learning: A Dual-Center Study. *Contrast Media Mol Imaging.* 2018; 2018:8923028.)

CT-based, PET-based, and PET/CT-based CNN models, respectively.[31]

Park and colleagues[32] showed a deep learning tumor segmentation model, trained with mixed neck and limb tumors, could delineate the GTV of neck tumors. They used a U-Net-architecture, CNN model on PET and CT of 155 patients (113 neck and 42 limb tumors). Different models were trained using the neck, limb, and combined neck and limb tumors. Each model was then tested on only neck cases. The GTV output of the model, which was trained with the combined dataset, showed accuracy similar to the model only trained with neck tumors (DSC = 0.66 and 0.69, respectively).

Recently, three-dimensional (3D) CNN models have been used for tumor segmentation purposes. As opposed to a 2D CNN model, a 3D model can gather information from a volume rather than a slice. However, the drawback is a significant increase in network sophistication and computational burden.

Guo and colleagues[33] proposed a deep learning model that automatically performed a GTV segmentation based on radiation planning PET/CT of 250 patients with head and neck cancer. They used 3D CNN models with Dense-Net and U-Net architectures, with ground truth being the manually delineated GTV drawn by radiation oncologists. They concluded the multimodality PET/CT Dense-Net model is superior to PET alone (DSC of 0.82 vs 0.60). Their Dense-Net model also outperformed the U-Net model (DSC of 0.80 vs 0.72).

Deep learning technology has been used in producing synthetic CT (sCT) from MR imaging that can be used in radiation dose calculation or PET attenuation correction.[34–36]

Olin and colleagues[37] proposed a CNN model to construct an sCT from in-phase and opposed-phase MR imaging sequences of the neck in patients with head and neck cancer. They used the output sCT from this model for both PET attenuation correction and radiation treatment dose calculation at the same time. They used transfer learning and fine-tuned a pretrained model. The sCT used for PET attenuation correction showed high agreement with CT-based attenuation correction. The difference between the CT- and sCT-based radiation dose calculations was insignificant (**Fig. 4**).

Lymph Node Detection

Location, size, and the number of involved lymph nodes are important factors in the staging and treatment of head and neck cancers.[3] Deep learning has shown fair accuracy (sensitivity and specificity of 73% and 52.5%, respectively) in detecting cervical lymph nodes on CT of patients with OPSCC.[38] However, combined PET and CT models demonstrated higher accuracy in such tasks, the example of which is a CNN model proposed by Dohopolski and colleagues[39] that achieved an AUC of 0.99, the sensitivity of 0.94, and specificity of 0.90 in the detection of metastatic lymph nodes in head and neck cancers. The

A

B   PET$_{CT}$ PET$_{sCT}$ Delineations

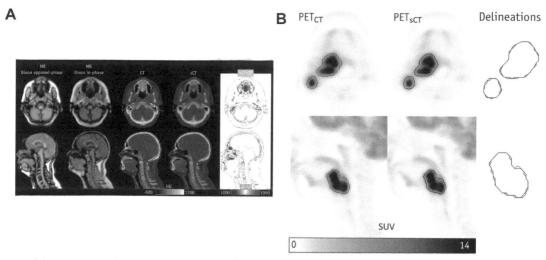

SUV

0   14

Fig. 4. (*A*) Patient sample exemplifying the quality of model input MR imaging and performance of generated synthetic computed tomography (CT) versus the reference CT image used for attenuation correction (AC) and radiation therapy (RT) purposes. (*B*) Patient sample exemplifying PET images reconstructed with either CT or sCT for attenuation correction, creating PET/CT and PET/sCT, respectively. (*From* Olin AB, Hansen AE, Rasmussen JH, et al. Feasibility of multiparametric positron emission tomography/magnetic resonance imaging as a one-stop-shop for radiation therapy planning for patients with head and neck cancer. *Int J Radiat Oncol Biol Phys.* 2020;108(5):1329-1338; with permission.)

dataset used in this model consisted of 791 lymph nodes from 129 patients with head and neck cancer labeled with pathologic results from surgical lymph node dissection. Kawauchi and colleagues[40] proposed a CNN model to classify the patients into benign, malignant, and equivocal categories based on the whole body FDG-PET maximum intensity projection images. In a region-based analysis, the prediction was correct with an accuracy of 97.3% for the head and neck region.

Lastly, another group conducted a study using PET/CT of 59 patients (236 lymph nodes) with head and neck cancer and built a model to predict lymph node metastasis. First, they used hand-crafted radiomic feature extraction combined with the support-vector machine prediction model, then used a separate 3D CNN architecture model. They ultimately proposed a hybrid model that could combine both models and predict the lymph node metastasis with higher accuracy (0.88) than both models alone (0.81 and 0.75)[41] (**Fig. 5**).

A

B

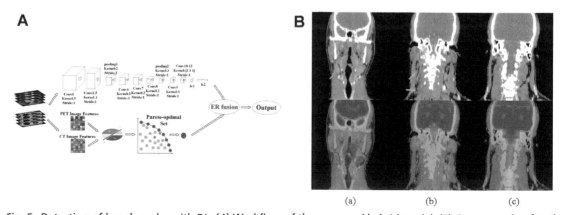

(a)   (b)   (c)

Fig. 5. Detection of lymph nodes with DL. (*A*) Workflow of the proposed hybrid model. (*B*) One example of each of CT and overlapped CT and PET images of normal, suspicious, and involved nodes. DL, deep learning. (*From* Chen L, Zhou Z, Sher D, et al. Combining many-objective radiomics and 3D convolutional neural network through evidential reasoning to predict lymph node metastasis in head and neck cancer. *Phys Med Biol.* 2019;64(7); with permission.)

Table 1
Use of machine learning in PET imaging of head and neck cancers

Author	Application	Modality	Feature Extraction	Prediction Model	Dataset (Train/Valid/Test)	Dataset	Result
Vallières et al,[22] 2017	Prediction of LR, DM, OS	FDG-PET/CT	Radiomics	Random forest	300 HNC (194 train/106 test)	Local	AUC: 0.69 for LR & 0.74 for OS
Haider et al,[23] 2021	Prediction of LRP	FDG-PET/CT	Radiomics	Random forest	190 HPV-associated OPSCC (190 primary tumors;266 lymph nodes)	Local + TCIA	C-index (IQR): 0.76 for LRP
Haider et al,[24] 2020	Prediction of PFS and OS	FDG-PET/CT	Radiomics	Random Forest	311 OPSCC patients (235 HPV-associated and 76 HPV-negative)	Local + TCIA	C-index: 0.63 for PFS
Folkert et al,[25] 2017	Prediction of LF, DM, ACM	FDG-PET/CT	Radiomics	Multiparameter logistic regression	174 OPSCC	Local	AUC:0.65 for ACM; 0.73 for LF; 0.66 for DM
Peng et al,[26] 2019	Prediction of DFS	FDG-PET/CT	Radiomics & CNN		707 NPC (470 train/237 test)	Local	C-index: 0.754 (training) and 0.722 (test)
Fujima et al,[28] 2020	Prediction of DFS	FDG-PET/CT	CNN (ResNet-101)	CNN (ResNet-101)	113 OCSCC (83 train/30 test)	Local	Accuracy: 0.8 Sensitivity: 0.8 Specificity: 0.8
Wang et al,[29] 2020	Treatment outcome	PET/CT	CNN (custom)	CNN (custom)	66 OPSCC (61train/5test)	Local	Predicted SUV_{mean} 99.8%/99.4% at GTV/CTV with 3D gamma test
Huang et al,[29] 2018	GTV	FDG-PET/CT	2D-CNN	2D-CNN	22 HNC	Local	DSC: 0.785
Moe et al,[30] 2019	GTV of tumor and LNs	FDG-PET/CT	2D-CNN (U-Net)	2D-CNN (U-Net)	197 HNC (142 train/15valid/40 test)	Local	DSC: 0.71 for PET/CT and 0.55 for CT

(continued on next page)

Table 1
(continued)

Author	Application	Modality	Feature Extraction	Prediction Model	Dataset (Train/Valid/Test)	Dataset	Result
Guo et al,[32] 2019	GTV	FDG-PET/CT	3D-CNN (Dense-Net)	3D-CNN (Dense-Net)	250 HNC (140 train/ 35 valid/75 test)	TCIA	DSC: 0.82 for PET/CT and 0.60 for PET
Park et al,[31] 2020	GTV	FDG-PET & CT	CNN (U-Net)	2D-CNN	113 H&N and 42 limb cancer patients Combinations of H&N, limb, and merged training dataset each with 1000 or 2000 train/ 300 test	TCIA	DSC: 0.66 for $N_M T_H$ and 0.69 for $N_H T_H$
Olin et al,[36] 2020	Synthetic CT (dose calculation and PET AC)	MR imaging	CNN (U-Net)	CNN (U-Net); transfer learning	8 HNC	local	Calculated dose within 1% of the reference
Dohopolski et al,[39] 2020	Prediction of MLNs	FDG-PET/CT	CNN (AlexNet)	CNN (AlexNet)	129 patients (479 train/125 valid/187 test)	Local	AUC:0.99, sensitivity:0.94 specificity:0.90 on the test dataset.
Kawauchi et al,[40] 2020	Prediction of presence or absence of MLNs	MIP of whole-body FDG-PET	CNN (ResNet)	CNN (ResNet)	3485 PET/CT	Local	Accuracy: 97.3% on region-based analysis for H&N
Chen et al,[41] 2019	Prediction of MLNs		Radiomic, 3D CNN	SVM, 3D CNN	59 HNC with 236 LNs (176 train/66 test)	Local	Accuracy: 0.88 for hybrid 3D CNN and radiomics model
Haider et al,[45] 2020	Prediction of tumor HPV status	FDG-PET/CT	Radiomics	Random forest	435 OPSCC and 741 MLNs	Local + TCIA	AUC: 0.78
Fujima et al,[46] 2020	Prediction of tumor HPV status	FDG-PET/CT	2D CNN (GoogleNet)	2D CNN (GoogleNet); transfer learning	120 OPSCC (training = 90 and test = 30)	Local	Sensitivity: 0.83; specificity: 0.83; and accuracy: 0.83

Abbreviations: ACM, all-cause mortality; AUC, area under the curve; DM, distant metastasis; DSC, Dice similarity index; GTV/CTV, gross tumor volume/clinical target volume; LF, local failure; LR, local recurrence; LRP, locoregional progression; MIP, maximum intensity projection; NHTH, model trained and tested with neck tumor dataset; NMTH, model trained with merged and tested with neck tumor datasets; OS, overall survival; PFS, progression-free survival.

Prediction of Tumor Markers

HPV-positive OPSCC has different biology and clinical characteristic from HPV-negative form—showing better response to chemoradiation therapy and overall more favorable outcomes and prognosis.[2] CT and PET findings can help differentiate HPV-positive OPSCCs from HPV-negative tumors.[42,43] AI predictive models based on CT radiomic features have been able to determine the HPV status of OPSCCs (AUC = 0.85 in training and AUC = 0.78 in the validation cohort).[44]

Haider and colleagues analyzed pretreatment PET/CT of 435 primary OPSCC and 741 metastatic lymph nodes and developed a model to predict the tumor HPV status using radiomic features extracted from combined PET/CT. They showed higher performance of combined PET/CT features compared with PET or CT alone (AUC = 0.78).[45]

Fujima and colleagues suggested a PET/CT-based CNN model can discriminate between the HPV-positive and HPV-negative OPSCC even better than radiologists. Their dataset consisted of 120 patients with OPSCC (90 training/30 test). They used transfer learning from a pretrained GoogleNet Inception v2 model. In the validation session, the deep learning diagnostic model revealed sensitivity of 0.83, specificity of 0.83, and diagnostic accuracy of 0.83, whereas the visual assessment by 2 radiologists revealed 0.78, 0.5, 0.7, 0.6, and 0.67 (reader 1) and 0.56, 0.67, 0.71, 0.5, and 0.6 (reader 2), respectively.[46]

Dataset

Most of the reviewed cohorts used their local institutional dataset. However, a few studies used The Cancer Imaging Achieve dataset alone or in combination with their institutional dataset[23,24,32,33,45] (Table 1).

DISCUSSION

There is a great promise in AI in radiology, particularly head and neck imaging, although few major obstacles currently preclude its full application.

The lack of large datasets necessary for training, validating, and testing the AI models and drawing meaningful results provides the most substantial barrier, as most research studies performed were conducted on small datasets. Outside of the medical field, models that achieved human-level accuracy were trained by massive datasets. For example, the DeepFace system, a famous face recognition model, used 4.4 million labeled faces for training.[47] The sample size issues can be partially overcome by applying "transfer learning" or "augmentation" methods. In transfer learning, a previously trained generic model can be used on a new smaller dataset while using all or most of the previously trained features. In augmentation, there is a transformation of data, such as rotation or mirror imaging, without affecting its relevant properties. The augmentation method is applied to increase the size of the dataset.

Heterogeneity of medical imaging data is another major challenge. AI models are easily susceptible to overfitting and lack generalizability if trained with a particular patient population or imaging setting. Therefore, AI models need to be locally evaluated, tuned, or even retrained before deployment. Large-scale multi-institutional cohorts with mixed heterogeneous populations, different settings, and equipment manufacturers can prevent overfitting of the models but are very difficult to coordinate due to data privacy and security risks. A potential solution to this problem is "federated learning," whereby different local models can share learned features with the exclusion of sensitive patient data.[48]

Annotations of medical imaging require expertise and a substantial investment of time. In addition, data that are labeled according to the opinion of a single radiologist are susceptible to systematic bias, which can be avoided by using consensus among a larger group of radiologists for defining the ground truth.

A more detailed discussion regarding the challenges of AI in radiology is beyond this current review's scope and can be found elsewhere in this issue.

Finally, the application of CNNs in the head and neck imaging may be more susceptible to data imbalance because of the inherently small regions of interest, occupying a smaller fraction of the entire image.[49]

SUMMARY

AI has many potential applications in head and neck cancer imaging and management. Prior studies have shown early success in applying machine learning in head and neck cancer imaging. There are likely many more potential applications that researchers may explore in the future. However, there are significant barriers in current practical application, most notably the absence of a large-scale dataset for training and validation. The acquisition of a robust dataset will permit AI-assisted radiology tools to pave the way toward precision medicine and improved outcomes.

CLINICS CARE POINTS

- AI has been used for prognostication, prediction of tumor markers, and radiation planning for head and neck cancers.
- A large-scale dataset for training and validation will permit AI-assisted radiology tools and pave the way toward precision medicine.

ACKNOWLEDGMENTS

Special thanks to Kyle J. Hunter, M.D. from the department of Radiology in MetroHealth Medical Center, Cleveland, OH, who contributed to the edition of this review.

DISCLOSURE

The authors have nothing to disclose.

REFERENCES

1. Siegel RL, Miller KD, Jemal A. Cancer statistics. CA Cancer J Clin 2016;66(1):7–30.
2. Pytynia KB, Dahlstrom KR, Sturgis EM. Epidemiology of HPV-associated oropharyngeal cancer. Oral Oncol 2014;50(5):380–6.
3. Amin MB, Greene FL, Edge SB, et al. The Eighth Edition AJCC Cancer Staging Manual: continuing to build a bridge from a population-based to a more "personalized" approach to cancer staging. CA Cancer J Clin 2017;67(2):93–9.
4. Wassef HR, Hanna N, Colletti P. PET/CT in head-neck malignancies: the implications for personalized clinical practice. PET Clin 2016;11(3):219–32.
5. Aiken AH, Hudgins PA. Neck imaging reporting and data system. Magn Reson Imaging Clin N Am 2018; 26(1):51–62.
6. Hsu D, Chokshi FH, Hudgins PA, et al. Predictive value of first posttreatment imaging using standardized reporting in head and neck cancer. Otolaryngol Head Neck Surg 2019;161(6):978–85.
7. Thrall JH, Li X, Li Q, et al. Artificial intelligence and machine learning in radiology: opportunities, challenges, pitfalls, and criteria for success. J Am Coll Radiol 2018;15(3 Pt B):504–8.
8. Obermeyer Z, Emanuel EJ. Predicting the future - big data, machine learning, and clinical medicine. N Engl J Med 2016;375(13):1216–9.
9. Kumar V, Gu Y, Basu S, et al. Radiomics: the process and the challenges. Magn Reson Imaging 2012;30(9):1234–48.
10. Gillies RJ, Kinahan PE, Hricak H. Radiomics: images are more than pictures, they are data. Radiology 2016;278(2):563–77.
11. Forghani R, Savadjiev P, Chatterjee A, et al. Radiomics and artificial intelligence for biomarker and prediction model development in oncology. Comput Struct Biotechnol J 2019;17:995–1008.
12. Rawat W, Wang Z. Deep convolutional neural networks for image classification: a comprehensive review. Neural Comput 2017;29(9):2352–449.
13. Pang S, del Coz JJ, Yu Z, et al. Deep learning and preference learning for object tracking: a combined approach. Neural Process Lett 2018;47(3): 859–76.
14. Simonyan K, Zisserman A. Very deep convolutional networks for large-scale image recognition. arXiv [csCV]. 2014. Available at: http://arxiv.org/abs/1409.1556.
15. Ren S, He K, Girshick R, et al. Faster R-CNN: towards real-time object detection with region proposal networks. IEEE Trans Pattern Anal Mach Intell 2017;39(6):1137–49.
16. Szegedy C, Vanhoucke V, Ioffe S, Shlens J, Wojna Z. Rethinking the inception architecture for computer vision. In: 2016 IEEE Conference on Computer Vision and Pattern Recognition (CVPR). Las Vegas, NV, USA: IEEE; 1 July 2016. doi:10.1109/cvpr.2016.308.
17. Krizhevsky A, Sutskever I, Hinton GE. ImageNet classification with deep convolutional neural networks. Commun ACM 2017;60(6):84–90.
18. He K, Zhang X, Ren S, Sun J. Deep residual learning for image recognition. In: 2016 IEEE Conference on Computer Vision and Pattern Recognition (CVPR). Las Vegas, NV, USA: IEEE; 26 June–1 July 2016. doi:10.1109/cvpr.2016.90.
19. Zhang H, Graham CM, Elci O, et al. Locally advanced squamous cell carcinoma of the head and neck: CT texture and histogram analysis allow independent prediction of overall survival in patients treated with induction chemotherapy. Radiology 2013;269(3):801–9.
20. Zhang L, Dong D, Li H, et al. Development and validation of a magnetic resonance imaging-based model for the prediction of distant metastasis before initial treatment of nasopharyngeal carcinoma: a retrospective cohort study. EBioMedicine 2019;40: 327–35.
21. Li S, Wang K, Hou Z, et al. Use of radiomics combined with machine learning method in the recurrence patterns after intensity-modulated radiotherapy for nasopharyngeal carcinoma: a preliminary study. Front Oncol 2018;8:648.
22. Vallières M, Kay-Rivest E, Perrin LJ, et al. Radiomics strategies for risk assessment of tumour failure in head-and-neck cancer. Sci Rep 2017;7(1): 10117.

23. Haider SP, Sharaf K, Zeevi T, et al. Prediction of post-radiotherapy locoregional progression in HPV-associated oropharyngeal squamous cell carcinoma using machine-learning analysis of baseline PET/CT radiomics. Transl Oncol 2021;14(1): 100906.

24. Haider SP, Zeevi T, Baumeister P, et al. Potential added value of PET/CT radiomics for survival prognostication beyond AJCC 8th edition staging in oropharyngeal squamous cell carcinoma. Cancers 2020;12(7):1–16.

25. Folkert MR, Setton J, Apte AP, et al. Predictive modeling of outcomes following definitive chemoradiotherapy for oropharyngeal cancer based on FDG-PET image characteristics. Phys Med Biol 2017;62(13):5327–43.

26. Peng H, Dong D, Fang M-J, et al. Prognostic value of deep learning PET/CT-based radiomics: potential role for future individual induction chemotherapy in advanced nasopharyngeal carcinoma. Clin Cancer Res 2019;25(14):4271–9.

27. Diamant A, Chatterjee A, Vallières M, et al. Deep learning in head & neck cancer outcome prediction. Sci Rep 2019;9(1):2764.

28. Fujima N, Andreu-Arasa VC, Meibom SK, et al. Deep learning analysis using FDG-PET to predict treatment outcome in patients with oral cavity squamous cell carcinoma. Eur Radiol 2020;30(11): 6322–30.

29. Wang C, Liu C, Chang Y, et al. Dose-distribution-driven PET image-based outcome prediction (DDD-PIOP): a deep learning study for oropharyngeal cancer IMRT application. Front Oncol 2020; 10:1592.

30. Huang B, Chen Z, Wu P-M, et al. Fully automated delineation of gross tumor volume for head and neck cancer on PET-CT using deep learning: a dual-center study. Contrast Media Mol Imaging 2018;2018:8923028.

31. Moe YM, Groendahl AR, Mulstad M, et al. Deep learning for automatic tumor segmentation in PET/CT images of patients with head and neck cancers. arXiv [eessIV]. 2019. Available at. http://arxiv.org/abs/1908.00841.

32. Park Y-I, Kang S-W, Kim K-H, et al. Feasibility study of deep learning tumor segmentation for a merged tumor dataset: head & neck and limbs. J Korean Phys Soc 2020;77(11):1049–54.

33. Guo Z, Guo N, Gong K, et al. Gross tumor volume segmentation for head and neck cancer radiotherapy using deep, dense multimodality network. Phys Med Biol 2019;64(20):205015.

34. Dinkla AM, Florkow MC, Maspero M, et al. Dosimetric evaluation of synthetic CT for head and neck radiotherapy generated by a patch-based three-dimensional convolutional neural network. Med Phys 2019;46(9):4095–104.

35. Farjam R, Tyagi N, Veeraraghavan H, et al. Multiatlas approach with local registration goodness weighting for MRI-based electron density mapping of head and neck anatomy. Med Phys 2017;44(7):3706–17.

36. Liu F, Jang H, Kijowski R, et al. A deep learning approach for 18F-FDG PET attenuation correction. EJNMMI Phys 2018;5(1):24.

37. Olin AB, Hansen AE, Rasmussen JH, et al. Feasibility of multiparametric positron emission tomography/magnetic resonance imaging as a one-stop-shop for radiation therapy planning for patients with head and neck cancer. Int J Radiat Oncol Biol Phys 2020;108(5):1329–38.

38. Ariji Y, Fukuda M, Nozawa M, et al. Automatic detection of cervical lymph nodes in patients with oral squamous cell carcinoma using a deep learning technique: a preliminary study. Oral Radiol 2020;6. https://doi.org/10.1007/s11282-020-00449-8.

39. Dohopolski M, Chen L, Sher D, et al. Predicting lymph node metastasis in patients with oropharyngeal cancer by using a convolutional neural network with associated epistemic and aleatoric uncertainty. Phys Med Biol 2020;65(22):225002.

40. Kawauchi K, Furuya S, Hirata K, et al. A convolutional neural network-based system to classify patients using FDG PET/CT examinations. BMC Cancer 2020;20(1):227.

41. Chen L, Zhou Z, Sher D, et al. Combining many-objective radiomics and 3D convolutional neural network through evidential reasoning to predict lymph node metastasis in head and neck cancer. Phys Med Biol 2019;64(7). https://doi.org/10.1088/1361-6560/ab083a.

42. Cantrell SC, Peck BW, Li G, et al. Differences in imaging characteristics of HPV-positive and HPV-Negative oropharyngeal cancers: a blinded matched-pair analysis. AJNR Am J Neuroradiol 2013;34(10):2005–9.

43. Tahari AK, Alluri KC, Quon H, et al. FDG PET/CT imaging of oropharyngeal squamous cell carcinoma: characteristics of human papillomavirus-positive and -negative tumors. Clin Nucl Med 2014;39(3): 225–31.

44. Bogowicz M, Riesterer O, Ikenberg K, et al. Computed tomography radiomics predicts HPV status and local tumor control after definitive radiochemotherapy in head and neck squamous cell carcinoma. Int J Radiat Oncol Biol Phys 2017; 99(4):921–8.

45. Haider SP, Mahajan A, Zeevi T, et al. PET/CT radiomics signature of human papillomavirus association in oropharyngeal squamous cell carcinoma. Eur J Nucl Med Mol Imaging 2020;47(13):2978–91.

46. Fujima N, Andreu-Arasa VC, Meibom SK, et al. Prediction of the human papillomavirus status in patients with oropharyngeal squamous cell carcinoma by FDG-PET imaging dataset using

deep learning analysis: a hypothesis-generating study. Eur J Radiol 2020;126:108936.

47. Taigman Y, Yang M, Ranzato M, et al. DeepFace: closing the gap to human-level performance in face verification. In: 2014 IEEE Conference on Computer Vision and Pattern Recognition. Columbus OH, USA: IEEE; 23-28 June 2014. doi:10.1109/cvpr.2014.220.

48. Li T, Sahu AK, Talwalkar A, et al. Federated learning: challenges, methods, and future directions. IEEE Signal Process Mag 2020;37(3):50–60.

49. Zhu W, Huang Y, Zeng L, et al. AnatomyNet: deep learning for fast and fully automated whole-volume segmentation of head and neck anatomy. Med Phys 2019;46(2):576–89.

Clinical Applications of Artificial Intelligence in Positron Emission Tomography of Lung Cancer

Katherine A. Zukotynski, MD, PhD, FRCPC, PEng[a,b,c],*,
Vincent C. Gaudet, PhD, PEng[d], Carlos F. Uribe, PhD[e], Katarina Chiam[f],
François Bénard, MD, FRCPC[g], Victor H. Gerbaudo, PhD, MSHCA[h]

KEYWORDS

- Lung cancer • Positron emission tomography • Pulmonary nodule • Cancer diagnosis
- Targeted therapy • Artificial intelligence

KEY POINTS

- AI is helpful to detect, segment, and characterize pulmonary nodules on CT and PET.
- AI is a helpful adjunct for PET as a predictive and prognostic biomarker in patients with lung cancer.
- Clinical applications of AI in PET of patients with lung cancer span the spectrum of initial and subsequent treatment strategy, including staging, detecting recurrence, and predicting outcomes.

LUNG CANCER, PRECISION MEDICINE, AND POSITRON EMISSION TOMOGRAPHY

Lung cancer is the second most diagnosed malignancy according to the American Cancer Society, accounting for 228,820 new cases and 135,720 deaths in the United States in 2020.[1] Although localized disease may be curable, systemic disease is the leading cause of cancer-related death, surpassing death from breast, prostate, and colorectal cancer combined.

Lung cancer is classified into 1. nonsmall cell lung cancer (NSCLC) and 2. small cell lung cancer (SCLC).[2] Treatment options include surgery, radiotherapy, chemotherapy, immunotherapy, and targeted medications including epidermal growth factor receptor (EGFR) inhibitors and others directed to genetic mutations (eg, ALK, ROS1), among others. Integration of clinical, genomic, and imaging findings may help personalize lung cancer management[2,3] and has the potential to identify appropriate treatment to maximize patient benefit while limiting toxicity.

Positron emission tomography (PET) plays a key role in lung cancer imaging, both at the time of initial staging and subsequent treatment planning. The true strength of PET lies in its ability to detect distant metastatic disease as well as to noninvasively characterize tumor heterogeneity

Please note that Dr K.A. Zukotynski, Dr V.C. Gaudet, Dr C.F. Uribe, Dr F. Bénard, Ms K. Chiam, and Dr V.H. Gerbaudo have nothing to disclose.

[a] Departments of Radiology and Medicine, McMaster University, 1200 Main St.W., Hamilton, ON L8N 3Z5, Canada; [b] School of Biomedical Engineering, McMaster University, 1280 Main St. W., Hamilton, ON L8S 4K1 Canada; [c] Edward S. Rogers Sr. Department of Electrical and Computer Engineering, University of Toronto, 10 King's College Rd., Toronto, ON M5S 3G8, Canada; [d] Department of Electrical and Computer Engineering, University of Waterloo, 200 University Ave.W., Waterloo, ON N2L 3G1, Canada; [e] PET Functional Imaging, BC Cancer, 600W. 10th Ave., Vancouver, V5Z 4E6, Canada; [f] Division of Engineering Science, University of Toronto, 40 St. George St., Toronto, ON M5S 2E4, Canada; [g] Department of Radiology, University of British Columbia, 2775 Laurel St., 11th floor, Vancouver, BC V5Z 1M9, Canada; [h] Department of Radiology, Brigham and Women's Hospital, Harvard Medical School, 75 Francis St., Boston, MA 02492, USA

* Corresponding author. Department of Radiology, McMaster University, 1200 Main St. W., Hamilton, ON L8N 3Z5, Canada.
E-mail address: katherine.zukotynski@utoronto.ca

throughout the body over time. It can provide predictive and prognostic insight into therapy response and identify sites of disease harboring clonal proliferation of cells resistant to treatment such that timely treatment changes can be made. Currently, PET scanners incorporate either computed tomography (CT) or magnetic resonance imaging (MRI). PET/CT is more common than PET/MR in routine clinical practice; however, both are helpful for the assessment of patients with lung cancer. Also, there are several radiopharmaceuticals that may be used to image lung cancer with PET. The most ubiquitous PET radiopharmaceutical in oncology is ^{18}F-labeled 2-fluoro-2-deoxy-D-glucose ([^{18}F]FDG), a glucose analog that is preferentially taken up by cancer cells.[4,5] Several other PET radiopharmaceuticals may be helpful for lung cancer imaging such as [^{18}F]fluoroazomycin arabinofuranoside (FAZA) and [^{18}F]fluoromisonidazole(1-(2-nitroimidazolyl)-2-hydroxy-3-fluoropropane) (FMISO) for targeting hypoxia, and the quinoline-based ligands for evaluating cancer-associated fibroblasts (fibroblast activating protein inhibitors or FAPI), among others.[6,7] To date, no radiopharmaceutical is specific for lung cancer and uptake can also occur in nonlung cancer malignancy or nonmalignant causes. Further, the intensity of uptake depends on several factors in addition to pathology, such as uptake time and other technical parameters. Ultimately, clinical context is a key for image interpretation.

AI applications may be helpful across the spectrum of lung cancer (from localized through widespread disease) both at the time of initial and subsequent treatment strategy, for several tasks including disease detection/staging, segmentation, and response prediction, among other tasks.

CURRENT CLINICAL VALUE OF PET AND AI IN PULMONARY NODULES AND LUNG CANCER STAGING

A solitary pulmonary nodule (SPN) is defined as being less than 3 cm in size and may be either solid or subsolid.[8] The risk that an incidentally detected SPN to be malignant is related to several factors, such as the patient age, smoking history, and appearance on CT. PET/CT is not included in the work-up of subsolid nodules, due to their low metabolic activity and risk of false-negative results. In this case, the Fleischner Society guidelines recommend follow-up with CT to check for lesion stability, and imaging surveillance for up to 5 years as needed.[9] However, one of the most common clinical indications for PET is the evaluation of a SPN

that is, indeterminate for malignancy based on clinical parameters and diagnostic imaging. [^{18}F]FDG-PET/CT is very accurate to characterize a solid SPN as malignant, with high negative predictive value to exclude cancer in nodules larger than 8 mm.[10–13] Also, if a nodule is known to be malignant, the more intensely [^{18}F]FDG-avid the nodule is, the more aggressive the disease tends to be. [^{18}F]FDG-PET/CT is also helpful for lung cancer staging. [^{18}F]FDG-PET/CT is used to 1) characterize indeterminate solitary solid pulmonary nodules over 8 mm on anatomic imaging; 2) localization of the site of most aggressive disease to guide the biopsy, and 3) evaluate disease extent including local, regional, and distant spread. Since certain lung cancer subtypes, such as carcinoid, may have low metabolic activity, while benign processes, such as infection or inflammation, may be intensely [^{18}F]FDG-avid, either follow-up imaging or tissue sampling is typically needed for further characterization. Ultimately, the post–[^{18}F]FDG-PET/CT risk of malignancy is used to guide clinical decisions such as CT surveillance, biopsy, and/or surgical resection. For example, an indeterminate SPN on CT with a low probability of lung cancer before PET/CT, and low [^{18}F]FDG avidity, indicates observation may be the most appropriate management. In contrast to this, an indeterminate SPN on CT but with intense [^{18}F]FDG uptake indicates biopsy is necessary, with surgical resection if this is the only site of malignant disease. According to the Society of Nuclear Medicine and Molecular Imaging (SNMMI), [^{18}F]FDG-PET/CT is helpful to 1) detect a potentially malignant SPN early permitting curative surgery in high-risk patients, 2) exclude malignancy in low-risk patients with a questionable lesion, and 3) improve outcomes by avoiding unnecessary surgery.[14]

In addition to lung nodule characterization, PET is helpful for lung cancer staging by providing complementary metabolic information to the anatomic information in CT.[15] [^{18}F]FDG-PET/CT helps detect malignant tissue differentiating it from adjacent benign findings.[16] For *lymph node disease* (N status), [^{18}F]FDG-PET/CT is more accurate than CT for evaluating disease spread.[17] False-negative results may be encountered, however, such as lesions that are too small to be detected by the scanner or those that are not metabolically active. On the other hand, false-positive results may occur with inflammation or infection. Therefore, tissue sampling is typically needed for lesion characterization.[18] The sensitivity, specificity, and accuracy of [^{18}F]FDG-PET/CT for detecting *distant metastases* (M status) are very high.[19,20]

Utility of Artificial Intelligence in Conjunction with Positron Emission Tomography in Lung Nodules and Lung Cancer

Research into the clinical applications of AI involving PET in patients with lung cancer has increased dramatically in recent years. This has largely resulted from improved electronics and software as well as access to databases containing large imaging datasets that can be used for the training of the AI models; for example, the Lung Image Database Consortium and Image Database Resource Initiative (LIDC-IRDI), the US National Lung Screening Trial (NLST), and the Dutch-Belgian Lung Cancer Screening trial (NELSON), among others.[21–24] Although these databases have made research more ubiquitous, the available data are still limited in many ways. For example, although the LIDC-IRDI database comprises chest CT studies with a spectrum of benign through malignant findings including lung cancer and metastatic disease, very few cases have histologic confirmation or a 2-year follow-up. In addition, for supervised AI algorithms, performance is tied to the gold standard, which is often the annotation of an expert (eg, a radiologist or a nuclear medicine physician), and as such remains imperfect.

Perhaps the most common clinical applications of AI in lung cancer are in the areas of nodule/disease detection. In general, these studies have concentrated on the use of CT, and have suggested that computer algorithms improve detection and assessment and may positively impact patient care.[25] However, there have been a few studies focused on the use of PET. Although often retrospective and including small numbers of subjects, these studies suggest that AI is helpful, albeit with performance closely tied to technical parameters. A retrospective study by Schwyzer and colleagues of 57 subjects with 92 [^{18}F]FDG-avid pulmonary nodules using deep learning algorithms, gave an area under the curve (AUC) for lung nodule detection of 0.796 [confidence interval (CI) 95%; 0.772 to 0.869] when ordered subset expectation maximization (OSEM) reconstruction was selected. The algorithm performance improved to an AUC = 0.848 (95%; CI: 0.828–0.869) with block sequential regularized expectation maximization (BSREM) reconstruction.[26] Another retrospective study by Schwyzer and colleagues of 100 subjects who had PET/CT, 50 with lung cancer ranging from stage I to stage IV disease and 50 without lung lesions, showed that a deep learning algorithm had a sensitivity of 95.9% and specificity of 91.5% to discriminate patients with lung cancer from normal controls. This decreased slightly with lower injected activity.[27] A deep learning approach based on individual convolutional neural networks (CNNs) for CT and PET, followed by the fusion of the results, was used for segmentation in lung cancer (Fig. 1).[28] Of note, accurate assessment of disease extent remains challenging when pathology abuts soft tissue of similar density, such as the pleura or blood vessels.

There have also been several studies using AI for lung cancer staging. For example, a study by Kirienko and colleagues of 472 patients imaged with PET/CT, of which 353 had T1-T2 disease and 119 T3-T4 tumors, achieved 69% accuracy using a CNN to classify subjects as having either T1-T2 disease or T3-T4 lung cancer.[29] A study by Tau and colleagues found the sensitivity, specificity and accuracy were 0.74 ± 0.32, 0.84 ± 0.16 and 0.80 ± 0.17, respectively, for predicting lymph node positivity and 0.45 ± 0.08, 0.79 ± 0.06, and 0.63 ± 0.05 for predicting distant metastases using a CNN in 264 subjects with nonsmall cell lung cancer.[30]

In addition, AI has been used for disease classification, localization, and volumetric assessment. Often, algorithm performance improves when more input data or data types are used. For example, Sibille and colleagues investigated a deep CNN to localize and classify [^{18}F]FDG uptake in patients with lung cancer, based on whole-body PET/CT.[31] In this study, the network structure (Fig. 2) combined convolutional and fully connected (dense) layers, and used several input modalities (PET, CT, maximum intensity projection (MIP), and atlas position), to produce 2 output decisions; node classification and localization. For patients with lung cancer, this approach gave 87% sensitivity and 99% specificity for classification, with localization accuracy of 97% (body part), 84% (organ/tissue), and 89% (subregion/nodal station). Hyun and colleagues compared several algorithms such as random forests, neural networks, and support vector machines, among others, to classify pathology in a sample of 396 subjects, 210 with adenocarcinoma and 186 with squamous cell carcinoma.[32] Interestingly, the authors found that a comparatively simple logistic regression model outperformed all other classifiers with accuracy estimated at 77%.

As certain features, such as heterogeneity, are associated with an increased risk of malignancy, work has also been conducted investigating the use of texture-based analysis to determine risk stratification. Sometimes, texture features are used to classify a lesion as benign or malignant.

Radiomics, in combination with AI, tries to identify previously unknown imaging features based on the review of mathematical patterns and pattern combinations. Further texture features that might

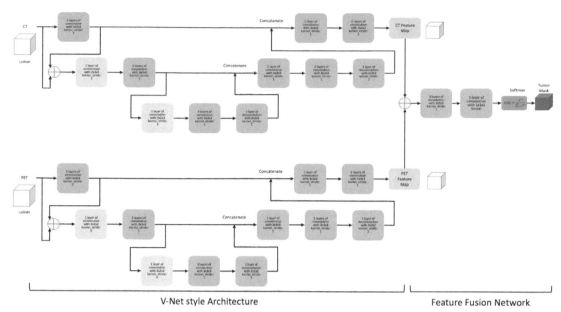

Fig. 1. Illustration of the network used by Zhao and colleagues to segment lung cancer based on PET/CT with V-net style 3D fully convolutional neural network (FCN) and feature fusion.[28] The CNNs create feature maps for each input (PET/CT). These feature maps are concatenated and undergo feature reextraction to produce a fused feature map.

not be easily quantifiable by the human eye can be extracted from images, quantified, and then used to aid with disease characterization and classification. A study by Zhang and colleagues of 135 patients with PET/CT used radiomic features on CT and metabolic parameters on PET to classify benign from malignant lung lesions across a spectrum of pathology. The authors found an AUC of 0.887 ± 0.046 with accuracy, sensitivity, and specificity of 0.815 ± 0.066, 0.814 ± 0.058, and 0.816 ± 0.079, respectively.[33] There is the suggestion that AI algorithms may reduce unnecessary follow-up.[34–38] Regardless of AI algorithm used, however, it is important to remember that tissue sampling remains key for disease confirmation.

Also, one of the challenges that remain is having access to sufficient data to capture the disease spectrum without overfitting for a specific cohort.

Understanding the genetic and pathobiological underpinnings of lung cancer contributes to precision medicine by optimizing the type of treatment and best surveillance method.[39,40] Ultimately large prospective studies are needed to confirm the utility of AI in clinical practice in this arena. Although standardization efforts for feature extraction have been made,[41] standardization in image acquisition, reconstruction, and segmentation, among other things, is also needed. We are in the early days of the application of AI to clinical practice and transparent reporting of the data used and algorithm

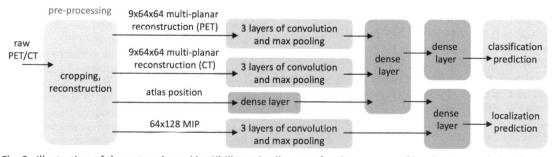

Fig. 2. Illustration of the network used by Sibille and colleagues for the purpose of localization and classification in patients with lung cancer or lymphoma.[31] Note that the model uses a combination of inputs (PET, CT, position of cropped region, maximum intensity projection (MIP)), and types of layers (convolutional, fully connected).

design remains essential for the assessment of reproducibility and to provide fair comparisons.[34,42]

CURRENT CLINICAL VALUE OF POSITRON EMISSION TOMOGRAPHY AND ARTIFICIAL INTELLIGENCE IN LUNG CANCER TREATMENT STRATEGY

PET is helpful to detect and characterize lung cancer, both at initial staging as well as for subsequent treatment strategy development. Metrics measured from PET images, such as baseline intensity and extent of radiopharmaceutical uptake as well as change in these metrics with therapy, can be used as *predictive biomarkers* of response to therapy as well as *biomarkers of prognosis*. According to the SNMMI, [18F]FDG-PET/CT is appropriate for 1) post-treatment restaging of lung

cancer, 2) recurrence detection, and 3) evaluation of treatment response.[43]

Utility of Artificial Intelligence in Conjunction with Positron Emission Tomography in Lung Cancer Follow-Up

Although preliminary investigations suggest that AI may be a helpful tool in the lung cancer treatment algorithm, to date, the available data remain limited. In this section, we highlight a few studies to illustrate the spectrum of what is being studied.

Buizza and colleagues used image features on PET/CT scans acquired at baseline and after 3 weeks of chemoradiotherapy in conjunction with linear support vector machines in 30 patients with NSCLC to predict survival.[44] Mattonen and colleagues also used image features on PET/CT

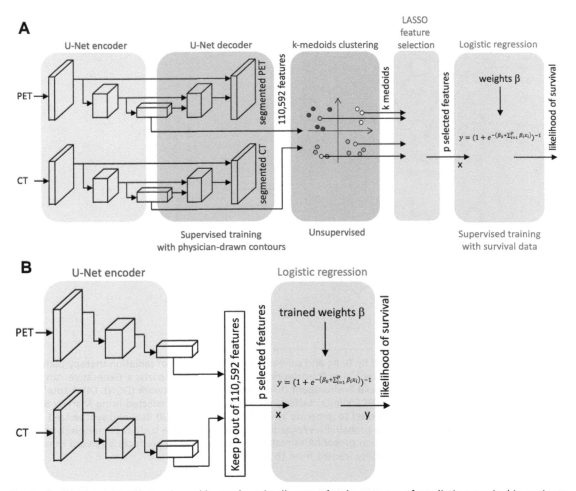

Fig. 3. Illustration of the network used by Baek and colleagues for the purpose of predicting survival in patients with nonsmall cell lung cancer.[46] (*A*) Simplified structure of a deep segmentation network to predict the likelihood of survival from NSCLC. The structure used for training included a U-Net (simplified here to 5 layers), k-medoids clustering, LASSO feature selection, and logistic regression. (*B*) The structure used for online operation, which includes the U-Net encoder, selection of p relevant features, and logistic regression.

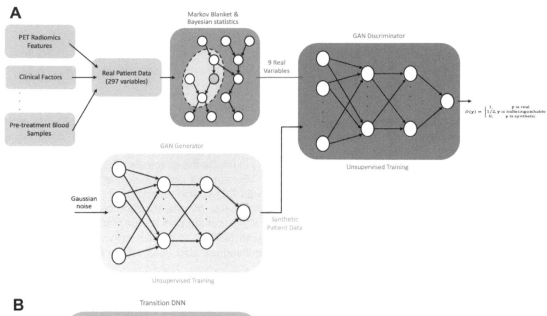

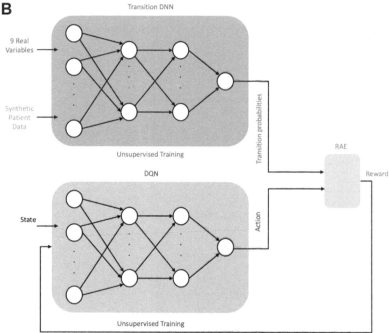

Fig. 4. Illustration of the network used by Tseng and colleagues for the purpose of radiation therapy planning in patients with nonsmall cell lung cancer.[47] The framework used consisted of 3 parts: a Generative Adversarial Network (GAN), a Radiotherapy Artificial Environment (RAE), and a Deep Q-Network (DQN). (A) A total of 297 variables were collected using the PET/CT, clinical factors, etc., with 9 variables selected using Markov Blankets and Bayesian statistics. The GAN was used to generate synthetic patient data. (B) Real and synthesized patient data were used to estimate transition probabilities regarding radiation response such as pneumonitis and local control prediction factors. The transition probabilities make up the RAE, which produces a reward in response to the action taken by the optimal policy learned from the DQN.

scans in conjunction with a linear regression model to predict survival in patients with NSCLC.[45] Although different algorithms have been assayed with varying results, ultimately multi-variable multi-step models may give among the best results. For example, a paper by Baek and colleagues appeared promising. In this paper, a sophisticated multi-step AI model (**Fig. 3**), referred to as a deep segmentation network, was trained to predict survival in patients with NSCLC.[46] Using cross-validation experiments on a data set with 96 NSCLC cases, the AUC was 0.88 when predicting 2-year overall survival, representing an improvement over other techniques that produce AUC values ranging from 0.60 to 0.83 over the same data set. The AI model consisted of supervised U-nets, followed by unsupervised k-medoids clustering, and then supervised logistic regression. Contrary to the more conventional approach wherebya CNN would be directly trained with survival data, in this paper, the U-nets were trained for segmentation using physician-drawn regions of interest (ROIs), and separate networks for CT and PET data. Intermediate results from the U-nets, taken from the middle encoded (ie, feature-space) layers were used as input to the clustering algorithm. The authors showed that by training the U-nets in this manner, the intermediate features conveyed more structural information than the textural information which is more prevalent in a network trained directly with survival data. Results from the k-medoids algorithm were used to identify key features that were then fed into the supervised logistic regression algorithm, trained using survival data.

Tseng and colleagues used generative adversarial networks (GANs) as part of the treatment planning for NSCLC to automate radiation adaptation to good effect (**Fig. 4**).[47]

SUMMARY

AI in conjunction with PET, though still in its infancy, has the potential to become an integral decision-making tool in the precision medicine algorithm of patients with lung cancer. PET coupled with either CT or magnetic resonance imaging provides anatomo-molecular insight during the course of lung cancer patient care. AI can use the information derived from this imaging to assist with staging, treatment planning, and outcome prediction.

REFERENCES

1. American Cancer Society. Key statistics for lung cancer 2020. Available at: http://www.cancer.org/cancer/lungcancer-non-smallcell/detailedguide/non-small-cell-lung-cancer-key-statistics. Accessed May 6, 2021.
2. Herbst RS, Morgensztern D, Boshoff C. The biology and management of non-small cell lung cancer. Nature 2018;553:446–54.
3. Mena E, Yanamadala A, Cheng G, et al. The current and evolving role of PET in personalized management of lung cancer. PET Clin 2016;11(3):243–59.

4. Warburg O, Wind F, Negelein E. The metabolism of tumours in the body. J Gen Physiol 1927;8(6):519–30.
5. Warburg O. On respiratory impairment in cancer cells. Science 1956;124(3215):269–70.
6. Kinoshita T, Fujii H, Hayashi Y, et al. Prognostic significance of hypoxic PET using (18)F-FAZA and (62)Cu-ATSM in non-small-cell lung cancer. Lung Cancer 2016;91:56–66.
7. Giesel FL, Adeberg S, Syed M, et al. FAPI-74 PET/CT using either 18F-AlF or cold-kit 68Ga-labeling: biodistribution, radiation dosimetry and tumor delineation in lung cancer patients. J Nucl Med 2021;62(2):201–7.
8. Gould MK, Tang T, Liu IL, et al. Recent trends in the identification of incidental pulmonary nodules. Am J Respir Crit Care Med 2015;192(10):1208–14.
9. MacMahon H, Naidich DP, Goo JM, et al. Guidelines for management of incidental pulmonary nodules detected on CT images: from the Fleischner society 2017. Radiology 2017;284(1):228–43.
10. Gould MK, Maclean CC, Kuschner WG, et al. Accuracy of positron emission tomography for diagnosis of pulmonary nodules and mass lesions: a meta-analysis. JAMA 2001;287:914–24.
11. Gambhir SS, Czernin J, Schwimmer J, et al. A tabulated summary of the FDG PET literature. J Nucl Med 2001;42:1S–93S.
12. Cronin P, Dwamena B, Kelly AM, et al. Solitary pulmonary nodules: meta-analytic comparison of cross-sectional imaging modalities for diagnosis of malignancy. Radiology 2008;246:772–82.
13. Garcia-Velloso MJ, Bastarrika G, de-Torres JP, et al. Assessment of indeterminate pulmonary nodules detected in lung cancer screening: diagnostic accuracy of FDG PET/CT. Lung Cancer 2016;97:81–6.
14. Fletcher JW, Djulbegovic B, Soares HP, et al. Recommendations on the use of ^{18}F-FDG PET in oncology. J Nucl Med 2008;49(3):480–508.
15. Lardinois D, Weder W, Hany TF, et al. Staging of non–small-cell lung cancer with integrated positron emission tomography and computed tomography. N Engl J Med 2003;348:2500–7.
16. Gerbaudo VH, Julius B. Anatomo-metabolic characteristics of atelectasis in F-18 FDG-PET/CT imaging. Eur J Radiol 2007;64(3):401–5.
17. Gould MK, Kuschner WG, Rydzak CE, et al. Test performance of positron emission tomography and computed tomography for mediastinal staging in patients with non-small-cell lung cancer: a meta-analysis. Ann Intern Med 2003;139:879–92.
18. Fischer BM, Mortensen J, Hansen H, et al. Multimodality approach to mediastinal staging in non-small cell lung cancer. Faults and benefits of PET-CT: a randomised trial. Thorax 2011;66(4):294–300.
19. Hellwig D, Ukena D, Paulsen F, et al. Onko-PET der Deutschen Gesellschaft Fur Nuklearmedizin. Meta-

analysis of the efficacy of positron emission tomography with F-18-Fluorodeoxyglucose in lung tumors. Basis for discussion of the german consensus conference on PET in Oncology 2000. Pneumologie 2001;55(8):367–77.

20. MacManus MP, Hicks RJ, Matthews JP, et al. High rate of detection of unsuspected distant metastases by PET in apparent stage III non-small-cell lung cancer: implications for radical radiation therapy. Int J Radiat Oncol Biol Phys 2001;50(2):287–93.

21. Uribe CF, Mathotaarachchi S, Gaudet V, et al. Machine learning in nuclear medicine: Part 1-introduction. J Nucl Med 2019;60(4):451–8.

22. Armato SG 3rd, McLennan G, Bidaut L, et al. The lung image database consorium (LIDC) and image database Resource initiative (IDRI): a completed reference database of lung nodules on CT scans. Med Phys 2011;38(2):915–31.

23. Aberle DR, Adams AM, Berg CD, et al. Reduced lung-cancer mortality with low-dose computed tomographic screening. N Engl J Med 2011; 365(5):395–409.

24. Zhao YR, Xie X, de Koning HJ, et al. NELSON lung cancer screening study. Cancer Imaging 2011;11. Spec No AS75-84.

25. Yang Y, Feng X, Chi W, et al. Deep learning aided decision support for pulmonary nodules diagnosing: a review. J Thorac Dis 2018;10(Suppl. 7):S867–75.

26. Schwyzer M, Martini K, Benz DC, et al. Artificial intelligence for detecting small FDG-positive lung nodules in digital PET/CT: impact of image reconstructions on diagnostic performance. Eur Radiol 2020;30(4):2031–40.

27. Schwyzer M, Ferraro DA, Muehlematter UJ, et al. Automated detection of lung cancer at ultralow dose PET/CT by deep neural networks – initial results. Lung Cancer 2018;126:170–3.

28. Zhao X, Li L, Lu W, et al. Tumor Co-segmentation in PET/CT using multi-modality fully convolutional neural network. Phys Med Biol 2020;64(1):015011.

29. Kirienko M, Sollini M, Silvestri G, et al. Convolutional neural networks promising in lung cancer T-parameter assessment on baseline FDG-PET/CT. Contrast Media Mol Imaging 2018;1382309.

30. Tau N, Stundzia A, Yasufuku K, et al. Convolutional neural networks in predicting nodal and distant metastatic potential of newly diagnosed non-small cell lung cancer on FDG PET images. AJR Am J Roentgenol 2020;215(1):192–7.

31. Sibille L, Seifert R, Avramovic N, et al. 18F-FDG PET/CT uptake classification in lymphoma and lung cancer by using deep convolutional neural networks. Radiology 2020;294:445–52.

32. Hyun SH, Ahn MS, Koh YW, et al. A machine-learning approach using PET-based radiomics to predict the histologic subtypes of lung cancer. Clin Nucl Med 2019;44(12):956–60.

33. Zhang R, Zhu L, Cai Z, et al. Potential feature exploration and model development based on 18F-FDG PET/CT images for differentiating benign and malignant lung lesions. Eur Radiol 2019;121:108735.

34. Zukotynski K, Gaudet V, Uribe CF, et al. Machine learning in nuclear medicine: Part 2-neural networks and clinical aspects. J Nucl Med 2021;62(1):22–9.

35. Kang G, Liu K, Hou B, et al. 3D multi-view convolutional neural networks for lung nodule classification. PLoS One 2017;12(11):e0188290.

36. Xie Y, Xia Y, Zhang J, et al. Knowledge-based collaborative Deep learning for benign-malignant lung nodule classification on chest CT. IEEE Trans Med Imaging 2019;38(4):991–1004.

37. Nibali A, He Z, Wollersheim D. Pulmonary nodule classification with deep residual networks. Int J Comput Assis Radiol Surg 2017;12(10):1799–808.

38. da Silva GLF, Valente TLA, Silva AC, et al. Convolutional neural network-based PSO for lung nodule false positive reduction on CT images. Comput Methods Programs Biomed 2018;162109–18.

39. Manafi-Farid R, Karamzade-Ziarati N, Vali R, et al. 2-[18F]FDG PET/CT radiomics in lung cancer: an overview of the technical aspect and its emerging role in management of the disease. Methods 2020;188: 84–97.

40. Yang SR, Schultheis AM, Yu H, et al. Precision medicine in non-small cell lung cancer: current applications and future directions. Semin Cancer Biol 2020;S1044-579X(20)30164-4.

41. Zwanenburg A, Vallières M, Abdalah MA, et al. The image biomarker standardization initiative: standardized quantitative radiomics for high-throughput image-based phenotyping. Radiology 2020;295(2): 328–38.

42. Park H, Sholl LM, Hatabu H, et al. Imaging of precision therapy for lung cancer: current state of the art. Radiology 2019;293:15–29.

43. Jadvar H, Colletti PM, Delgado-Bolton R, et al. Appropriate use criteria for 18F-FDG PET/CT in restaging and treatment response assessment of malignant disease. J Nucl Med 2017;58(12): 2026–37.

44. Buizza G, Toma-Dasu I, Lazzeroni M, et al. Early tumor response prediction for lung cancer patients using novel longitudinal pattern features from sequential PET/CT image scans. Phys Med 2018;54:21–9.

45. Mattonen SA, Davidzon GA, Benson J, et al. Bone marrow and tumor radiomics at 18F-FDG PET/CT: impact on outcome prediction in non-small cell lung cancer. Radiology 2019;293(2):451–9.

46. Baek S, He Y, Allen BG, et al. Deep segmentation networks predict survival of non-small cell lung cancer. Sci Rep 2019;9:17286.

47. Tseng HH, Luo Y, Cui S, et al. Deep reinforcement learning for automated radiation adaptation in lung cancer. Med Phys 2017;44(12):6690–705.

Artificial Intelligence and Cardiac PET/Computed Tomography Imaging

Robert J.H. Miller, MD[a], Ananya Singh, MSc[b], Damini Dey, PhD[b], Piotr Slomka, PhD[b],*

KEYWORDS

• Artificial intelligence • AI • PET • Positron emission tomography • Machine learning • Deep learning

KEY POINTS

• Understanding the methods used for training and testing artificial intelligence is crucial when assessing applicability to new populations.
• Artificial intelligence can be used for image reconstruction, potentially allowing improved image quality, a decreased radiation dose, or both.
• Artificial intelligence can be applied to attenuation correction imaging to extract useful anatomic information or alternatively provide synthetic attenuation correction.
• The diagnostic and prognostic potential of PET imaging can be optimized by using artificial intelligence algorithms.

INTRODUCTION

Artificial Intelligence (AI) is an increasingly important technology, with rapidly expanding applications for all cardiac imaging, including PET.[1,2] As an introduction, we review common AI terminology including methods for training and testing. Next, we highlight the potential applications of AI to improve PET image acquisition, reconstruction, and segmentation. Computed tomography (CT) imaging is commonly acquired in conjunction with PET and various AI methods have been proposed to better use these scans, including methods to automatically extract anatomic information or alternatively to generate synthetic attenuation correction images. Lastly, we review methods to automate disease diagnosis or risk stratification. This summary highlights current and future clinical applications of AI to PET imaging.

INTRODUCTION TO ARTIFICIAL INTELLIGENCE TERMINOLOGY

Classification of Artificial Intelligence Algorithms

Recently there has been growing interest in clinical applications of AI; however, the terminology remains a barrier to better understanding for many clinicians and researchers. AI is used to describe algorithms that perform tasks normally characteristic of human intelligence such as recognizing images and learning patterns.[1,2] Machine learning (ML) is a subset of AI which includes deep learning (DL).

Classical ML algorithms assess existing observations to determine which features are predictive of outcomes and then use this information to predict the outcomes of future observations. ML algorithms use precoded data (such as clinical

Dr. Slomka is Funded by: NIHHYB. Grant number(s): R01HL135557 and R01HL089765.
a Department of Cardiac Sciences, University of Calgary, GAA08 HRIC, 3230 Hospital Drive NW, Calgary AB, T2N 4Z6, Canada; b Departments of Imaging and Medicine, Cedars-Sinai Medical Center, 8700 Beverly Blvd, Suite Metro 203, Los Angeles, CA 90048, USA
* Corresponding author. 127 S. San Vicente Boulevard, Advanced Health Sciences Pavilion, Suite A3100, Los Angeles, CA 90048-1860, USA.
E-mail address: Piotr.Slomka@cshs.org

PET Clin 17 (2022) 85–94
https://doi.org/10.1016/j.cpet.2021.06.011

variables or results of image quantification), but are not explicitly programmed with assumptions about the importance of the different features.[3,4] Additionally, they are inherently capable of identifying variable interactions and nonlinear relationships.[3,4] These algorithms are well-suited to integrating clinical, stress, and imaging information from nuclear cardiology studies to improve disease diagnosis or risk prediction.[2]

DL is a subset of ML that refers to algorithms characterized by a multilayer learning approach with artificial neural networks. Each layer can be thought of as a container that receives weighted input, transforms it with a set function, and then passes the resulting values to the next layer. Each layer contains a number of neurons (or nodes) that, similar to biologic neurons, receive signals, extract meaningful representations from the input data, and pass the output along to neurons in the following layer. Convolutional neural networks (CNN) are an example of DL that is commonly applied to imaging data.[1,5] Typically, when using a CNN each input image pixel is connected to 1 neuron in the first layer of the network. In a classical artificial neural network, each neuron is connected to every neuron in the subsequent layer. In a CNN, the neurons from adjacent layers are only connected to other nearby neurons. This strategy preserves the spatial relationships of the image and is conceptually similar to a convolutional filter commonly used in imaging where only neighboring pixels are used by the filter. A graphical representation of a classical artificial neural network and CNN are shown in **Fig. 1**. CNN are well-suited for image interpretation and segmentation, because they capture and recognize the spatial structure of the input image.[6,7] Additionally, because the CNN is not specifically directed regarding the importance of image features, it may identify aspects of images that are not immediately apparent to human observers.[8] It is also possible to combine the CNN layers with some fully connected layers—usually as the late layers of the network to allow connections between all features.[5,9,10]

In addition to describing model architecture, AI models are further classified as having supervised or unsupervised learning.[11] Supervised learning is performed using a ground truth, for instance, the presence of obstructive coronary artery disease, as the target output for the algorithm.[11] Supervised learning, where models are tasked with predicting a ground truth, is frequently used when the goal task is classification or segmentation.[11,12] Unsupervised learning is performed without a specified output, with the AI model instead learning the inherent structure of the data.[11] Principal component analysis and

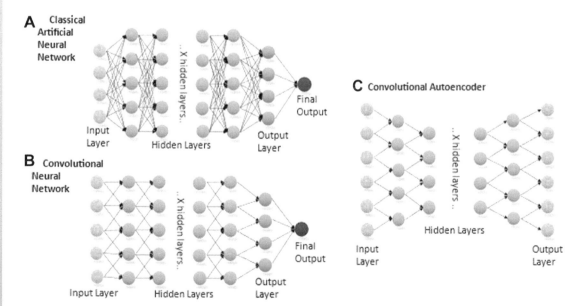

Fig. 1. Three DL architectures. Classical artificial neural networks (*A*) are composed of input (*yellow*) and output (*blue*) layers with hidden inner layers (*green*). Each neuron, or node, is connected to many neurons in the following layer, with all information moving forward through the network. In CNNs (*B*), neurons only connect to local (spatially related) neurons in the next layer. Convolutional autoencoders (*C*) are an example of unsupervised learning with layers connected in a similar fashion to CNNs. They are characterized by inner hidden layers with fewer dimensions than either the input or output layer.

autoencoders are 2 examples of unsupervised learning. In principal component analysis, the algorithm condenses the information from a large set of variables into a few "principal component" variables.[13] An autoencoder is a neural network tasked with copying the input layer to the output layer. However, the model architecture has inner hidden layers, which have fewer dimensions than either the input or output layers. As a result, the algorithm only extracts the most important information from the image that can be applied to denoise images.[14,15] A graphical representation of a convolutional autoencoder is also shown in **Fig. 1.**

Training Artificial Intelligence Algorithms

All AI algorithms require data to learn patterns, which can then be applied to predicting future outcomes. Training datasets should be large, heterogenous and ideally representative of the population in which it will eventually be applied. The process of identifying features and determining their relative importance for predicting the outcome of interest is referred to as training. Hyperparameters are variables that control the learning process and are specific to the particular AI technique. For example, these variables can be the learning rate and number of layers in a CNN,[16] or the number of iterations in classical ML method.[17] Optimization of model hyperparameters is called "tuning." It is critical that the data used for training and tuning the model are not used during model testing.[18] For example, if additional tuning of the model parameters is required, this process cannot be done with the testing dataset and a set of the training samples (sometimes referred to as a validation dataset) should be kept separate for tuning. Similarly, any feature selection should be performed during the training stage with only training data used to establish the feature importance.

Testing Artificial Intelligence Algorithms

Testing is the process in which an AI model, which has already been trained and tuned (if required) on separate data to set the model parameters, is applied to a new dataset to evaluate its performance. This procedure can be performed once or multiple times and may be applied to a random set of the study population or in patients selected by a specific grouping factor (such as site). Two commonly used procedures, k-fold internal testing and external testing, are depicted in **Fig. 2.** In k-fold internal testing, the population is randomly divided into k-folds (or sets of data), with one fold held out from model training to be used for

testing.[19] Typically, 5 or 10 such folds are used and consequently the process is repeated 5 or 10 times with a different fold being held out for testing each time. Repeated testing decreases the variance in estimating the model accuracy and is preferred to testing in a single random sample.[20]

In external testing, patients are selected to be used as the testing set based on a specific factor, such as site. External testing can be using multiple groups for testing (termed repeated external testing).[21] External testing provides an estimate of the model performance when applied in a new, unrelated population.[21] Similar to repeated internal testing, repeated external testing will decrease the variability related to the random selection of the final external site for testing.

When assessing AI applications in cardiovascular PET, it is critical to understand the method used for training and testing the AI model. In addition to clear separation of testing and training data, the training population should ideally reflect the characteristics of the planned application. These considerations are important when determining the expected performance when these algorithms are applied prospectively to clinical practice.

CLINICAL APPLICATIONS
Improving PET Instrumentation

A central technical aspect of PET imaging is determining the exact origin of the photon annihilation with high spatial resolution. Knowledge of the depth of interaction in the crystal detectors of the PET scanner can reduce parallax errors for photons originating from off-center positions.[22] Gradient tree boosting, a type of ML, can be used to estimate depth of interaction with similar spatial resolution to traditional estimation methods but with more uniform performance across detector crystals.[22] Peng and colleagues[23] demonstrated that a DL model could be used to account for Compton scatter within the PET detector crystal. This method for Compton scatter correction can be combined with neural networks trained to accurately decode interaction positions.[24] PET detector modules integrating these 2 DL methods achieve high count sensitivity with a spatial resolution of 1.1 ± 0.1 mm.[24] Lastly, CNN have also been used to estimate time-of-flight, demonstrating an approximately 20% better timing resolution compared with leading edge discrimination or constant fraction discrimination.[25] It seems likely that 1 or more AI algorithms will be integrated to improve instrumentation in future PET camera system designs.

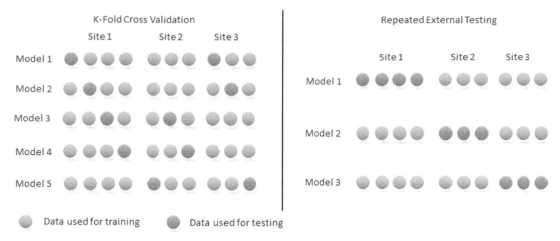

Fig. 2. Comparison of K-fold internal testing and repeated external testing. In k-fold cross validation, the dataset is randomly divided into k sets (in this case 5). Each set is sequentially held-out from model training to be used for testing by a specific model built from the training data. In repeated external testing, datasets are grouped according to specific factors such as site. Each site is sequentially held out from model training to be used for testing.

Improving Image Quality During Reconstruction

AI can be integrated within the image reconstruction process to improve image quality. Gong and colleagues embedded a CNN within an iterative reconstruction process for brain and lung fluorodeoxyglucose PET reconstruction to improve contrast recovery and decrease image noise compared with standard reconstruction methods in combination with standard postprocessing or CNN denoising for postprocessing.[26] Liu and colleagues[27] developed a conditional generative adversarial network to reconstruct brain PET data from sinograms with a lower bias and variance compared with maximum likelihood–expectation maximum reconstruction. These techniques can be extended to cardiovascular PET imaging. Wang and Liu[28] trained a 2 component DL model to first reconstruct cardiac PET images from a sinogram and then denoise the same images. Another approach uses a CNN to directly map sensor data to image domains, providing direct image reconstruction.[29] Xie and colleagues[30] used a 3-dimensional convolutional sparse coding model to reconstruct brain PET images, accounting for anatomic priors without a need for image registration, with superior contrast resolution recovery compared with other reconstruction methods. AI algorithms can also be used during postprocessing to improve image quality, which potentially can be used to reduce radiation exposure, shorten imaging times, or both. Wang and colleagues[31] applied an artificial neural network that integrated both raw myocardial perfusion images and reconstructed images to improve image contrast and detection of defects on PET myocardial perfusion imaging (MPI). Lassen and colleagues[32] demonstrated image denoising with a DL algorithm could be applied to substantially decrease ^{18}F sodium fluoride scan times. Images from this study are shown in **Fig. 3**. Ladefoged and colleagues[33] evaluated the potential of denoising fluorodeoxyglucose PET images with a DL model, simulating dose decreases as low as 1% of the injected dose. Convolutional autoencoders have also been applied to denoise dynamic ^{11}C-raclopride images.[34] Generative adversarial networks, where a generator network and a discriminator network are trained simultaneously to compete with each other -and generate (by the generator) simulated full-dose images from low-dose input images which are virtually indistinguishable (by the discriminator) from the real full-dose PET images, have also be applied to improve image quality.[35,36] Given the potential for improved image quality with decreased radiation exposure it is likely that AI will increasingly be used during image reconstruction.

Left Ventricular Image Segmentation

Accurate myocardial segmentation is critical to the precision of subsequent image quantitation and interpretation in PET.[37] Although existing classic image processing approaches achieve high performance in segmentation of PET and single photon emission CT (SPECT) images,[38,39] efforts are ongoing to use DL for this task to further reduce the frequency with which manual corrections required. Wang and colleagues[40] described

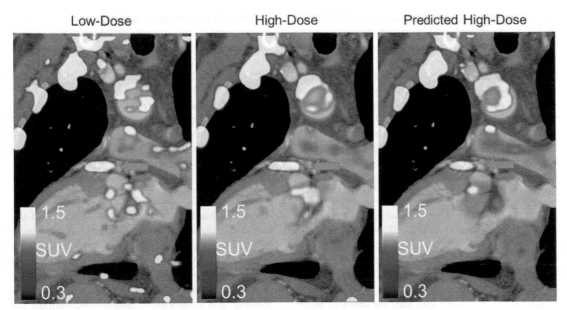

Fig. 3. Example of image de-noising for 18F-NaF images to improve image quality with shorter acquisition times. The convolutional neural network was used to predict full dose images (right) from low dose (10% of acquired counts) images (left). The resulting images were similar to actual full-dose images (middle). Blue arrow points to coronary 18F-NaF activity. This research was originally published in JNM. From Lassen ML, Commandeur F, Kwiecinski J et al. 10-fold reduction of scan time with deep learning reconstruction of Coronary PET images. Journal of Nuclear Medicine 2019;60:244 © SNMMI.

a DL-algorithm, which could segment the left ventricular myocardium by delineating its endocardial and epicardial surfaces after SPECT. The CNN was trained with contours delineated by expert interpreters, and in 56 patients demonstrated excellent precision for left ventricular myocardium volume (mean error, 1.1 ± 3.7%).[40] This application could readily be extended to PET. Similar methods could be applied to improve segmentation of dynamic PET cardiac data, which can be particularly technically challenging.

Motion Correction

One of the key problems in cardiac PET images is the degrading effect of patient motion, which can affect quantitative values in flow imaging and the quality of the attenuation correction owing to shifts between PET images and the associated CT attenuation scans. AI could potentially be used to optimize motion correction algorithms or correct for residual errors. Guo and colleagues[41] developed an AI algorithm to identify irregular breathing patterns that could be used to apply patient-specific respiratory corrections. Although the study was applied to abdominal PET imaging, it could readily be translated to cardiac PET. Unsupervised nonrigid image registration by DL can also be used to correct for respiratory motion in cardiac PET images with lower normalized root mean

square error compared with iterative registration based correction.[42] Su and colleagues used an ensemble learning method to correct for partial volume errors in the arterial input function that could be used to improve the accuracy of myocardial blood flow estimation.[43] Given these promising results, it is possible that AI will be increasingly used for motion correction in cardiac PET.

Applications to Attenuation Correction Imaging

During cardiac PET imaging, a CT attenuation correction scan is obtained to correct PET emission images for photon attenuation. Yu and colleagues[44] developed an unsupervised DL model to improve registration between whole body PET and CT attenuation correction imaging with a high degree of accuracy. As an alternative to separately acquired CT attenuation correction images, AI can be used to generate synthetic attenuation correction maps. Liu and colleagues[45] trained a CNN to generate synthetic CT scan images from magnetic resonance images, which could then be used to provide attenuation correction for PET. Yang and colleagues[46] used a CNN to provide scatter and attenuation correction for brain PET images for circumstances where CT attenuation correction imaging is not available, with similar results reported for applications in whole body PET.[47] More recently, Shi and colleagues recently trained a DL algorithm to predict CT-attenuation maps from cardiac SPECT alone.[48] Alternatively, DL could be used to predict attenuation correction images directly from non–attenuation correction images.[49] AI assisted attenuation correction could be used to improve the image quality of the original PET images without the radiation exposure associated with CT attenuation correction.

Extracting Anatomic Information from a Computed Tomography Scan

Hybrid cardiovascular PET is almost always obtained in conjunction with a CT scan during the same patient visit. These CT scans can include a simple CT scan obtained for attenuation correction, noncontrast electrocardiography-gated CT scans obtained for calcium scoring or CT coronary angiography scans. AI can also be used to automatically extract additional anatomic information from these CT scans, such as coronary artery calcification (CAC). One approach to automatically extract CAC information used a 2-stage CNN developed to detect CAC from low-dose chest CT scans, demonstrating excellent agreement with manual scoring.[50] This approach has subsequently been demonstrated to have high accuracy in a large study incorporating a variety of types of CT scans.[51] In patients undergoing PET MPI, Isgum and colleagues[52] showed a good correlation between CAC scores derived automatically with DL from noncontrast CT attenuation correction maps and dedicated gated CAC scans. In

addition to having good correlation with manually determined CAC scores, automatically derived CAC scores are independently associated with risk of major adverse cardiovascular events in a range of patient populations,[53] including in CAC scores derived from PET CT attenuation correction maps.[54] DL can be also used to detect calcium in the thoracic aorta and heart valves,[55] or quantify epicardial adipose tissue volumes.[56,57] An example of automated CAC segmentation using DL is shown in **Fig. 4**.

Improving Disease Diagnosis

AI can be trained to predict the likelihood of disease, such as obstructive coronary artery disease using the image data. Initially, improved detection of coronary artery disease has been demonstrated from SPECT imaging using ML,[58] and DL algorithms,[9] where large repositories of data for AI training are available.[59] Similar techniques can also be applied to cardiovascular PET imaging. Clerc and colleagues[60] used ML to predict the presence of stress perfusion defect on PET by incorporating clinical parameters and CAC with a high degree of accuracy (area under the curve of 0.86). Santarelli and colleagues[61] developed a DL model that was tasked with differentiating transthyretin cardiac amyloidosis and light chain cardiac amyloidosis from control patients undergoing 18F-Florbetapir imaging. The proposed DL model achieved high diagnostic accuracy, with an overall accuracy of 94% and 97% for light chain and transthyretin amyloidosis, respectively.[61] Additionally, CNNs have also

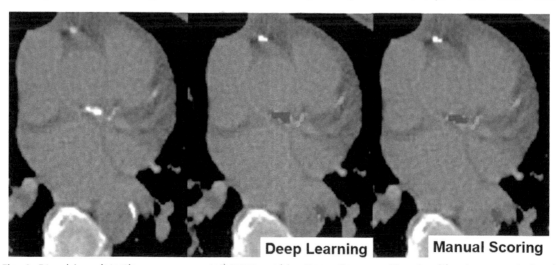

Fig. 4. DL calcium detection on a computed tomographic attenuation scan. The algorithm is a convolutional long–short–term memory network, which imitates a clinician's approach to identifying calcification by integrating information from adjacent slices. The identification of CAC by DL (*middle*) demonstrates good agreement with manual calcium scoring (*right*). *Red*, left main; *green*, left anterior descending; *yellow*, right coronary artery; *blue*, aorta.

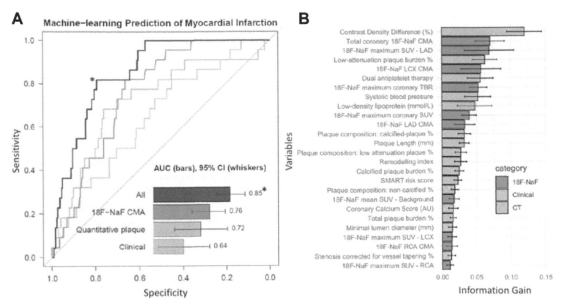

Fig. 5. Kwiecinski et al. developed a machine learning algorithm that integrated clinical factors, computed tomographic plaque characteristics, and 18F-NaF positron emission tomography quantitation to predict risk of myocardial infarction (69). The ML model incorporating all available information had higher accuracy compared to any of the imaging components in isolation (Panel A, p<0.01). Panel B outlines feature importance, highlighting the potential gains in accuracy from combining clinical and multimodality imaging variables. This research was originally published in JNM. (From Kwiecinski J, Tzolos E, Meah M et al. Machine-learning with 18F-sodium fluoride PET and quantitative plaque analysis on CT angiography for the future risk of myocardial infarction. Journal of nuclear medicine : official publication, Society of Nuclear Medicine 2021; jnumed.121.262283.)

been applied to PET studies in patients with suspected cardiac sarcoidosis, demonstrating improved sensitivity and specificity compared with maximum standardized uptake value and coefficient of variation-based classifications.[62]

Improving Risk Prediction

The prediction of cardiovascular events is another classification task that can be performed by AI with a high degree of accuracy. These methods have been rigorously evaluated with SPECT imaging[17,63,64]; however, they can readily be applied to PET as well. Recently, a DL model was developed to predict the risk of adverse cardiovascular events directly from polar maps of rest and stress myocardial blood flow and myocardial perfusion reserve.[65] The DL model demonstrated higher accuracy compared with other risk models, with an area under the curve of 0.90 for the prediction of the combined outcome of death, myocardial infarction, revascularization, or heart failure.[65] For coronary PET imaging, Kwiecinski and colleagues[66] described an ML algorithm that integrated clinical characteristics, quantitative coronary CT plaque characteristics, and ^{18}F-NaF PET quantitation to predict risk of myocardial infarction in patients undergoing hybrid imaging.

The ML model incorporating all available information had higher accuracy (c-statistic 0.85) compared with clinical characteristics (c-statistic 0.64) or quantitative plaque characteristics alone (c-statistic 0.72).[66] Results from this study are shown in **Fig. 5**.

FUTURE POSSIBILITIES

We have outlined many recent applications of AI to PET imaging; however, there are numerous potential applications that could be explored in the future. For example, the ability to accurately quantify myocardial blood flow provides robust diagnostic and prognostic information to PET MPI but is technically demanding.[67] AI methods could potentially be used to automatically detect, and flag for the physicians and technologists, abnormalities in time–activity curves, which are potentially related to technical issues.[68] Given the diverse array of variables associated with a PET MPI study, AI could be used to further improve the diagnostic and prognostic accuracy. These algorithms could incorporate clinical characteristics, CAC from CT attenuation correction imaging (automatically derived with DL), and PET quantitative parameters including relative perfusion and absolute myocardial blood flow. These models could also potentially be trained to predict benefit from revascularization.[69] Additionally, future AI algorithms could incorporate methods to explain these predictions to clinicians to promote clinical adoption.[17] With the recent growth in both cardiovascular PET and AI, we will probably see new efforts to further optimize PET image quality, image analysis, disease detection and risk prediction with the use of the AI tools.

SUMMARY

The potential applications of AI in cardiac PET imaging are broad, including important roles in image acquisition, reconstruction, and interpretation. We reviewed common terminology in AI, including the importance of training and testing methods. AI may be able to improve PET instrumentation by allowing for improved knowledge of depth of interaction and Compton scatter correction. Additionally, there is a clear role for AI methods to improve image segmentation and denoising. AI has been applied extensively to CT imaging, which is frequently acquired in conjunction with cardiovascular PET, to automatically extract additional anatomic information with a high degree of accuracy. Alternatively, synthetic attenuation correction imaging can be generated with AI to improve image quality without additional radiation exposure. Last, AI can be used to improve disease diagnosis or risk prediction either directly from images or by combining clinical, stress, and imaging data. Clinicians should be aware of the multiple, diverse applications of AI to PET, which will no doubt continue to grow in the future.

CLINICS CARE POINTS

- Understanding the methods and data used for training and testing AI is crucial when assessing its applicability to new populations
- AI can be used to improve image reconstruction, allowing improved image quality, a decreased radiation dose, or both.
- AI can be used to improve registration with computed tomographic imaging, extract additional anatomic information, or generate synthetic attenuation correction images
- Methods to automatically detects obstructive coronary artery disease with AI may be superior to quantitative analysis or expert interpretation

DISCLOSURE

The authors have no relevant disclosures.

REFERENCES

1. Dey D, Slomka PJ, Leeson P, et al. Artificial intelligence in cardiovascular imaging: JACC state-of-the-art review. J Am Coll Cardiol 2019;73:1317–35.
2. Slomka PJ, Miller RJ, Isgum I, et al. Application and translation of artificial intelligence to cardiovascular imaging in nuclear medicine and noncontrast CT. Semin Nucl Med 2020;50:357–66.
3. Obermeyer Z, Emanuel EJ. Predicting the future - big data, machine learning, and clinical medicine. N Engl J Med 2016;375:1216–9.
4. Banerjee M, Reynolds E, Andersson HB, et al. Tree-based analysis. Circ Cardiovasc Qual Outcomes 2019;12:e004879.
5. Krittanawong C, Tunhasiriwet A, Zhang H, et al. Deep learning with unsupervised feature in echocardiographic imaging. J Am Coll Cardiol 2017;69: 2100–1.
6. Razavian S, Azizpour H, Sullivan J, et al. Cnn features off-the-shelf: An astounding baseline for recognition. Comp Vis Pattern Recog Workshop 2014; 512-519.
7. Krizhevsky A, Sutskever I, Hinton GE. Imagenet classification with deep convolutional neural networks. Advance Neural Info Process System 2012; 25:1097–105.
8. Zech JR, Badgeley MA, Liu M, et al. Variable generalization performance of a deep learning model to detect pneumonia in chest radiographs: a cross-sectional study. Plos Med 2018;15:e1002683.
9. Betancur J, Commandeur F, Motlagh M, et al. Deep learning for prediction of obstructive disease from fast myocardial perfusion SPECT: a multicenter study. JACC Cardiovasc Imaging 2018;11:1654–63.
10. Betancur J, Hu LH, Commandeur F, et al. Deep learning analysis of upright-supine high-efficiency SPECT myocardial perfusion imaging for prediction of obstructive coronary artery disease: a multicenter study. J Nucl Med 2019;60:664–70.
11. Deo RC. Machine learning in medicine. Circulation 2015;132:1920–30.
12. Uddin S, Khan A, Hossain ME, et al. Comparing different supervised machine learning algorithms for disease prediction. BMC Med Inform Decis Mak 2019;19:281.
13. Martis RJ, Acharya UR, Mandana KM, et al. Application of principal component analysis to ECG signals for automated diagnosis of cardiac health. Expert Syst Appl 2012;39:11792–800.
14. Lundervold AS, Lundervold A. An overview of deep learning in medical imaging focusing on MRI. Z Med Phys 2019;29:102–27.

15. Chen C, Qin C, Qiu H, et al. Deep learning for cardiac image segmentation: a review. Front Cardiovasc Med 2020;7:25.

16. Graham BM, Adler A. Objective selection of hyperparameter for EIT. Physiol Meas 2006;27:S65–79.

17. Hu LH, Miller RJH, Sharir T, et al. Prognostically safe stress-only single-photon emission computed tomography myocardial perfusion imaging guided by machine learning: report from REFINE SPECT. Eur Heart J Cardiovasc Imaging 2021;22:705–14.

18. Xu Y, Goodacre R. On splitting training and validation set: a comparative study of cross-validation, Bootstrap and systematic sampling for estimating the generalization performance of supervised learning. J Anal Test 2018;2:249–62.

19. Jung Y, Hu J. A K-fold averaging cross-validation procedure. J Nonparametr Stat 2015;27:167–79.

20. Cawley GC, Talbot NLC. On Over-fitting in model selection and subsequent selection bias in performance evaluation. J Mach Learn Res 2010;11:2079–107.

21. Riley RD, Ensor J, Snell KI, et al. External validation of clinical prediction models using big datasets from e-health records or IPD meta-analysis: opportunities and challenges. BMJ 2016;353:i3140.

22. Muller F, Schug D, Hallen P, et al. A novel DOI positioning algorithm for monolithic scintillator crystals in PET based on gradient tree boosting. IEEE Trans Radiat Plasma Med Sci 2019;3:465–74.

23. Peng P, Judenhofer MS, Jones AQ, et al. Compton PET: a simulation study for a PET module with novel geometry and machine learning for position decoding. Biomed Phys Eng Express 2018;5:015018.

24. Peng P, Judenhofer MS, Cherry SR. Compton PET: a layered structure PET detector with high performance. Phys Med Biol 2019;64:10LT01.

25. Berg E, Cherry SR. Using convolutional neural networks to estimate time-of-flight from PET detector waveforms. Phys Med Biol 2018;63:02LT01.

26. Gong K, Wu D, Kim K, et al. EMnet: an unrolled deep neural network for PET image reconstruction. Med Imaging 2019.

27. Liu Z, Chen H, Liu H. Deep learning based framework for direct reconstruction of PET images. In: Shen D, Liu T, Peters TM, et al, editors. Medical image computing and computer assisted Intervention – MICCAI 2019. Cham: Springer International Publishing; 2019. p. 48–56.

28. Wang B, Liu H. FBP-Net for direct reconstruction of dynamic PET images. Phys Med Biol 2020.

29. Zhu B, Liu JZ, Cauley SF, et al. Image reconstruction by domain-transform manifold learning. Nature 2018;555:487–92.

30. Xie N, Gong K, Guo N, et al. Penalized-likelihood PET image reconstruction using 3D structural convolutional sparse coding. IEEE Trans Biomed Eng 2020.

31. Wang X, Yang B, Moody JB, et al. Improved myocardial perfusion PET imaging using artificial neural networks. Phys Med Biol 2020;65:145010.

32. Lassen ML, Commandeur F, Kwiecinski J, et al. 10-fold reduction of scan time with deep learning reconstruction of Coronary PET images. J Nucl Med 2019;60:244.

33. Ladefoged C, Hasbak P, Hansen J, et al. Low-dose PET reconstruction using deep learning: application to cardiac imaged with FDG. J Nucl Med 2019;60:573.

34. Klyuzhin IS, Cheng JC, Bevington C, et al. Use of a Tracer-specific deep artificial neural net to denoise dynamic PET images. IEEE Trans Med Imaging 2020;39:366–76.

35. Wang Y, Yu B, Wang L, et al. 3D conditional generative adversarial networks for high-quality PET image estimation at low dose. Neuroimage 2018;174:550–62.

36. Zhao K, Zhou L, Gao S, et al. Study of low-dose PET image recovery using supervised learning with CycleGAN. PLoS One 2020;15:e0238455.

37. Slomka PJ, Moody JB, Miller RJH, et al. Quantitative clinical nuclear cardiology, part 2: evolving/emerging applications. J Nucl Med 2021;62:168–76.

38. Nakazato R, Berman DS, Dey D, et al. Automated quantitative Rb-82 3D PET/CT myocardial perfusion imaging: normal limits and correlation with invasive coronary angiography. J Nucl Cardiol 2012;19:265–76.

39. Germano G, Kavanagh PB, Fish MB, et al. "Same-patient processing" for multiple cardiac SPECT studies. 1. Improving LV segmentation accuracy. J Nucl Cardiol 2016;23:1435–41.

40. Wang T, Lei Y, Tang H, et al. A learning-based automatic segmentation and quantification method on left ventricle in gated myocardial perfusion SPECT imaging: a feasibility study. J Nucl Cardiol 2020;27:976–87.

41. Guo Y, Dvornek N, Lu Y, et al. Deep Learning based Respiratory Pattern Classification and Applications in PET/CT Motion Correction. 2019 IEEE Nuclear Science Symposium and Medical Imaging Conference (NSS/MIC), 2019;1–5.

42. Li T, Zhang M, Qi W, et al. Motion correction of respiratory-gated PET images using deep learning based image registration framework. Phys Med Biol 2020;65:155003.

43. Su KH, Lee JS, Li JH, et al. Partial volume correction of the microPET blood input function using ensemble learning independent component analysis. Phys Med Biol 2009;54:1823–46.

44. Yu H, Zhou X, Jiang H, et al. Learning 3D non-rigid deformation based on an unsupervised deep learning for PET/CT image registration. Biomed Appl Molec Structur Function Imaging SPIE 2019. 109531X.

45. Liu F, Jang H, Kijowski R, et al. Deep learning MR imaging-based attenuation correction for PET/MR imaging. Radiology 2018;286:676–84.

46. Yang J, Park D, Gullberg GT, et al. Joint correction of attenuation and scatter in image space using deep convolutional neural networks for dedicated brain (18)F-FDG PET. Phys Med Biol 2019;64:075019.

47. Dong X, Lei Y, Wang T, et al. Deep learning-based attenuation correction in the absence of structural information for whole-body positron emission tomography imaging. Phys Med Biol 2020;65:055011.

48. Shi L, Onofrey JA, Liu H, et al. Deep learning-based attenuation map generation for myocardial perfusion SPECT. Eur J Nucl Med Mol Imaging 2020;47:2383–95.

49. Mostafapour S, Gholamiankhah F, Maroofpour S, et al. Deep learning-based attenuation correction in the image domain for myocardial perfusion SPECT imaging. arXiv preprint arXiv:210204915 2021.

50. Lessmann N, van Ginneken B, Zreik M, et al. Automatic calcium scoring in low-dose chest CT using deep neural networks with Dilated Convolutions. IEEE Trans Med Imaging 2018;37:615–25.

51. van Velzen SG, Lessmann N, Velthuis BK, et al. Deep learning for automatic calcium scoring in CT: validation using multiple cardiac CT and chest CT protocols. Radiology 2020;295:66–79.

52. Isgum I, de Vos BD, Wolterink JM, et al. Automatic determination of cardiovascular risk by CT attenuation correction maps in Rb-82 PET/CT. J Nucl Cardiol 2018;25:2133–42.

53. Zeleznik R, Foldyna B, Eslami P, et al. Deep convolutional neural networks to predict cardiovascular risk from computed tomography. Nat Commun 2021;12:715.

54. Dekker M, Waissi F, Bank IEM, et al. The prognostic value of automated coronary calcium derived by a deep learning approach on non-ECG gated CT images from (82)Rb-PET/CT myocardial perfusion imaging. Int J Cardiol 2021;329:9–15.

55. Sprem J, de Vos BD, Lessmann N, et al. Coronary calcium scoring with partial volume correction in anthropomorphic thorax phantom and screening chest CT images. PLoS One 2018;13:e0209318.

56. Commandeur F, Goeller M, Razipour A, et al. Fully automated CT quantification of epicardial adipose tissue by deep learning: a multicenter study. Radiol Artif Intell 2019;1:e190045.

57. Eisenberg E, McElhinney PA, Commandeur F, et al. Deep learning-based quantification of epicardial adipose tissue volume and attenuation predicts major adverse cardiovascular events in asymptomatic subjects. Circ Cardiovasc Imaging 2020;13:e009829.

58. Arsanjani R, Xu Y, Dey D, et al. Improved accuracy of myocardial perfusion SPECT for the detection of coronary artery disease using a support vector machine algorithm. J Nucl Med 2013;54:549–55.

59. Slomka PJ, Betancur J, Liang JX, et al. Rationale and design of the REgistry of fast myocardial perfusion imaging with NExt generation SPECT (REFINE SPECT). J Nucl Cardiol 2020;27:1010–21.

60. Clerc O, Caobelli F, Haaf P, et al. Prediction of coronary artery disease in positron emission tomography using machine learning algorithms with clinical data and calcium score. Eur Heart J Cardiovasc Imaging 2021;22(S1). jeaa356.384.

61. Santarelli MF, Genovesi D, Positano V, et al. Deep-learning-based cardiac amyloidosis classification from early acquired pet images. Int J Cardiovasc Imaging 2021;37(7):2327–35.

62. Togo R, Hirata K, Manabe O, et al. Cardiac sarcoidosis classification with deep convolutional neural network-based features using polar maps. Comput Biol Med 2019;104:81–6.

63. Betancur J, Otaki Y, Motwani M, et al. Prognostic value of combined clinical and myocardial perfusion imaging data using machine learning. JACC Cardiovasc Imaging 2018;11:1000–9.

64. Hu LH, Betancur J, Sharir T, et al. Machine learning predicts per-vessel early coronary revascularization after fast myocardial perfusion SPECT: results from multicentre REFINE SPECT registry. Eur Heart J Cardiovasc Imaging 2020;21:549–59.

65. Juarez-Orozco LE, Martinez-Manzanera O, van der Zant FM, et al. Deep learning in quantitative PET myocardial perfusion imaging: a study on cardiovascular event prediction. JACC Cardiovasc Imaging 2020;13:180–2.

66. Kwiecinski J, Tzolos E, Meah M et al. Machine learning with 18F-sodium fluoride PET and quantitative plaque analysis on CT angiography for the future risk of myocardial infarction. J Nucl Med 2021. doi: 10.2967/jnumed.121.262283.

67. Murthy VL, Bateman TM, Beanlands RS, et al. Clinical quantification of myocardial blood flow using PET: joint position paper of the SNMMI Cardiovascular Council and the ASNC. J Nucl Med 2018;59:273–93.

68. Pang G, Shen C, Cao L, Hengel Avd. Deep learning for anomaly detection: a review. arXiv preprint arXiv:200702500 2020.

69. Azadani PN, Miller RJH, Sharir T, et al. Impact of early revascularization on major adverse cardiovascular events in relation to automatically quantified Ischemia. JACC Cardiovasc Imaging 2021;14:644–53.

Artificial Intelligence in Vascular-PET:
Translational and Clinical Applications

Sriram S. Paravastu, BA[a,b,c], Elizabeth H. Theng, BA[a,b,c],
Michael A. Morris, MD, MS, DABR, DABNM[a,d,e], Peter Grayson, MD, MSc[f],
Michael T. Collins, MD[b], Roberto Maass-Moreno, PhD, DABR[a],
Reza Piri, MD[g,h], Oke Gerke, MSc, PhD[g,h],
Abass Alavi, MD, MD (Hon), PhD (Hon), DSc (Hon)[i],
Poul Flemming Høilund-Carlsen, MD, DMSc, Prof (Hon)[g,h],
Lars Edenbrandt, MD, DMSc[j,k], Babak Saboury, MD, MPH, DABR, DABNM[a,d,i],*

KEYWORDS

• Vascular disease • Artificial intelligence • Atherosclerosis • Vasculitis • Inflammation • Calcification
• Segmentation

KEY POINTS

• Despite the well-documented utility of PET imaging in the diagnosis, prognosis, and treatment monitoring of vascular disease, full-force translation to clinical routine has not yet occurred.

• The main bottleneck in the clinical adoption of PET for daily use as an objective, quantitative tool is the time and effort burden for the manual segmentation of the vasculature.

• AI-based segmentation can cut down the pre-analysis processing steps in PET quantification from hours to a minute or less, potentially serving as an avenue for clinical translation of a robust research literature surrounding vascular PET.

• This clinical translation of PET will bring forth a revolution of vascular medicine and medicine in general, allow for monitoring of vascular disease progression at earlier stages, and increase the ability to phenotype vascular diseases based on PET appearance and patterns. In addition, fast, robust PET imaging quantification and phenotyping could be the key to vascular disease discovery and characterization.

S.S. Paravastu and E.H. Theng contributed equally.
[a] Department of Radiology and Imaging Sciences, Clinical Center, National Institutes of Health (NIH), Bethesda, MD 20892, USA; [b] Skeletal Disorders and Mineral Homeostasis Section, National Institute of Dental and Craniofacial Research, National Institutes of Health (NIH), Bethesda, MD 20892, USA; [c] School of Medicine, University of Missouri-Kansas City, 2411 Holmes Street, Kansas City, MO 64108, USA; [d] Department of Computer Science and Electrical Engineering, University of Maryland, Baltimore County, Baltimore, MD, USA; [e] Institute for Data Science, Department of Diagnostic Radiology and Nuclear Medicine - University of Miami Miller School of Medicine, Miami, FL, USA; [f] National Institute of Arthritis and Musculoskeletal and Skin Diseases, National Institutes of Health, 10 Center Dr, Building 10 Room 12S-253, Bethesda, MD 20892, USA; [g] Department of Nuclear Medicine, Odense University Hospital, 5000 Odense C, Denmark; [h] Department of Clinical Research, University of Southern Denmark, Odense, Denmark; [i] Department of Radiology, Perelman School of Medicine, University of Pennsylvania, Philadelphia, PA, USA; [j] Region Västra Götaland, Sahlgrenska University Hospital, Department of Clinical Physiology, Gothenburg, Sweden; [k] Department of Molecular and Clinical Medicine, Institute of Medicine, SU Sahlgrenska, 413 45 Göteborg, Sweden
* Corresponding author. Department of Radiology and Imaging Sciences, Clinical Center, National Institutes of Health, 9000 Rockville Pike, Building 10, Room 1C455, Bethesda, MD 20892, USA
E-mail address: babak.saboury@nih.gov

PET Clin 17 (2022) 95–113
https://doi.org/10.1016/j.cpet.2021.09.003
1556-8598/22/© 2021 Elsevier Inc. All rights reserved.

pet.theclinics.com

INTRODUCTION

Vascular imaging by positron emission tomography (PET) using ^{18}F-fluorodeoxyglucose (^{18}F-FDG) or ^{18}F-sodium fluoride (^{18}F-NaF) radiotracers is a broad topic that covers applications in both vessels and the organs they perfuse. After examining the current use of PET in vascular diseases, this review explores how artificial intelligence (AI) based quantification has had and may soon have significant clinical impact by facilitating the acquisition, the segmentation and then the comparison of crucial disease parameters to qualitative assessment (gross visual assessment) or operator dependent image processing. In effect, AI increases diagnostic accuracy with high processing speed, improved characterization of disease activity, and spatial information.

The use of PET alongside computed tomography (CT) or computed tomography angiography (CTA) (PET/CT or PET/CTA) allows the physicians to extract information on the vascular mural thickness or luminal changes beyond what PET alone can offer. In most applications, this dual-modal application allows the physician to place molecular information derived from PET into the anatomic context derived from CT or CTA. In addition, the combination of data from PET and CT/CTA augments the segmentation performance beyond the structural segmentation-registration approach (using structural data alone for the delineation of the vessel and subsequently transferring the segmented structure from the CT image domain to the PET image domain using mutual information registration methods).[1]

In the context of this article, we refer to large vessels (the major branches of the aorta, the carotid arteries, and the main pulmonary vessels) when using the term "vasculature". This distinction between macrovascular and meso-/microvascular analyses can be conceptualized by the level of segmentation required for analysis as well. For meso-/microvascular disease quantification, it may be more practical to use an organ-level segmentation strategy and quantify changes in that space. However, for macrovasculature, there is adequate spatial resolution to allow for vessel-level segmentation and therefore we consider the macrovasculature in the context of this article. We allow other sections in this journal edition to define and conceptualize AI-based segmentation of other structures.

After a brief discussion on the emerging role of PET in large vessel disorders and image quantification methods for global disease assessment, we will delve into the transformative role of AI in the reinvention and redesign of the workflow. Abundance of empirical data during the last 3 decades demonstrates the importance of the "global disease assessment" paradigm.[2] This necessity primed the field to demand such a technical revolution, with inevitable integration. Let's go back to the future and evaluate the practical advantages of this hybrid technology (AI and PET) for vascular diseases.

EMERGING APPLICATIONS OF POSITRON EMISSION TOMOGRAPHY IN LARGE VESSEL PATHOLOGY

In this section, we discuss two major vascular diseases in which PET imaging has been applied (atherosclerosis and vasculitis) and discuss the current limitations to the translation of PET to daily clinical use. Current uses of PET in vascular disease are summarized in **Table 1**. In addition to atherosclerosis and vasculitis, the applications of vascular PET include assessing infectious causes of arterial inflammation, venous thromboembolisms, and exploring pulmonary atherosclerosis, among many others; the former two of these examples are also briefly shown in **Table 1**.

Atherosclerosis

The burden of atherosclerotic disease is well-established as it is the leading cause of morbidity and mortality globally. In the face of a widespread disease, PET radiotracers such as ^{18}F-FDG[7] and ^{18}F-NaF[8] offer the potential to reframe how this disease is understood and to identify disease at an earlier stage. Broadly, atherosclerosis pathophysiology begins with arterial wall inflammation and plaque formation, followed by microcalcification of the plaque. Provided that the plaque does not rupture, the microcalcifications may coalesce into stable macrocalcifications.[9] Although the exact interplay between these events as inciter, mediator, stabilizer, or destabilizer remains elusive, processes of inflammation, microcalcification, and macrocalcification are captured by ^{18}F-FDG-PET, ^{18}F-NaF-PET, and CT respectively.[8,10] Currently, clinical practice relies on these later stages of stable macrocalcification, as evidenced by the practical use of calcium scoring (**Fig. 1**). In an effort to assess disease at an earlier and more active stage for intervention, we turn toward molecular imaging. Of these 2 radiotracers, ^{18}F-FDG and ^{18}F-NaF, ^{18}F-NaF demonstrates increased specificity and consistent correlation with CT calcium burden and recognized atherosclerotic disease risk factors as a marker of active calcium turnover.[11-14] Moving beyond individual plaques, understanding of atherosclerotic disease is

Table 1
Current utility of vascular PET imaging

	Vascular Pathology			
	Atherosclerosis	Large Vessel Vasculitides	Venous Thromboembolism	Vascular grafts
Problem	• Current clinical approaches focus on end-stage disease processes (e.g. as calcifications on CT) and individual lesions (e.g. high-risk plaques) because the characterization of early-stage disease is challenging by means of conventional imaging and laboratory testing.	• Challenges in diagnosis and management are due to variable clinical presentations, nonspecific biochemical profiles, and feasibility of histologic confirmation of diagnosis • Challenge of accurately attributing clinical symptoms to ongoing active inflammation vs prior vascular damage • Clinically difficult to capture the spatio-temporal heterogeneity of disease	• Current practice requires high clinical suspicion for VTE diagnosis and does not detect nonocclusive thrombi well • Difficulty in identifying new clots from chronic clots by US and venography • Limited evaluation of anatomic spaces of the body cavity, pelvic veins, or distal veins	• Deteriorating vascular grafts are difficult to characterize solely by morphology on conventional assessments (e.g. CTA), as infection can precede structural changes
Solution PET offers	• ^{18}F-PET allows for the specific and sensitive visualization of pathology at an earlier time point in the disease course • PET can assess the vessel *in toto* (lumen, arterial wall, calcification)	• Whole-body assessment by ^{18}F-FDG-PET can capture the heterogeneity of disease and find novel patterns of disease - Readout of vascular inflammation in relationship to structural damage • Improved diagnosis/management of disease	• Metabolic activity on PET can differentiate between new and chronic clots • Whole-body evaluation allows assessment of atypical veins	• FDG-PET can better characterize vascular grafts by identifying areas of abnormally increased inflammation for infection detection and management
Example of study exploring PET solution	Paydary et. al., 2021[3] Global microcalcification in the thoracic aorta as measured by 18F-FDG-PET increases with age, and is found to have a high correlation in patients with classic CVD risk factors. The Alavi-Carlsen	Grayson et. al., 2018[4] FDG-PET is used to differentiate LVV from mimics (eg, atherosclerosis) with 85% sensitivity and 83% specificity. PET Vascular Activity Score (PETVAS), a summative qualitative score, derived from total	Rondina et. al., 2012[5] FDG-PET/CT accurately detected DVT of the lower limbs with a sensitivity of 87.5% and a specificity of 100%. There was a negative correlation between maximum metabolic activity	Husmann et al., 2015[6] In the clinical course of patients with known vascular graft infection, the use of FDG-PET/CT during follow-up influenced clinical decision making in more than a third of cases, in the presence of an

(continued on next page)

Table 1
(continued)

	Vascular Pathology			
	Atherosclerosis	Large Vessel Vasculitides	Venous Thromboembolism	Vascular grafts
	score of the whole thoracic aorta and individual segment was a stronger predictor of FRS risk than SUV_{mean} or SUV_{max}.	body arterial FDG uptake, was independently associated with glucocorticoid use, clinical disease activity status, BMI, and disease duration. High PETVAS Scores were associated with relapse.	in thrombosed veins and time from DVT symptom onset, suggesting a means to differentiate acute from chronic clots	otherwise normal CRP.
Population & methods of study	• 124 patients (44 patients with chest pain, 80 controls) • Manual segmentation of hearts	• 170 PET/CTs of 115 patients (56 affected, 59 control patients) • Manual segmentation of focal arterial wall uptake	• 36 patients (12 symptomatic of DVT, 24 control subjects) • Manual segmentation of thrombosed veins	• 266 PET/CTs of 68 patients • Semiautomated identification of the site of highest FDG uptake

Abbreviations: CRP, C-reactive protein; CTA, computed tomographic angiography; ESR, erythrocyte sedimentation rate; FDG-PET, [18]fluorodeoxyglucose PET; ^{18}F-NaF-PET, [sodium] [18]fluoride PET; FRS, Framingham risk score; GCA, giant-cell arteritis; LVV, large-vessel vasculitis; ROC curve, receiver operating characteristic curve; SUV_{mean}, mean standardized uptake value; SUV_{max}, maximal standardized uptake value; TAK, Takayasu arteritis; VTE, venous thromboembolism.

shifting away from a lesion-based paradigm toward one of total disease burden, as evidenced by the diminishing utility of high-risk plaque identification.[15]

In the same spirit, total body PET assessment of atherosclerosis is promising; for example, a study of the thoracic aorta has shown the Alavi–Carlsen Calcium Score (ACCS) to be a better predictor of classic cardiovascular disease (CVD)/Framingham risk score factors than maximal standardized uptake value (SUV_{max}) or mean standardized uptake value (SUV_{mean}).[3] However, translation into the clinical space will rely on AI-based interpretation to bypass the technically challenging and tedious labor of manual segmentation. AI methods for segmentation are desperately needed to greatly advance atherosclerosis understanding via PET imaging.

Large-Vessel Vasculitides

Noninfectious vasculitides are inflammatory diseases of the blood vessel linings whose downstream sequelae can involve any system.[16] Current understanding of vasculitides is based on the size of predominantly affected vessels,

appropriately termed large, medium, and small vessel-disease, even though the inflammation extends beyond vessel size or type.[16] Nonspecific definitions of vasculitis, variable clinical

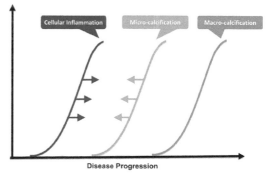

Fig. 1. The likely sequence of biological processes in atherosclerosis is depicted visually. Because endothelial inflammation and vascular microcalcification occur before macrocalcification, 18F-FDG and 18F-NaF PET might identify the illness in its early stages in asymptomatic patients. (*From* Moghbel M, Al-Zaghal A, Werner TJ, Constantinescu CM, Høilund-Carlsen PF, Alavi A. The Role of PET in Evaluating Atherosclerosis: A Critical Review. Semin Nucl Med. 2018;48(6):488–497.)

presentations, elusive biochemical profiles, and challenges in histologic confirmation result in less-than-certain diagnoses and nonuniformity in the management of these patients.[17–19]

PET has emerged as a robust clinical tool for diagnosis and management of the large-vessel vasculitides (LVV), including giant cell arteritis (GCA) and Takayasu's arteritis (TAK).[4,17,20] Specific parameters of ^{18}F-FDG-PET such as SUV_{max} have demonstrated reasonable sensitivity and specificity for early diagnosis (**Fig. 2** illustrates the early detection capability conferred by ^{18}F-FDG-PET imaging in vasculitis) in cranial GCA with negative biopsy, noncranial GCA, for prognosis, and for assessment of acute response to therapy.[20]

Although it is difficult to provide concordant histologic evidence to corroborate PET findings due to the invasive nature of blood vessel biopsy, evidence suggests that subclinical vascular inflammation detected on ^{18}F-FDG-PET can predict the risk of clinical relapse.[4,18,21] Over a median 15-month follow-up period, Grayson and colleagues found that LVV patients with a high global burden of arterial FDG uptake were at a significant risk of clinical recurrence.[4] Using a summative qualitative score based on global arterial uptake, PET vascular activity score (PETVAS), Grayson and colleagues[4] were able to distinguish clinically active large-vessel vasculitis disease from controls. This global score was independently associated with disease activity, duration, body-mass index, and glucocorticoid treatment; additionally, these qualitative global scores were associated with relapse and may have prognostic value, whereas before, the gross visual assessment of PET was unable to predict relapse.[20,22]

The value of ^{18}F-FDG-PET to potentially identify vascular inflammation in the early phases of disease before the development of irreversible vascular damage cannot be understated. Vasculitides can be quite insidious diseases affecting many systems throughout the body, wreaking often irreversible havoc. Most of the time, patients with vasculitides are diagnosed at the later stages

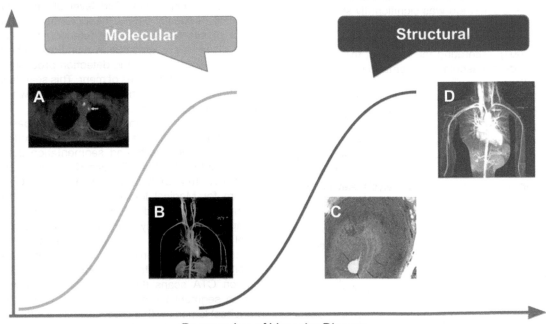

Progression of Vascular Disease

Fig. 2. ^{18}F-FDG-PET gives a molecular signal of vascular inflammation that is an early sign of disease. Over time, inflammation in arteries progresses to cause structural damage which can be detected by histopathology or CT or MR. (A) ^{18}F-FDG-PET, yellow arrow is pointing to the area of vascular wall ^{18}F-FDG uptake greater than in the liver; this indicates active vasculitis (B) Baseline MRA (pictured here) or CTA may look normal despite the detection of molecular level inflammation on ^{18}F-FDG-PET early in the course of vascular disease (C) Structural changes can be seen on histopathology after the progression of vascular disease. (D) Structural changes can be seen on MRA or CTA (CTA pictured here) as the vascular disease progresses. (*Modified from* Newman KA, Ahlman MA, Hughes M, Malayeri AA, Pratt D, Grayson PC. Diagnosis of Giant Cell Arteritis in an Asymptomatic Patient. Arthritis Rheumatol. 2016;68(5):1135 and Moghbel M, Al-Zaghal A, Werner TJ, Constantinescu CM, Høilund-Carlsen PF, Alavi A. The Role of PET in Evaluating Atherosclerosis: A Critical Review. Semin Nucl Med. 2018;48(6):488–497.)

of the disease, even though early diagnosis and treatment may prevent the severe, potentially fatal complications that can lead to organ failure.[20] Currently, a prohibitive factor in further research on PET-based phenotyping of vasculitides as well as clinical adoption is the arduous nature of manual segmentation of the blood vessels.

Roadblocks to the Clinical Translation of Positron Emission Tomography

In virtually all of the papers discussed in the realm of atherosclerosis and vasculitis, a key rate-limiting step to the analysis of vascular PET imaging is the manual segmentation of the aorta and major branches. Manual segmentation of the aorta may take as long as 2 hours if not more,[23] the labor of which is collectively recognized by Fantazzini and colleagues who note that ground truth acquisition by the manual segmentation of 10 CTAs took 150 hours. The resulting AI-based algorithm was able to complete segmentation of the aorta in a mere 25 seconds.[24] Yu and colleagues reported that the measurement time using the DL method was significantly shorter than that of the manual method (21.7 ± 1.1 [20.0–23.5] vs 82.5 ± 16.1 [60–100] minutes per case, $P < .001$), reiterating the fact that the DL-based methods of vascular segmentation may be labor and time saving.[25]

There has not been a translation of the literature surrounding the utility of PET to clinical diagnosis and prediction because the workflow of the average physician does not allow for a minimum of 2 hours per patient for imaging analysis. AI-based segmentation of vasculature is an important advance that can make this analysis relevant to the clinician. For example, AI-based segmentation of all the vasculature could allow for the easy development of a global disease burden score for virtually any vascular disease which can be assessed by PET. The predictive utility of these global scoring methods has been discussed previously and supports the practical utility of this approach.[4,26,27]

Segmentation of the large vessels is a crucial prerequisite for the advanced quantification of PET to evaluate the burden of disease, from atherosclerosis to vasculitides.[28,29] The manual delineation of the vessels is the bottleneck of the workflow and a prohibitive step in the analysis of vascular disease. Automatic segmentation of the large vessels is the key step in disseminating this methodology from academic centers to mainstream clinical practice and to implement this quantitative task into the daily workflow (from byte to bedside).

CURRENT METHODS FOR ARTIFICIAL INTELLIGENCE-BASED SEGMENTATION OF VASCULATURE

Several large vessel segmentation methods have been explored. Some methods of segmentation include manual segmentation by a reader, Hounsfield unit (HU) threshold-based segmentation, edge-based segmentation, texture features methods, watershed, statistical shape models, region-growing, and deep learning (DL) methods.[30] A detailed table of DL-based vascular segmentation methods can be found in **Table 2**. Comprehensive reviews on AI in aortic disease are also available from Hahn and colleagues[31] and Raffort and colleagues.[32] Additional reviews by Jin and colleagues,[33] Lesage and colleagues.[34] and Pepe and colleagues[35] discuss aortic lumen and aortic dissection segmentation, respectively.

A key point to keep in mind when discussing segmentation is the requirement for the *detection* of an object of interest before segmentation takes place. The objective of *detection* is to find a subspace in an image scene that contains a certain object class with a specified level of certainty. This task frequently entails the localization of an object of interest. Often, the detection process takes place in a segmentation workflow without the user being aware of the detection process or being notified of the figures of merit. This seamless detection and segmentation approach is known as an "end-to-end" approach.[36]

Currently, few solutions exist for the AI-based segmentation of the vasculature. In this section, we discuss two end-to-end segmentation solutions of interest. Other DL-based methods are listed in **Table 2**. Of these, only the Research Consortium for Medical Image Analysis (RECOMIA) segmentation method[23,48] is designed for PET/CT applications. Lareyre and colleagues used a novel hybrid method using a rule-based AI for the training of a convolutional neural network (CNN) which segmented the abdominal vasculature on CTA scans (**Fig. 3**).[38] This model was able to segment the abdominal aorta and major branches' lumens with a Dice similarity coefficient of 0.90 (**Fig. 4**).[38] The authors reported a time of 25 to 40 minutes per scan for manual segmentation; however, the computational time using the automated method ranged from 5 seconds to 1 minute, highlighting the immense workflow benefit of AI-based segmentation of the vasculature.[38]

Recently, Piri and colleagues described the use of the RECOMIA[48] AI-based PET/CT segmentation platform to segment boundaries of the aortic wall in ^{18}F-NaF-PET/CT scans.[23] In both the manual and CNN-based segmentation performed

Table 2
Deep learning-based aortic segmentation methods

Author	Input/Output	Method Used	FoM	Clinical Application Detail	Scans/Patients
Adam et al,[37] 2021	Input: CTA Output: Segmented entire aorta	V-net based CNN, referred to as Augmented Radiology for Vascular Aneurysm (ARVA) by authors	DSC = 0.84 for healthy aortas, 0.95 for diseased aorta, and 0.93 for diseased aortas after endovascular treatment	Measured the maximum aortic diameter.	Training: 489 CTAs Validation: 62 CTAs Testing: NOT PERFORMED
Lareyre et al,[38] 2021	Input: CTA Output: Segmented abdominal vascular tree	Supervised DL vascular segmentation technique based on hybridization of a CNN with a knowledge-based model	DSC = 0.89,0.86 for DL and expert systems respectively	Abdominal vascular tree segmentation itself even in the presence of AAA.	Training: 40 CTAs Validation: 58 CTAs Testing: NOT PERFORMED
Piri et al,[23] 2021	Input: ^{18}F-NaF-PET/CT Output: Segmented entire aorta	Two CNN: first one to segment similarly shaped objects like the vertebrae, second one segmented the aorta	DSC = 0.87	Aorta segmentation itself; noted that the segmentation time was reduced from 1.5-2 h to 1 min than manual segmentation	Training/ Validation: 339 CTs, 80% training, 20% validation Testing: 49 patients (20 angina pectoris patients, 29 controls)
Yu et al,[25] 2021	Input: CTA Output: Segmented entire aorta	CNN that segments and measures the entire aorta and true and false lumens in type B AD	DSC = 0.958	Segmentation of true and false lumens in Type B aortic AD and then diameter measurement of the AD; noted that segmentation was reduced from 83 to 22 min	Training: 99 CTA Validation: 15 CTA Testing: 25 CTA
Zhong et al. (2021)[39]	Input: CTA Output: Segmented the entire aorta with the labeling of the ascending root, ascending aorta, arch, and descending aorta	Attention-gated CNN; the CNN learns to suppress background tissue and focus on tissue of interest.	DSC = 0.966, HD = 0.189	Aorta segmentation itself	Training: 89 CTA Validation:15 CTA Testing: 90 CTA

(continued on next page)

Table 2
(continued)

Author	Input/Output	Method Used	FoM	Clinical Application Detail	Scans/Patients
Fantazzini et al,[24] 2020	Input: CTA Output: Segmented entire aorta with branch vessels of the aortic arch and abdominal segment	DL (first CNN to detect and coarsely segment, then 3 single-view CNNs to segment from the axial, sagittal, and coronal planes under higher resolution).	DSC = 0.93, MSD = 0.80	Segmentation of aortas with AAA in preoperative CTAs for surgical planning.	Training: 64 CTA Validation: 6 CTA Testing: 10 CTA All preoperative CTAs from AAA patients
Berhane et al,[40] 2020	Input: 4D-flow MR Output: Segmented entire aorta with branch vessels of the aortic arch	CNN; 3D U-Net network with DenseNet-based dense blocks replacing the original convolution layers	DSC = 0.951, HD = 2.8, MSD = 0.176	Aorta segmentation itself; noted that segmentation of the aorta took < 1 s	Training: 499 4D-flow MR Validation: 101 4D-flow MR Testing: 418 4D-flow MR
Chen et al,[41] 2020	Input: CTA Output: Segmented the entire aorta to the aortic bifurcation and dual lumens in type B AD	Multi-stage learning: 3-D patch-based CNN segmentation of entire aorta, then aorta simplification by straightening and then CNN segmentation of true and false lumens	DSC >0.89	Segmented the entire aorta to the iliac bifurcations and dual lumens in type B AD for better preoperative visualization.	Training: 80 CTA Validation:20 CTA Testing: 20 CTA All patients had type B AD
Hepp et al,[42] 2020	Input: MR Output: Segmented the thoracic aorta	U-net-based CNN	DSC = 0.85	Thoracic aorta shape analysis was performed and could be applied to TAA detection	Training: 70 MR Validation: 30 MR Testing: NOT PERFORMED 100 patients with MR from the German National Cohort (GNC) study.

(continued on next page)

Table 2
(continued)

Author	Input/Output	Method Used	FoM	Clinical Application Detail	Scans/Patients
Hahn et al,[43] 2020	Input: CTA Output: Segmentation of total aortic lumen, true lumen, and false lumen in type B AD	Two CNN pipeline; derives the aortic centerline, generates MPRs in relation to the centerline, and segments the false and true lumens	DSC = 0.873 for total aortic lumen	True and false lumen segmentation in type B AD for surgical planning	Training: 103 CTA Validation: 22 CTA Testing: 28 CTA
Cao et al,[44] 2019	Input: CTA Output: Segmentation of total aortic lumen, true lumen, and false lumen in type B AD	U-net-based CNN	DSC = 0.93 for total aortic lumen	Fully automatic segmentation of type B AD for extraction of lumen diameters	Training: 246 CTA of patients with type B AD Validation: 30 CTA of patients with type B AD
Lu et al,[45] 2019	Input: 3D CTA and noncontrast CT Output: Segmented abdominal aorta with or without AAA	3D U-net-based CNN which accepts series with varying numbers of images	DSC = 0.89	Aorta segmentation itself	Training: 153 CTA, 168 noncontrast CT Validation: 57 CTs Testing: NOT PERFORMED
Li et al,[46] 2019	Input: CT Output: Segmentation of total aortic lumen and true and false lumens in AD	Cascaded U-net-based CNN	DSC = 0.989 for total aorta lumen	True and false lumen segmentation in AD, to enhance visibility	Training: 45 AD CT Validation: Five-fold cross-validation on same 45 cases Testing: NOT PERFORMED
Trullo et al,[47] 2017	Input: CT Output: Segmentation of the trachea, esophagus, aorta, and a portion of the heart	FCN and SharpMask feature fusion architecture; features from early layers of FCN and high-level features from deep layers are used to improve segmentation results.	DSC = 0.86	Aorta segmentation itself	Training: 25 CT Validation: 5 CT

Abbreviations: abdominal aortic aneurysm (AAA), abdominal aortic thrombus (AAT); aortic dissection (AD), computed tomography (CT); computed tomography angiography (CTA), convolutional neural network (CNN); deep learning (DL), figures of merit (FoM); fully convolutional network (FCN), magnetic resonance (MR); magnetic resonance angiography (MRA), Pearson correlation score (R); thoracic aortic aneurysm (TAA), All the models in this example were *end-to-end* segmentation models; due to automatic detection and localization of the aorta before segmentation, without any outward representation of these processes.

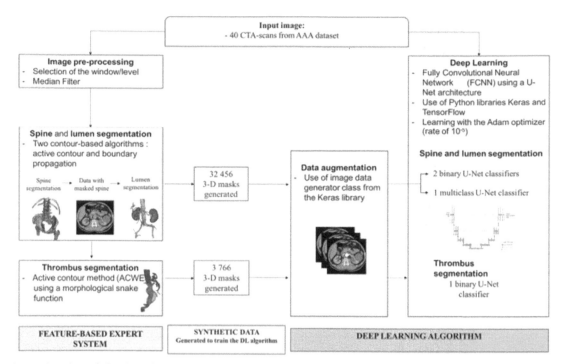

Fig. 3. Creation of the deep learning (DL) algorithm. A feature-based expert system pipeline is applied to the input CTA images, comprising of three consecutive steps: image preprocessing, spine and lumen segmentation, and thrombus segmentation. The DL algorithm is trained using synthetic data supplied by the expert system. To segment the lumen and spine, the DL method utilizes either a mixture of two binary U-Net classifiers or a multi-class U-Net classifier. For thrombus segmentation, a binary U-Net classifier is utilized. (*From* Lareyre F, Adam C, Carrier M, Raffort J. Automated Segmentation of the Human Abdominal Vascular System Using a Hybrid Approach Combining Expert System and Supervised Deep Learning. J Clin Med Res. 2021;10(15).)

in this study, there was first a surface segmentation of the aorta, and then an expansion of the inner surface to include 3 mm (mm) of the proposed aortic wall, and an expansion of the outer surface to include 2 mm of the proposed aortic wall. In total, a wall thickness of 5 mm was segmented (**Fig. 5**). In the RECOMIA web-based platform, two CNNs help with CT-based segmentation. The first CNN is responsible for bones that must be split into several instances, such as vertebrae, whereas the second is responsible for all other single instance labels. The CNNs are loosely based on the U-Net architecture commonly used by medical image segmentation models.

Piri and collegues performed a head to head comparison between manual segmentation of the aorta and segmentation using the RECOMIA platform and found that on average, the manually segmented volumes were 13% to 17% larger than volumes segmented using CNNs, and SUV_{max} and SUV_{total} values were similarly 15% to 16% and 13% to 16% higher in manually segmented volumes than CNN segmented volumes.[23] However the SUV_{mean} values were virtually identical between the 2 methods.[23] This was due to the propensity for manual segmenters to inadvertently clip some of the vertebral columns which has higher SUV values than the aorta, as part of their volume of interest. This was not an issue in CNN segmentation. The CNN method had a 100% repeatability versus manual segmentation which had a maximal 6% deviation at repeated manual segmentation. Interestingly, the training dataset was acquired from a different scanner than the dataset used in the study, and the model performed extremely well on the study dataset, pointing to potential high robustness across scanners. The AI-based segmentation took a total of 1 minute versus 1.5 to 2 hours for the manual segmentation of the aorta. Taken together, AI-based segmentation can greatly improve the reproducibility, efficiency, accuracy, and precision of segmentation, all of which are crucial to downstream analysis. The 3D results of segmentation are shown in **Fig. 6**.

A Feature-based expert system

1
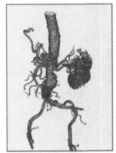

2
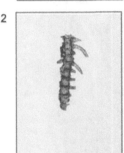

3
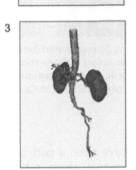

B Hybrid Method using the Deep Learning algorithm (2D U-Net)

1
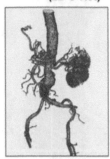

2
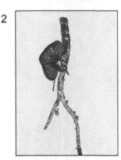

3
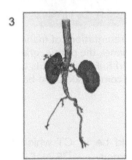

Fig. 4. Representative 3D lumen segmentation results using (A) a feature-based expert system and (B) a hybrid algorithm based on U-Net. (1) The AAA database was used to acquire representative images. (2) and (3) are representative images acquired using the AMI database after accurate segmentation by the expert system and the hybrid approach. The expert system fails to recognize the vascular system in low-contrast images, but the hybrid technique detects it accurately. (*From* Lareyre F, Adam C, Carrier M, Raffort J. Automated Segmentation of the Human Abdominal Vascular System Using a Hybrid Approach Combining Expert System and Supervised Deep Learning. J Clin Med Res. 2021;10(15). (Under open access Creative Commons license http://creativecommons.org/licenses/by/4.0/)

FUTURE OF VASCULAR POSITRON EMISSION TOMOGRAPHY IMAGING IN THE WORLD OF ARTIFICIAL INTELLIGENCE

In this section, we discuss some of the improvements to come in AI-based vascular segmentation to make it more relevant to the clinical practice of medicine. We start with the discussion of improving the technical robustness of AI-based vascular segmentation. Later, we explore the concept of vascular atlas to facilitate the global disease assessment (GDA).

Artificial Intelligence Segmentation of Vasculature: Future Technical Aspects

Segmentation of vasculature can be a difficult task due to the immense level of variability between patients as well as within patients. The aging patient's aorta looks considerably different on imaging than that of a younger patient. Over a lifetime, the aorta endures a large amount of wear and tear leading to a decrease in elastic fibers in the vessel wall, causing stiffness and even ballooning of the aorta.[49] This also leads to different appearances over time on PET/CT imaging due to the interplay between molecular, functional, and structural effects of disease which is still being actively understood.[50,51] In those patients with coarctation of the aorta there may be difficulty in automatic segmentation, due to a potential sudden difference in lumen thickness along the length of the aorta.[52] In addition mural thrombosis, blood vessel tortuosity, and differing levels of calcification between patient populations can cause variability in segmentation capacity.

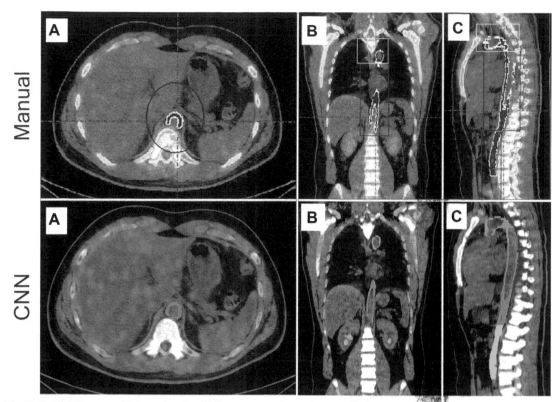

Fig. 5. Axial (*A*), coronal (*B*), and sagittal (*C*) representations of manually (top panel) and DL segmented (bottom panel) aortas in a single patient. In the bottom panel, the purple, orange, and light green colors indicate thoracic arch, and abdominal aorta respectively. (*From* Piri R, Edenbrandt L, Larsson M, et al. Aortic wall segmentation in 18F-sodium fluoride PET/CT scans: Head-to-head comparison of AI-based vs manual segmentation. J Nucl Cardiol. Published online May 12, 2021.)

AI algorithms to segment the aorta should be age-aware and should accommodate for segmentation difficulties as a result of the variability found in the vasculature. The current algorithms can take into account the information contained within one scan to segment the aorta, but the concept of using previous scans to segment the current scan should be used; this is the concept of prior-aware segmentation (**Fig. 7**). Rather than registering the old scan with the new scan, prior-aware segmentation recognizes the similar patterns between multiple scans from the same patient and uses this awareness when segmenting the newer of the scans as demonstrated by Zhou et Al.[53] This is particularly important in the case of prior scans with higher resolution than the current scan of interest. Potentially, this could also minimize the problem of interscanner and interscan quality and resolution variability.

Another nuance in the deployment of prior-aware imaging is the utilization of multimodality information to segment the vasculature. For example, to segment the aorta on a low-dose CT which may originally have been a part of an 18F-NaF-PET/CT scan, a model which is prior-aware of an already captured CTA may be very useful in segmenting not only the aortic wall, but also in segmenting the lumen of the aorta with much greater accuracy.

Similarly, MR imaging may be able to better detect mural edema in the aorta (**Fig. 8**),[54] so this information can be used in segmentation of the large vessels in CT to better define areas of mural edema which can be suggestive of GCA or TAK. Similarly, the use of modalities such as CTA or MRA can be very useful in segmenting the lumen of the large vessels as discussed above. The combination of information from multiple modalities when segmenting can be very useful in compiling various data that can be obtained in different modalities to analyze the patient's vascular disease.

In medium and smaller sized vessels (eg, coronary arteries), empirical evidence suggests vessel-level quantification fails to capture the disease process due to motion-induced smearing of the activity;[55] other quantitative techniques could

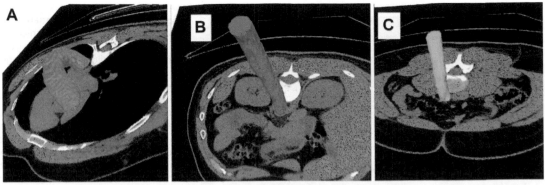

Fig. 6. 3D representation of the deep learning-based segmentation of the arch of the aorta (*A*), thoracic aorta (*B*), and abdominal aorta (*C*) (*From* Piri R, Edenbrandt L, Larsson M, et al. Aortic wall segmentation in 18F-sodium fluoride PET/CT scans: Head-to-head comparison of AI-based vs manual segmentation. J Nucl Cardiol. Published online May 12, 2021.)

provide more accurate and biologically relevant measurements.[26] For example, in measuring the progression of coronary artery disease and calcification, a global heart calcification score using ^{18}F-NaF-PET maybe more efficient and accurate than a method in which all the coronary arteries are segmented and then individually analyzed.[26] In calculating the ACCS, the whole heart is segmented, and then a global score is assigned to reflect the severity of disease (**Fig. 9**). This score can then be compared across timepoints.[26] Similar to the ACCS methodology, the concept of vascular partial volume correction (PVC) can be utilized to calculate the vessel wall activity (PVC-VWA) by PET imaging. To calculate PVC-VWA, the aorta is first segmented. Then, the delineated

boundary is expanded to include spill-over counts. The degree of expansion depends on spatial resolution of PET scanner (i.e. width of the point spread function, which is defined as its full width at half maximum (FWHM)). Within this new volume of interest, all the activity is measured and then the activity from the blood pool (representative of the background activity) is subtracted from that value to derive the recovered activity of the vessel wall. All these steps can be automated using deep learning automatic segmentation and automation of PVC-VWA calculation; this can enable the widespread use of a relatively simple and easily interpretable methodology to measure vascular wall activity over time. Potentially, this can be used to track vascular response to therapy or vascular

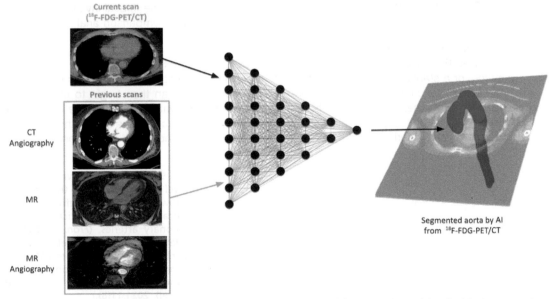

Fig. 7. Prior-aware segmentation. Information from prior, multimodality scans is combined with the current scan information to segment a structure of interest (aorta) which can be visualized on all the scans. Aorta segmentation cinematic rendering for this figure was created using the RECOMIA platform.[48]

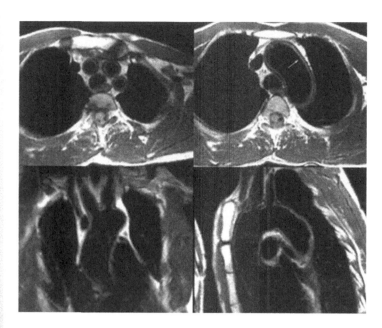

Fig. 8. MR images of a patient with TAK show increased mural thickness in the aorta. Axial (*top*) and longitudinal-oblique (*bottom*) images of the thoracic aorta reveal pathologic aortic mural thickening and widening of the aorta (*arrow*). (*From* Tso E, Flamm SD, White RD, Schvartzman PR, Mascha E, Hoffman GS. Takayasu arteritis: utility and limitations of magnetic resonance imaging in diagnosis and treatment. Arthritis Rheum. 2002;46(6):1634 to 1642.)

disease progression over time.[56,57] In addition, segmentation of major vasculature can be useful in mapping out the vasculature to create an "atlas" along which nuances in disease-specific activity can be tracked.

The Vascular Atlas: Roadmap to Vascular Disease Characterization, Understanding, and Discovery

The vascular structures are continuous, tubular structures that can be thought of as a "roadway" of sorts spanning the whole body. Much like we can understand the relative location of a car on a roadway using a map, it is not unreasonable to translate vascular PET findings into a standard common space, or a standardized vascular atlas, on which to pinpoint vascular lesions and characterize the landscape of disease within a particular region. Creating an average statistical atlas (ASA) may allow for better characterization of the spatial

heterogeneity along the length of the atlas. The "common space" for the statistical atlas can be obtained by averaging vessel segment length (for example, the descending thoracic aorta would be an average of the descending thoracic aorta of all patients evaluated). The common length of each vascular segment should be derived separately so that the integrity of each segment is preserved during the resampling process. An individual's spatial data is then converted into a relative continuum and mapped to the common space, normalizing the spatial involvement which allows for relative comparison analysis over time (**Fig. 10**).

Atlas Applications: Phenomics

In consistently mapping out patterns into a common space, we can then begin to classify patterns of disease with some measure of scientific certainty. In practice, this is simply the extension of common phenotyping by history, physical

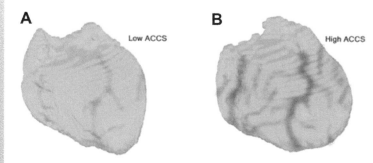

A Low ACCS   **B** High ACCS

Fig. 9. ACCS Score derived by organ-level segmentation of the heart to allow for meaningful, efficient quantification of microcalcification in the coronary arteries. (*From* Saboury B, Edenbrandt L, Piri R, et al. Alavi-Carlsen Calcification Score (ACCS): A Simple Measure of Global Cardiac Atherosclerosis Burden. Diagnostics (Basel). 2021;11(8).)

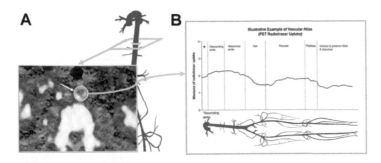

Fig. 10. Vascular atlas concept. (*A*) An axial view of the aorta with accompanying region-of-interest (*arrow*). Radiotracer uptake within the region of interest is sequentially captured across the length of aorta and distal vasculature and mapped out into a graphical representation of a common, standardized space (*B*). The image in box A is a slice from an ^{18}F-NaF-PET/CT scan.

examination, and biochemical profiles, into the molecular space in such a way that captures quantitative, spatial, and temporal information. Such a map will serve as a launch point in redefining our understanding of vascular disease, and will perhaps enable disease discovery. For instance, in evaluating TAK, investigators noticed consistently extravascular uptake in the thyroid, lymph node, and bone marrow of vertebrae and pelvis.[58] The significance of these findings remains unknown and not yet attributed to known pathophysiology; however, these reports may increase our understanding of inflammatory processes within TAK.

The use of a vascular atlas may also identify a particularly sensitive region to pathology, thus refining models to predictive regions for disease prognosis or to the assessment of treatment response. On the other hand, the atlas may separate out diseases once thought to be closely related and cluster those previously considered distant.

For instance, differentiating types of vasculitis rely heavily on the anatomic size of the most commonly involved vessels. Substantial clinical heterogeneity exists within patients with LVV, and clinical overlap with other systemic inflammatory diseases can occur. In one example, a symptomatic patient diagnosed with TAK was found to have underlying concomitant sarcoidosis diagnosed by ^{18}F-FDG radiotracer uptake in the mediastinal and hilar lymph nodes, demonstrating the ability of molecular imaging to identify a more complete spectrum of disease extent and thereby inform novel methods of disease classification (**Fig. 11**).[59] In the face of positive imaging findings,

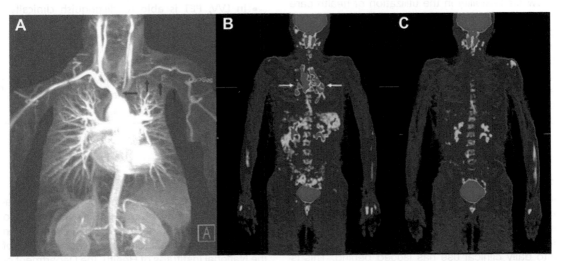

Fig. 11. A 32-year-old symptomatic woman with TAK was incidentally diagnosed with sarcoidosis. (*A*) Maximum intensity projection on magnetic MRA showed a narrowed left common carotid and left subclavian arteries (*red arrows*), which could be observed from the time of diagnosis. (*B*) High level of ^{18}F-FDG avidity in several enlarged mediastinal and hilar lymph nodes (*yellow arrows*). This pattern is suggestive of sarcoidosis with (*C*) spontaneous resolution on follow-up imaging after one year. (*From* Betancourt BY, Ahlman MA, Grayson PC. Sarcoidosis Concomitant With Takayasu Arteritis, Identified by Advanced Molecular Imaging. Arthritis Rheumatol. 2019;71(6):990.)

authors discussed the possibility of a closer phenotypic relationship between sarcoidosis and LVV than previously thought, in addition to the body of genotyping work in the field which has traced linkages between these 2 diseases.[60,61]

Another example is the fact that patients with GCA and polymyalgia rheumatica (PMR) are theoretically inclined to develop malignancies due to immune system dysregulation. However, conflicting reports studying the association of malignancies and GCA/PMR may lead to clinician hesitation when screening for malignancy. Emamifar and colleagues[19] demonstrated that ^{18}F-FDG-PET can can highlight previously undetected cancer earlier in its course with a high negative predictive value, and specifically beneficiary for PMR/GCA patients with nonspecific symptoms. In both of these examples, the use of PET is critical in providing clinical clarity.

Atlas Applications: Delta Radiomics

The use of a common space lends itself toward delta radiomics, which deals with serial changes in images. In standardizing the data for each patient, localizing specific lesions or perhaps the global disease, one can create subtracted matrices of information from two time points of the same patient to assess response. Establishing temporal patterns will be crucial in linking and definitively describing the "natural history course" of vascular inflammation on ^{18}F-FDG-PET, microcalcification on ^{18}F-NaF-PET, and macro-calcific phenotypes on CT. With time, this knowledge will allow for flexibility in the utilization of health care resources, as we will be able to confidently limit certain types of imaging to yield the most relevant information at different ages. For example, in addition to management of classic atherosclerotic risk factors, middle-aged patients may undergo early screening of ^{18}F-NaF-PET to characterize early-disease plaques, reserving CTs and CTAs for acute, late-disease events.

SUMMARY

Apart from cancer diagnoses, metastases surveillance, and mostly qualitative monitoring of therapy, most applications of PET imaging have expanded our understanding of disease manifestation in the scientific context, whereas translation into daily clinical use has lagged behind. This is despite the fact that in several domains it would be rational for PET to compete with or replace conventional imaging of CT or MRI, which due to inherent limitations show mainly late phase structural tissue changes when the disease has spread and become more difficult to treat. However, the absence of fast and reliable quantification tools has been a major obstacle for this transition. Consequently, AI-based analysis that addresses this need is anticipated to become a significant game-changer.

AI will have the capability to help the field of PET imaging overcome some of the practical and logistical limitations that hinder its full translation from the scientific literature into the clinic. AI-based interpretation of CT and PET is currently already available; with the right approach, it can enable ultra-rapid detection and reliable measurements of vascular diseases in their early stages, when presumably more sensitive to intervention than when later occurring structural tissue changes make them visible by conventional imaging. We anticipate that in the future, AI-based solutions will in addition help ensure more targeted referral to PET, improved treatment triage, more effective treatment response evaluation, and refined prognostication of patients with vascular disorders.

CLINICS CARE POINTS

- PET has the potential to redefine clinical approaches to vascular diseases.
- In atherosclerosis, PET allows for the specific and sensitive visualization of pathology at an earlier time point in disease course.
- In LVV, PET is able to distinguish clinically active disease, assess response to treatment, predict the risk of clinical relapse, and even identify occult malignancy in LVV patients with equivocal symptoms.
- AI-based segmentation approaches will expedite translation of these applications into the clinical space.

ACKNOWLEDGMENTS

This research was supported by the Intramural Research Program of the NIH Clinical Center and NIDCR. The opinions expressed in this publication are the author's own and do not reflect the views of the National Institutes of Health, the Department of Health and Human Services, or the United States government.

DISCLOSURE

The authors have nothing to disclose.

REFERENCES

1. Saboury B, Moghbel M, Basu S, et al. Modern quantitative techniques for PET/CT/MR hybrid imaging. In: Schaller B, editor. Molecular imaging. IntechOpen; 2012. https://doi.org/10.5772/33882.

2. Høilund-Carlsen PF, Edenbrandt L, Alavi A. Global disease score (GDS) is the name of the game! Eur J Nucl Med Mol Imaging 2019;46(9):1768–72.

3. Paydary K, Revheim M-E, Emamzadehfard S, et al. Quantitative thoracic aorta calcification assessment by 18F-NaF PET/CT and its correlation with atherosclerotic cardiovascular disorders and increasing age. Eur Radiol 2021;31(2):785–94.

4. Grayson PC, Alehashemi S, Bagheri AA, et al. 18 F-Fluorodeoxyglucose-positron emission tomography as an imaging biomarker in a prospective, longitudinal cohort of patients with large vessel vasculitis. Arthritis Rheumatol 2018;70(3):439–49.

5. Rondina MT, Lam UT, Pendleton RC, et al. 18)F-FDG PET in the evaluation of acuity of deep vein thrombosis. Clin Nucl Med 2012;37(12):1139–45.

6. Husmann L, Sah B-R, Scherrer A, et al. 18F-FDG PET/CT for therapy control in vascular graft infections: a first Feasibility study. J Nucl Med 2015; 56(7):1024–9.

7. Yun M, Yeh D, Araujo LI, et al. F-18 FDG uptake in the large arteries: a new observation. Clin Nucl Med 2001;26(4):314–9.

8. Derlin T, Richter U, Bannas P, et al. Feasibility of 18F-sodium fluoride PET/CT for imaging of atherosclerotic plaque. J Nucl Med 2010;51(6):862–5.

9. Wang Y, Osborne MT, Tung B, et al. Imaging cardiovascular calcification. J Am Heart Assoc 2018;7(13). https://doi.org/10.1161/JAHA.118.008564.

10. Dweck MR, Chow MWL, Joshi NV, et al. Coronary arterial 18F-sodium fluoride uptake: a novel marker of plaque biology. J Am Coll Cardiol 2012;59(17):1539–48.

11. Derlin T, Tóth Z, Papp L, et al. Correlation of inflammation assessed by 18F-FDG PET, active mineral deposition assessed by 18F-fluoride PET, and vascular calcification in atherosclerotic plaque: a dual-tracer PET/CT study. J Nucl Med 2011;52(7): 1020–7.

12. Blomberg BA, de Jong PA, Thomassen A, et al. Thoracic aorta calcification but not inflammation is associated with increased cardiovascular disease risk: results of the CAMONA study. Eur J Nucl Med Mol Imaging 2017;44(2):249–58.

13. Morbelli S, Fiz F, Piccardo A, et al. Divergent determinants of 18F-NaF uptake and visible calcium deposition in large arteries: relationship with Framingham risk score. Int J Cardiovasc Imaging 2014;30(2):439–47.

14. Arani LS, Zirakchian Zadeh M, Saboury B, et al. Assessment of atherosclerosis in multiple myeloma and smoldering myeloma patients using 18F- sodium fluoride PET/CT. J Nucl Cardiol 2021 Jan 3. https://doi.org/10.1007/s12350-020-02446-0.

15. Arbab-Zadeh A, Fuster V. The myth of the "vulnerable plaque": transitioning from a focus on individual lesions to atherosclerotic disease burden for coronary artery disease risk assessment. J Am Coll Cardiol 2015;65(8):846–55.

16. Jennette JC, Falk RJ, Bacon PA, et al. 2012 Revised international chapel hill consensus conference nomenclature of vasculitides. Arthritis Rheum 2013; 65(1):1–11.

17. Nikpanah M, Katal S, Christensen TQ, et al. Potential applications of PET scans, CT scans, and MR imaging in inflammatory diseases: Part II: cardiopulmonary and vascular inflammation. PET Clin 2020; 15(4):559–76.

18. Emamifar A, Ellingsen T, Hess S, et al. The utility of 18F-FDG PET/CT in patients with clinical suspicion of polymyalgia rheumatica and giant cell arteritis: a prospective, observational, and cross-sectional study. ACR Open Rheumatol 2020;2(8): 478–90.

19. Emamifar A, Hess S, Ellingsen T, et al. Prevalence of newly diagnosed malignancies in patients with polymyalgia rheumatica and giant cell arteritis, comparison of 18F-FDG PET/CT scan with chest X-ray and abdominal ultrasound: data from a 40 week prospective, exploratory, single centre study. J Clin Med Res 2020;9(12). https://doi.org/10.3390/jcm9123940.

20. Danve A, O'Dell J. The role of 18F fluorodeoxyglucose positron emission tomography scanning in the diagnosis and management of systemic vasculitis. Int J Rheum Dis 2015;18(7):714–24.

21. Newman KA, Ahlman MA, Hughes M, et al. Diagnosis of giant cell arteritis in an asymptomatic patient. Arthritis Rheumatol 2016;68(5):1135.

22. Blockmans D, de Ceuninck L, Vanderschueren S, et al. Repetitive 18F-fluorodeoxyglucose positron emission tomography in giant cell arteritis: a prospective study of 35 patients. Arthritis Rheum 2006;55(1):131–7.

23. Piri R, Edenbrandt L, Larsson M, et al. Aortic wall segmentation in 18F-sodium fluoride PET/CT scans: head-to-head comparison of artificial intelligence-based versus manual segmentation. J Nucl Cardiol 2021. https://doi.org/10.1007/s12350-021-02649-z.

24. Fantazzini A, Esposito M, Finotello A, et al. 3D automatic segmentation of aortic computed tomography angiography combining multi-view 2D convolutional neural networks. Cardiovasc Eng Technol 2020; 11(5):576–86.

25. Yu Y, Gao Y, Wei J, et al. A three-dimensional deep convolutional neural network for automatic segmentation and diameter measurement of type B aortic dissection. Korean J Radiol 2021;22(2):168–78.

26. Saboury B, Edenbrandt L, Piri R, et al. Alavi-carlsen calcification score (ACCS): a Simple measure of

global cardiac atherosclerosis burden. Diagnostics (Basel) 2021;11(8). https://doi.org/10.3390/diagnostics11081421.

27. Pournazari K, Jahangiri P, Muser D, et al. Coronary molecular calcification calculated by Alavi-Carlsen score (ACS) and its correlation with aging and cardiovascular risk factors as assessed by 18F-sodium fluoride PET/CT. J Nucl Med 2019;60(supplement 1): 449. Available at: https://jnm.snmjournals.org/content/60/supplement_1/449. Accessed September 18, 2021.

28. Saboury B, Ziai P, Alavi A. Detection and quantification of molecular calcification by PET/computed tomography: a new paradigm in assessing atherosclerosis. PET Clin 2011;6(4):409–15.

29. Mehta NN, Torigian DA, Gelfand JM, et al. Quantification of atherosclerotic plaque activity and vascular inflammation using [18-F] fluorodeoxyglucose positron emission tomography/computed tomography (FDG-PET/CT). J Vis Exp 2012;(63):e3777.

30. Foster B, Bagci U, Mansoor A, et al. A review on segmentation of positron emission tomography images. Comput Biol Med 2014;50:76–96.

31. Hahn LD, Baeumler K, Hsiao A. Artificial intelligence and machine learning in aortic disease. Curr Opin Cardiol 2021. https://doi.org/10.1097/HCO.0000000000000903.

32. Raffort J, Adam C, Carrier M, et al. Artificial intelligence in abdominal aortic aneurysm. J Vasc Surg 2020;72(1):321–33.e1.

33. Jin Y, Pepe A, Li J, et al. AI-based aortic vessel tree segmentation for cardiovascular diseases treatment: status Quo. 2021. Available at: http://arxiv.org/abs/2108.02998.

34. Lesage D, Angelini ED, Bloch I, et al. A review of 3D vessel lumen segmentation techniques: models, features and extraction schemes. Med Image Anal 2009;13(6):819–45.

35. Pepe A, Li J, Rolf-Pissarczyk M, et al. Detection, segmentation, simulation and visualization of aortic dissections: a review. Med Image Anal 2020;65:101773.

36. Yousefirizi F, Jha AK, Brosch-Lenz J, et al. Toward high-throughput artificial intelligence-based segmentation in Oncological PET imaging. PET Clin 2021;16(4):577–96.

37. Adam C, Fabre D, Mougin J, et al. Pre-surgical and post-surgical aortic aneurysm Maximum diameter measurement: full automation by artificial intelligence. Eur J Vasc Endovasc Surg 2021. https://doi.org/10.1016/j.ejvs.2021.07.013.

38. Lareyre F, Adam C, Carrier M, et al. Automated segmentation of the human abdominal vascular system using a hybrid approach combining expert system and supervised deep learning. J Clin Med Res 2021;10(15). https://doi.org/10.3390/jcm10153347.

39. Zhong J, Bian Z, Hatt CR, et al. Segmentation of the thoracic aorta using an attention-gated U-Net.

Medical imaging 2021: Computer-Aided diagnosis, 11597. SPIE; 2021. p. 147–53. https://doi.org/10.1117/12.2581947.

40. Berhane H, Scott M, Elbaz M, et al. Fully automated 3D aortic segmentation of 4D flow MRI for hemodynamic analysis using deep learning. Magn Reson Med 2020;84(4):2204–18.

41. Chen D, Zhang X, Mei Y, et al. Multi-stage learning for segmentation of aortic dissections using a prior aortic anatomy simplification. Med Image Anal 2021;69:101931.

42. Hepp T, Fischer M, Winkelmann MT, et al. Fully automated segmentation and shape analysis of the thoracic aorta in non-contrast-enhanced magnetic resonance images of the German National Cohort study. J Thorac Imaging 2020;35(6):389–98.

43. Hahn LD, Mistelbauer G, Higashigaito K, et al. CT-based true- and false-lumen segmentation in type B aortic dissection using machine learning. Radiol Cardiothorac Imaging 2020;2(3):e190179.

44. Cao L, Shi R, Ge Y, et al. Fully automatic segmentation of type B aortic dissection from CTA images enabled by deep learning. Eur J Radiol 2019;121: 108713.

45. Lu J-T, Brooks R, Hahn S, et al. DeepAAA: clinically applicable and generalizable detection of abdominal aortic aneurysm using deep learning. In: Shen D., Yap P.-T., Liu T., et al., eds. 22nd International Conference on medical image Computing and Computer-Assisted intervention, MICCAI 2019. Vol 11765 LNCS. Springer Science and Business Media Deutschland GmbH; 2019:723-731. doi:10.1007/978-3-030-32245-8_80

46. Li Z, Feng J, Feng Z, et al. Lumen segmentation of aortic dissection with cascaded convolutional network. In: Statistical atlases and computational models of the heart. Atrial segmentation and LV quantification challenges. Springer International Publishing; 2019. p. 122–30. https://doi.org/10.1007/978-3-030-12029-0_14.

47. Trullo R, Petitjean C, Ruan S, et al. Segmentation of organs at risk in thoracic CT images using a Sharp-Mask architecture and Conditional random fields. In: 2017 IEEE 14th International Symposium on Biomedical imaging (ISBI 2017). Melbourne, VIC, Australia; 18-21 April, 2017:1003-1006. doi:10.1109/ISBI.2017.7950685

48. Trägårdh E, Borrelli P, Kaboteh R, et al. RECOMIA-a cloud-based platform for artificial intelligence research in nuclear medicine and radiology. EJNMMI Phys 2020;7(1):51.

49. Ohyama Y, Redheuil A, Kachenoura N, et al. Imaging insights on the aorta in aging. Circ Cardiovasc Imaging 2018;11(4):e005617.

50. Moghbel M, Al-Zaghal A, Werner TJ, et al. The role of PET in evaluating atherosclerosis: a critical review. Semin Nucl Med 2018;48(6):488–97.

51. Fan C, Hernandez-Pampaloni M, Houseni M, et al. Age-related changes in the metabolic activity and distribution of the red marrow as demonstrated by 2-deoxy-2-[F-18]fluoro-D-glucose-positron emission tomography. Mol Imaging Biol 2007;9(5):300–7.

52. Law MA, Tivakaran VS. Coarctation of the aorta, . StatPearls. StatPearls Publishing; 2021. Available at: https://www.ncbi.nlm.nih.gov/pubmed/28613663.

53. Zhou Y, Li Z, Bai S, et al. Prior-aware neural network for partially-supervised multi-organ segmentation. In: 2019 IEEE/CVF International conference on computer vision (ICCV). IEEE; 2019. doi:10.1109/iccv.2019.01077

54. Tso E, Flamm SD, White RD, et al. Takayasu arteritis: utility and limitations of magnetic resonance imaging in diagnosis and treatment. Arthritis Rheum 2002; 46(6):1634–42.

55. Dinges J, Nekolla SG, Bundschuh RA. Motion artifacts in oncological and cardiac PET imaging. PET Clin 2013;8(1):1–9.

56. Hofheinz F, Langner J, Petr J, et al. A method for model-free partial volume correction in oncological PET. EJNMMI Res 2012;2(1):1–12.

57. Santamarina A, Maass-Moreno R, Ahlman M. Guidance from F-18 FDG Vascular Lesion Image Simulations for the Design of Procedures for Vascular Lesion Quantification. J Nucl Med 2017; 58(supplement 1):1314-1314.

58. Tsuchiya J, Tezuka D, Maejima Y, et al. Takayasu arteritis: clinical importance of extra-vessel uptake on FDG PET/CT. Eur J Hybrid Imaging 2019;3(1):12.

59. Betancourt BY, Ahlman MA, Grayson PC. Sarcoidosis concomitant with Takayasu arteritis, identified by advanced molecular imaging. Arthritis Rheumatol 2019;71(6):990.

60. Fischer A, Ellinghaus D, Nutsua M, et al. Identification of immune-relevant factors conferring sarcoidosis genetic risk. Am J Respir Crit Care Med 2015;192(6):727–36.

61. Saruhan-Direskeneli G, Hughes T, Aksu K, et al. Identification of multiple genetic susceptibility loci in Takayasu arteritis. Am J Hum Genet 2013;93(2): 298–305.

Applications of Artificial Intelligence in ¹⁸F-Sodium Fluoride Positron Emission Tomography/Computed Tomography:
Current State and Future Directions

Sriram S. Paravastu, BA[a,b], Navid Hasani, BS[a,c], Faraz Farhadi, BS[a,d],
Michael T. Collins, MD[b], Lars Edenbrandt, MD, DMS[e],
Ronald M. Summers, MD, PhD[a], Babak Saboury, MD, MPH, DABR, DABNM[a,f,g],*

KEYWORDS

• Artificial intelligence • Positron emission tomography • Computed tomography • Sodium fluoride
• Bone • Deep learning

KEY POINTS

- As it stands currently, the analysis of ¹⁸F-NaF-PET/CT is subjective and cumbersome due to the initial bottleneck of segmentation of bone.
- Methods of bone segmentation have previously been used such as manual segmentation, threshold-based segmentation, and others. However, a deep learning-based segmentation method may confer advantages in speed and accuracy of segmentation.
- A potential deep learning platform for bone segmentation on ¹⁸F-NaF-PET/CT is the RECOMIA online platform.
- Currently, no ¹⁸F-NaF-PET-based bone segmentation algorithms exist; larger databases of ¹⁸F-NaF-PET scans are required to develop these.

INTRODUCTION

¹⁸F- sodium fluoride (¹⁸F-NaF)-positron emission tomography (PET)/ computed tomography (CT) is extremely valuable for bone disease evaluation. However, the quantification of these scans remains a relatively cumbersome task. The subjective nature of this task necessitates the use of more quantitative methods to assess diseases of the skeleton and improve patient care. Segmentation of ¹⁸F-NaF-PET/CT also can be a very time-consuming process for the radiologist's workflow. Deep learning (DL) methodologies to analyze medical imaging are increasingly being

[a] Department of Radiology and Imaging Sciences, Clinical Center, National Institutes of Health (NIH), 9000 Rockville Pike, Building 10, Room 1C455, Bethesda, MD 20892, USA; [b] Skeletal Disorders and Mineral Homeostasis Section, National Institute of Dental and Craniofacial Research, National Institutes of Health (NIH), 30 Convent Dr., Building 30, Room 228 MSC 4320, Bethesda, MD 20892, USA; [c] University of Queensland Faculty of Medicine, Ochsner Clinical School, New Orleans, LA 70121, USA; [d] Geisel School of Medicine at Dartmouth, Hanover, NH 03755, USA; [e] Department of Clinical Physiology, Sahlgrenska University Hospital, Göteborg, Sweden; [f] Department of Computer Science and Electrical Engineering, University of Maryland- Baltimore County, Baltimore, MD, USA; [g] Department of Radiology, Perelman School of Medicine, University of Pennsylvania, Philadelphia, PA, USA
* Corresponding author. Department of Radiology and Imaging Sciences, Clinical Center, National Institutes of Health, 9000 Rockville Pike, Building 10, Room 1C455, Bethesda, MD 20892, USA.
E-mail address: babak.saboury@nih.gov

PET Clin 17 (2022) 115–135
https://doi.org/10.1016/j.cpet.2021.09.012

developed due to their increased objectivity, automaticity, and speed over other methods of analysis. However, this approach has not yet been adapted to ^{18}F-NaF-PET/CT imaging. The widespread application of DL methodology to ^{18}F-NaF-PET/CT will bring with it the potential to make clinical use of ^{18}F-NaF-PET/CT bone scans more objective and efficient.

CT is important in ^{18}F-NaF-PET/CT imaging to give spatial resolution to the ^{18}F-NaF uptake on PET. ^{18}F-NaF-PET/CT imaging also relies on the use of the CT scan for segmentation and labeling of the bone due to the relative abundance of CT bone segmentation algorithms. Currently, there are some DL-based solutions that allow the accurate and automated segmentation of bone on whole-body CT. Although well developed, there is still room for improvement in whole-body CT bone segmentation. There is variation in segmentation accuracy based on the specific bone being segmented, and few of the methods currently described in the literature accurately label all the bones, including individual vertebrae and ribs. Achieving a level of granularity of labeling on CT that includes all individual bones is crucial in automating ^{18}F-NaF-PET/CT analysis and biomarker evaluation. In addition, fully automated segmentation of bone on whole-body CT will make it simpler to automate and quantify bone disease burden downstream on ^{18}F-NaF-PET/CT studies.

Here, we discuss the current state of artificial intelligence (AI) in ^{18}F-NaF-PET/CT imaging and the potential applications to come in diagnosis, prognostication, and improvement of care in patients with bone diseases. Additionally, we emphasize the role of AI algorithms in CT bone segmentation, relying on their prevalence in medical imaging and utility in the extraction of spatial information in combined PET/CT studies.

We define some terms related to AI-based analysis of ^{18}F-NaF-PET/CT in **Box 1**:

CURRENT STATE OF ARTIFICIAL INTELLIGENCE IN ^{18}F-SODIUM FLUORIDE POSITRON EMISSION TOMOGRAPHY/COMPUTED TOMOGRAPHY IMAGING

In this section, we review the current state of applications of DL in ^{18}F-NaF-PET/CT imaging and comment on the strengths and limitations of the current methods. We examine 3 different approaches to ^{18}F-NaF-PET/CT segmentation: (1) bone segmentation is first performed on the CT portion of the study and carried over to the ^{18}F-NaF-PET image, (2) segmentation is performed on the ^{18}F-NaF-PET portion of the study, and (3) multi-modal processing is performed using an end-to-end approach (all available data are used simultaneously in a DL algorithm to analyze ^{18}F-NaF-PET/CT studies).

Deep Learning Analysis of ^{18}F-Sodium Fluoride Positron Emission Tomography/Computed Tomography Images Using Initial Computed Tomography Segmentation

Skeletal segmentation on computed tomography studies

Many DL algorithms have been reported in the literature for bone segmentation on CT. Because of the availability of these algorithms, the use of CT bone segmentation methods is a rational approach to bone segmentation in ^{18}F-NaF-PET/CT studies. Therefore, in this section, we describe studies that use DL to segment bone on stand-alone CT studies.

Previously, attempts to segment bone on CT have included manual segmentation, edge-based, region growing, texture features, watershed, Hounsfield unit (HU) threshold-based, and statistical shape segmentation methods.[1,2] These all rely on local gray values for segmentation, and have been less successful due to the various, irregular shapes of healthy bones and their heterogeneous internal structure. DL techniques provide an

---

Box 1
Glossary

Segmentation	Delineation of the bones of interest using the voxels or pixels in which they are visible.
Multiclass Segmentation	Segmentation of bones which identifies distinct bones into different classes.
Labelling	Parsing of the image to group pixels of the same class under a common name that is recognizable anatomically.
Landmark	Discrete points in an image that are expected to correspond to anatomical structures.
Surface Unwrapping (extended Curved Planar Reformation)	Topological transformation mapping the surface of a 3-dimensional object to a 2-dimensional plane.

Table 1
CT bone segmentation algorithms discussed in this article

Purpose and Outcome	Input Images	Training Dataset	Validation Dataset	Testing Dataset	FoM
Algorithms for Segmentation without Labeling					
Vertebral Segmentation					
Fully automated CNN to quantify body composition; seg. muscle, bone (L3,L4 vertebrae), fat on abd CT; unlabelled bones[4]	Single 2D axial slices of abd CT at L3 vertebral level	2430 2D gastrointestinal cancer, pancreatic cancer, renal cell CA, transitional cell CA patient slices at L3 level	Validated on 270 axial gastrointestinal cancer, pancreatic cancer, renal cell CA, transitional cell CA patient slices;	2369 HCC axial L3 and L4 slices	DC: 0.95; JI: 0.91; TPF: 0.99; FPF:0.10
Total Skeleton Segmentation					
Fully automatic bone seg. on whole-body CT scans of patients with multiple myeloma; seg. but did not label head, upper body, pelvic, leg bones.[5]	2D axial slices on whole-body CT	Sixfold cross-validation on the dataset of 18 expert annotated CT from PET/CT for multiple myeloma. 12 for training, 3 for validation, and 3 for testing	Sixfold cross-validation on the dataset of 18 expert annotated CT from PET/CT for multiple myeloma. 12 for training, 3 for validation and 3 for testing	Sixfold cross-validation on the dataset of 18 expert annotated CT from PET/CT for multiple myeloma. 12 for training, 3 for validation, and 3 for testing	DC: 0.95; JI: 0.91; SN: 0.91; SP: 1.00; PPV: 0.94; Accuracy: 1.00
Algorithms for Multiclass Segmentation and/or Labeling					
Vertebral Multiclass Segmentation and/or Labeling					
Seg. lumbar vertebrae from spine CTs; seg. and labeled L1-L5 vertebrae.[6]	3D spine CT	Five-fold cross-validation on same 15 spine CT images with ground truth seg	Five-fold cross-validation on same 15 spine CT images with ground truth seg 5 times;	Tested on 1 Spine CT	DC: 0.96; JI: 91.9; HD:4.32 mm

(continued on next page)

Table 1
(continued)

Purpose and Outcome	Input Images	Training Dataset	Validation Dataset	Testing Dataset	FoM
Seg. vertebrae on spine CT using a instance-by-instance segmentation approach; seg. and labeled T1-L5 vertebrae.[7]	3D spine CT	Training and validation on 5 datasets: lumbar spine CTs with compression fracture, healthy spine CTs, NCI low-dose CT lung CA screening dataset	Training and validation on 5 datasets: lumbar spine CTs with compression fracture, healthy spine CTs, NCI low-dose CA screening dataset	30 scans: 5 lumbar spine CT with compression fractures, 10 low-dose chest CT, 10 healthy lumbar spine CT, and 5 thoracolumbar spine CT.	DC: 0.96 normal dose CT ~0.92 low-dose CT; T1-L5 was labeled with an accuracy of 93%
Pelvic Multiclass Segmentation and/or Labeling					
Automated seg. of pelvic muscles, fat, and bone from pelvic CT for body composition assessment; seg pelvic bones and vertebra in 2D.[8]	2D axial CT images	180 2D axial CT images at the supra-acetabular level	20 2D axial CT images at the supra-acetabular level	No testing dataset	DC: ~0.93
Fully automatic seg. of all the pelvic bones from CT; seg. But did not label right pelvic bone, left pelvic bone, lumbar spine, sacrum.[2]	3D pelvic CT	665 pelvic CT	222 pelvic CT	236 pelvic CT	DC: 0.99; HD: 5.5 mm
Multi-regional Multiclass Segmentation and/or Labeling					
Seg. bone in chest/ abd/pelvic CT; seg. and labeled broadly as femoral,hip, sacral, sternal, vertebral, and costal bones.[1]	3D chest/abd/ pelvic CT	Trained on 21 chest/abd/ pelvic CT from first rib to femoral neck	Validated on 1 chest/ abd/pelvic CT	Tested on 4 chest/abd/ pelvic CT	DC: 0.93; PPV: 0.96

DL based method for axial skeleton seg. on CT; Seg. and labeled 49 bones of the axial skeleton.[9]	3D CTs from PET/CT scans	100 CTs from PET/CT scans taken on Biograph 64 TruePoint (Siemens Healthineers)	N/A	46 CTs from PET/CT scans obtained by a Discovery VCT 64 (GE Health Care)	DC: 0.95
Bone seg. on whole-body CT; seg. but did not label axial skeleton excluding cervical spine and skull.[10]	Various 3D CTs with various views	Threefold cross-validation of 32 whole-body CT scans that were obtained in 16 patients and performed at authors' institution.	Threefold cross-validation of 32 whole-body CT scans that were obtained in 16 patients and performed at authors' institution.	3 whole-body CTs from a public dataset	DC: 0.98; JI:0.97; SN: 0.98; PPV: 0.98
Perform deep-learning-based basic organ segmentations on CT; Seg. and labeled 77 bones head to toe.[11]	CT from PET/CT scans	Approximately 10,400 manual organ segmentations in 319 images	Approximately 2600 manual organ segmentations in 68 images	10 CTs from PET/CT scans	DC: 0.90; PPV: 0.87

Abbreviations: FoM, figures of merit; seg., segmented/segmentation/segmented; 2D, two-dimensional; 3D, three-dimensional; abd, abdominal; CA, carcinoma; CNN, convolutional neural network; DC, dice coefficient; FCN, fully convolutional network; FPF, false positive fraction; HCC, hepatocellular carcinoma; HD, hausdorff distance; JI, jaccard index; PPV, positive predictive value; SN, sensitivity; SP, specificity; TPF, true positive fraction.

avenue for more reliable and robust segmentation of bone on CT scans, with a streamlined workflow for analysis and continual improvement of the model after initial training.[3] There are some studies in the current literature that use DL methodology to automate this process; these studies investigate the segmentation of bone at various regions depending on the task of interest (Table 1). The main areas that have been focused on are the vertebrae, pelvis, and axial skeleton due to the wider availability of CT scans that encapsulate these bones. More recently, multiregional and total-skeletal DL bone segmentation methods have been described.

Some DL methods for skeletal segmentation on CT focus on delineating bone from other tissue types without labeling each individual bone within a skeletal area of interest. Multiclass skeletal segmentation aims to delineate bone from other tissue types as well as identify individual bones. Labeling individual bones or groups of bones within the skeletal area of interest is very important as well. In the first subsection 'Bone segmentation methods on free-standing computed tomography studies' we discuss methodologies that only segment the bone. We focus on multiclass segmentation and labeling in the subsection 'Multiclass segmentation and labeling methods on free-standing computed tomography studies'.

Bone segmentation methods on free-standing computed tomography studies In this section, we discuss various DL methods described in the literature for the segmentation of bone on CT without labeling the specific bones.

Vertebral bone segmentation The objective of vertebral segmentation is to accurately delineate the boundary of each vertebra. The vertebrae are closely linked objects that within spinal sections may look very similar or have similar features. As such, the segmentation needs to consider the context surrounding each spinal level. At the same time, the segmentation should be accurate, even in cases of spinal degeneration, to accommodate a wider repertoire of patients and reflect the natural heterogeneity of disease as well as healthy bone CT phenotypes.

Vertebral bone segmentation has traditionally been used in body composition analysis on a single two-dimensional slice at the L3 level. Weston and colleagues trained an AI algorithm to segment L3-level CT two-dimensional slices and were able to use this algorithm to segment other vertebral bodies. The authors trained a U-Net-based convolutional neural network (CNN) to perform abdominal segmentation on 2430 single CT transverse

images taken at the L3 vertebral level for patients with transitional cell carcinoma, renal cell carcinoma, gastrointestinal cancer, and pancreatic cancer.[4] When this model was validated on a dataset of 270 abdominal CT scans of patients with the same cancers as the training dataset, the bone segmentation performance achieved a Dice score of 0.98 versus a semiautomated approach with manual correction.[4] Finally, this method was tested on a dataset of 2369 abdominal L3 and L4 level CT scans from patients with hepatocellular carcinoma and achieved a mean Dice score of 0.97. The model was only trained at the L3 level and did not label bone due to its application to body composition measurement. However, the model was able to accurately segment the bone as well as other organs, including previously unseen organs such as lungs, bladder, and pelvis, suggesting that the model is learning organ characteristics that could potentially be applied to the three-dimensional segmentation of bone using a model trained on a lower number of two-dimensional slices. This method can be applied to structures that are similarly shaped such as the vertebrae and ribs, however may be more limited with more complex bony structures.

In a recent body composition study by Borrelli and colleagues, an AI-based 3D method was trained to quantify muscle and fat in CT.[12] The authors used the method to analyze the relation between traditional body composition values at the L3 vertebral level and corresponding 3D volumes from the same patients. Predicting a patient's muscle and fat volume from a 2D-based measurement typically resulted in an inaccuracy of approximately 20%.[12] Their results show that there may be a disadvantage to using 2D methods to describe 3D objects, however, this has yet to be validated in the context of bone.

Total-skeleton segmentation Segmenting the whole skeleton is important in quantifying total bone disease burden among other bone disease metrics on ^{18}F-NaF-PET/CT. Toward achieving this, Klein and colleagues developed a model which aimed to segment the total skeleton including the axial as well as the appendicular skeleton (Fig. 1). This group trained the model to segment whole-body CT from PET/CT studies using two-dimensional axial slices.[5] The authors mentioned the difficulty in segmenting the skull due to the irregular shapes of these bones. In addition, most of the patients in their training datasets had tooth crowns, which created metal artefacts in the CT. When evaluated on an external dataset, this model had a Dice coefficient of 0.92. However, multiclass segmentation is required to perform

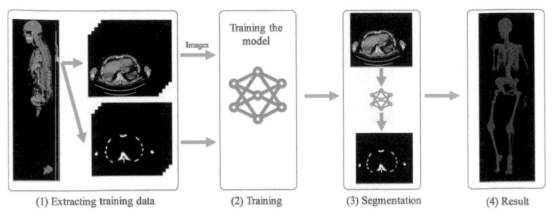

(1) Extracting training data   (2) Training   (3) Segmentation   (4) Result

Fig. 1. Schematic of method described by Klein et al. (*Modified from* Klein A, Warszawski J, Hillengaß J, Maier-Hein KH. Automatic bone segmentation in whole-body CT images. Int J Comput Assist Radiol Surg. 2019;14(1):21-29.)

further skeletal regional analyses downstream of CT bone segmentation such as the identification and analysis of radiological biomarkers.

Multiclass segmentation and labeling methods on free-standing computed tomography studies

In this section we describe published methods of multiclass segmentation and labeling of bone in CT scans (eg, methods that both segment and label bones)

Vertebral bone multiclass segmentation and labeling Multiclass segmentation of the vertebra should aim to identify the vertebral components (eg, body, pedicles, lamina, processes) as distinct objects. The methods should also label the location of the vertebra (eg, T4: fourth thoracic vertebra). Multiclass segmentation and labeling of the vertebra are very important because it is crucial to identify the individual vertebra along the vertebral column for the accurate localization of disease on ^{18}F-NaF-PET/CT. The vertebrae can also serve as landmarks for adjacent anatomic structures, including the ribs.

Recently, Sekuboyina and colleagues approached this task using the VerSe '20 database; a database of 374 abdominal CT scans that is publicly available.[13] The authors used a detection fully convolutional network (FCN) to create a probabilistic heat map masking the vertebrae.[14] Then, the spine was cropped automatically, and sagittal and coronal maximum intensity projections were sent to the Btrfly-Net labeling network.[15] Finally, the heat map was used to localize 3D vertebra patches around the vertebrae, which were segmented using a U-Net based network (**Fig. 2**). This method's strengths lie in the fact that it is fully automated and is available in a free, web-based platform. In addition, the use of both sagittal and coronal views is a good data augmentation technique that strengthened the performance of the model.

Lessmann and colleagues introduced iterative instance segmentation to segment vertebral bone (**Fig. 3**). In this segmentation method, a three-dimensional patch slides in a top-down or bottom-up fashion over the vertebral column on the CT until a vertebral bone fragment is detected. Then, the vertebra is centered in the center of the patch and the vertebra is segmented and labeled. The authors refer to the segmentation of one vertebra as an instance. The instance is then added to the instance memory neural network, which remembers voxels that have already been labeled. The patch progresses downward on the vertebral column until the next vertebra is detected, then the centering process occurs again on the next vertebra, and using the memory of the previous instance, the next instance of the vertebral column is segmented and labeled. This occurs until all the vertebrae are segmented.[7] Using this stored memory data, the CNN only segments the next nonsegmented vertebra and ignores the already segmented vertebrae. A separate subnetwork anatomically labels each detected vertebra [7]. The authors were able to label the detected vertebrae from T1 to L5 with 93% accuracy.[7] A limitation of this paper is that the authors manually cropped the image and restricted the field of view to the vertebrae. This method is inherently not fully automated, as it requires a manual cropping step, which can be time-consuming, especially among

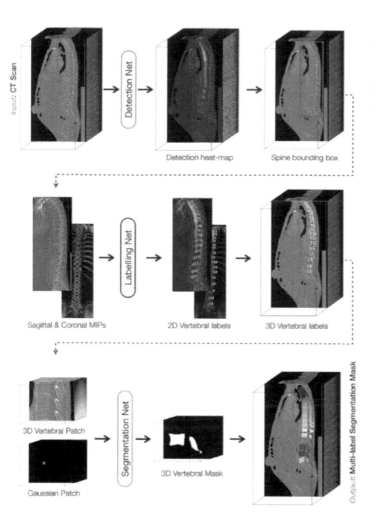

Detection heat-map   Spine bounding box

Sagittal & Coronal MIPs   2D Vertebral labels   3D Vertebral labels

3D Vertebral Patch

3D Vertebral Mask

Gaussian Patch

Output: Multi-label Segmentation Mask

Fig. 2. Use of probabilistic heat maps created by a detection network for labeling via Btrfly Net and segmentation by U-Net based algorithm.[14] (*From* Sekuboyina A, Husseini ME, Bayat A, et al. VerSe: A Vertebrae labeling and segmentation benchmark for multi-detector CT images. *Med Image Anal.* 2021;73:102166.)

many scans that require the radiologist's attention at a time. In addition, bone segmentation should ideally occur in the CT scan in the context of other organs that surround it so the algorithm can be generalizable to CT scans that have not been manually cropped.

Pelvic bone multiclass segmentation and labeling Segmentation of the bones in the pelvis can be difficult and inaccurate due to the complex shape of the bones and the presence of interfering material such as bowel contents and contrasted vessels. Given these difficulties, previous pelvic CT bone segmentation methods are mostly semiautomatic or manual. DL can greatly improve the efficiency and accuracy of pelvic bone segmentation over these previous time-intensive methods. Recently, a DL based method for automatic pelvic bone multi-class segmentation was described by Liu and colleagues which achieved

an average Dice coefficient of 0.99 for metal-free scans, and was able to segment the lumbar spine, right hip bone, left hip bone, and sacrum.[2] In the context of pelvic bone fracture, it is also important to segment the bone fragments that belong to the larger bone entity. Importantly, Liu and colleagues introduced a postprocessor (process after neural network multi-class segmentation to correct error) based on the signed distance function (SDF). SDF postprocessing allows for the measurement of a bone fragment's distance from its parent bone as well as the consideration of the fragment's size to link it to its parent bone. Compared with a traditional postprocessor, maximum connected region (MCR), the SDF maintained greater fidelity to the ground truth, reducing Hausdorff distance by 15.1%.[2] The SDF postprocessor was able to classify the broken fragments of the hip bone as parts of the bone (**Fig. 4**).

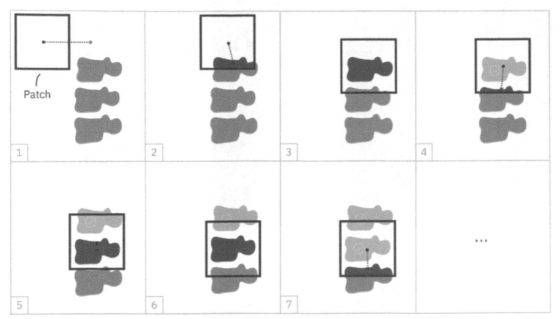

Fig. 3. Visualization of iterative instance segmentation method.[7] 1. The 3D patch slides top-down over the image. 2. A fragment of the vertebral bone is detected. 3. The fragment is centered in the patch, this repeats until the whole vertebra is within the patch. 4. The vertebra is segmented. The next fragment of the vertebra is detected, and the patch continues to slide down to the next vertebrae, while ignoring all voxels of the previous vertebra. (5–7) The patch is centered around the next vertebra and the process repeats until all vertebrae are segmented. (*From* Lessmann N, van Ginneken B, de Jong PA, Išgum I. Iterative fully convolutional neural networks for automatic vertebra segmentation and identification. Med Image Anal. 2019;53:142-155.)

Skeletal segmentation on ^{18}F-sodium fluoride positron emission tomography/computed tomography studies

In ^{18}F-NaF-PET/CT, it is critical to be able to segment and label all the bones on CT with a single algorithm to easily localize and quantify the PET signal in the context of the bone; this will allow for greater capability to quantify bone disease burden and identify radiological biomarkers of various bone diseases downstream on ^{18}F-NaF-PET/CT. We discuss here studies describing DL methodologies to segment bone on the CT image from ^{18}F-NaF-PET/CT studies.

Lindgren-Belal and colleagues proposed a U-Net-based model for bone segmentation which was able to accurately segment 49 bones of the axial skeleton.[9] This group also noted difficulty in segmenting similarly shaped bones such as the ribs and vertebrae. Lindgren-Belal and colleagues devised an elegant method using the detection of landmarks such as the rib joints to differentiate between similar bones such as the ribs and vertebrae.[9] These landmarks were detected by the CNN using a probability map which applied a "blob" at high-value regions, which were the landmarks (**Fig. 5**A). Each segmented bone had either

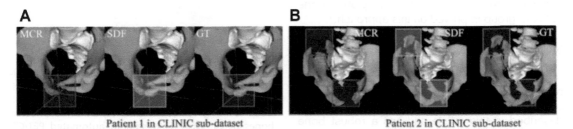

Patient 1 in CLINIC sub-dataset   Patient 2 in CLINIC sub-dataset

Fig. 4. Comparison of MCR and SDF postprocessing methods. SDF method is closer to the ground truth. GT, ground truth; MCR, maximum connected region, SDF, signed distance function.[2] (*From* Liu P, Han H, Du Y, et al. Deep learning to segment pelvic bones: large-scale CT datasets and baseline models. Int J Comput Assist Radiol Surg. 2021;16(5):749-756.)

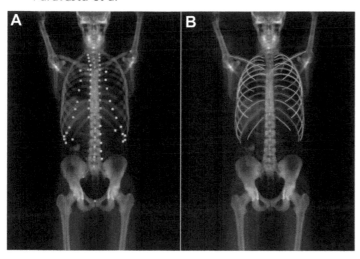

one or zero landmarks. The CNN identified the positions of landmarks that were close together. A second network was trained to detect rib centerlines and then track ribs from the rib joint landmark to the end of the rib (**Fig. 5**B). The positions of the centerlines of the ribs and the transverse processes of the vertebrae were the landmark pairs (**Fig. 5**A) fed to the final CNN as a five-dimensional mask along with the original image to help the CNN correctly identify adjacent similarly shaped bones such as the ribs and vertebra. Postprocessing of the segmentation was performed by binary hole filling and deletion of spurious voxels. This study used CT scans from patients of various genders, ages, and diagnoses to train the model. The method was focused on segmenting the ribs, thoracic and lumbar vertebrae, sternum, clavicles, scapula, and pelvic bones and did not include the segmentation of the cervical vertebrae or skull (**Fig. 6**).[9] However, because of the novelty of landmark-based segmentation of the previously difficult to segment ribs and vertebrae, as well as the high accuracy attained by this approach, this segmentation is an essential initial step toward complete skeleton segmentation. In the Research Consortium for Medical Image Analysis (RECOMIA) platform, the authors' group improved on this approach.[11]

The RECOMIA platform provides DL-based tools that can perform basic organ segmentation in CT, including 77 bones and 23 soft tissue organs (**Fig. 7**).[11] This platform includes an update of the bone segmentation model developed in the paper by Lindgren-Belal and colleagues previously described in this article and has a robust bone segmentation capability, including the segmentation of both the axial and appendicular skeleton from head to toe.[9,11] The model used on the RECOMIA platform was trained on low-dose CT,

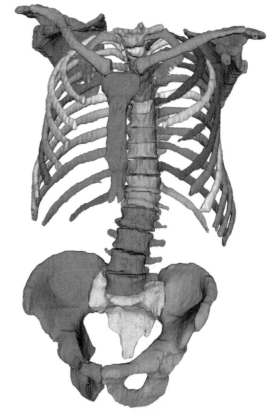

Fig. 6. Lindgren-Belal et al. segmentation results.[9] Ribs, thoracic and lumbar vertebrae, sternum, clavicles, scapula, and pelvic bones were segmented. (*From* Lindgren Belal S, Sadik M, Kaboteh R, et al. Deep learning for the segmentation of 49 selected bones in CT scans: First step in automated PET/CT-based 3D quantification of skeletal metastases. Eur J Radiol. 2019;113:89-95: under open access Creative Commons license http://creativecommons.org/licenses/by/4.0/)

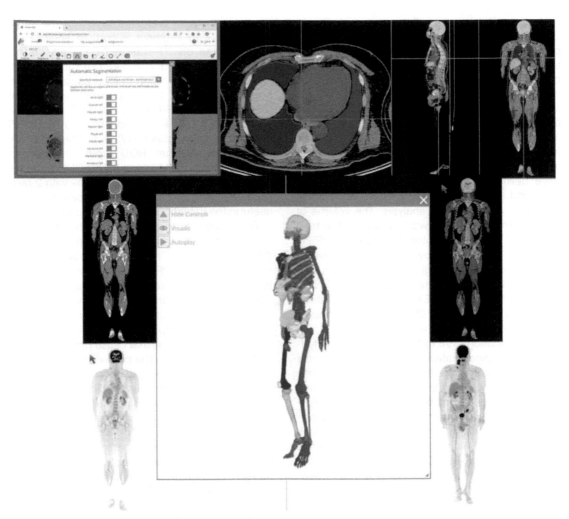

Fig. 7. RECOMIA platform. 77 bones and 23 soft tissue organs are segmented and labeled using the RECOMIA segmentation platform. The automated segmentation results can be viewed as an overlay (top right) or in 3D (bottom).[11] (*From* Trägårdh E, Borrelli P, Kaboteh R, et al. RECOMIA-a cloud-based platform for AI research in nuclear medicine and radiology. EJNMMI Phys. 2020;7(1):51: used under an open access Creative Commons license http://creativecommons.org/licenses/by/4.0/)

therefore, it is easily translatable to ^{18}F-NaF-PET/CT studies, in which the CT portion is usually low-dose. Across all bones, the RECOMIA platform achieved a Dice index of 0.90 when compared with expert manual segmentation. RECOMIA is a web-based platform that has browser-accessible DL-based tools for organ segmentation. These segmentation volumes can also be quantified and easily exported in a browser. This web-based AI segmentation model should be applied to future clinical segmentation systems to make whole skeletal multiclass segmentation much more accessible to clinicians.

DL-based segmentation of both the bone and soft tissue organs in a single platform will allow for more robust isolation of bone for ^{18}F-NaF-PET/CT analysis, as all soft tissue can be identified and excluded. Potentially, this also means that the FCN used can detect ectopic calcifications as distinct entities from both the bone and the soft tissue organs, as both of those will be segmented. More detailed classification and naming of the bones are still to come and will be important to measure global bone disease burden as well as identify potential radiological biomarkers of bone disease.

CT-based bone segmentation of ^{18}F-NaF-PET/CT studies and downstream analysis of the ^{18}F-NaF-PET image

In this subsection, we describe studies in which the CT bone segmentation mask is applied to the ^{18}F-NaF-PET image in the ^{18}F-NaF-PET/CT study.

Lindgren-Belal and colleagues used DL to segment ^{18}F-NaF-PET/CT bone scans for the purpose of segmenting prostate cancer bone metastases on ^{18}F-NaF-PET to measure bone tumor burden.[16] First, 49 bones of the axial skeleton were segmented on the CT as described by the same group in a paper discussed previously in this review.[9] Subsequently, this mask was transferred to the ^{18}F-NaF-PET image. After this, using a simple thresholding segmentation method with an SUV threshold of 15, the bone metastases were delineated as "hotspots" on the ^{18}F-NaF-PET, and all hotspots outside of the bone mask were excluded from the analysis. The volume of all segmented hotspots was divided by the total volume of bone segmented to derive the "PET/CT index" which was shown to predict survival in these patients.[16] Although this was a novel and elegant way to automate analysis of ^{18}F-NaF-PET/CT, the ^{18}F-NaF-PET portion of the study was not analyzed using DL methodology; this is an area that is still being explored.

The application of AI to the detection and identification of degenerative spinal osteophytes has also been explored due to the importance of identifying osteophytes in the diagnosis of many spine diseases. Detection of osteophytes on ^{18}F-NaF-PET/CT is a time-consuming process, and AI can help expedite this. In 2017, Wang and colleagues developed a CNN to detect spine osteophytes based on ^{18}F-NaF-PET/CT scans. First, the vertebral column was segmented using simple thresholding. The group then used their previously published four-part vertebral model (**Fig. 8**A), to segment the vertebral body separately from the rest of the spine and the surrounding bones.[17] The authors further trained the CNN to extract the periosteal and endosteal layers of the vertebrae on CT to segment a cortical shell of the bone volume on ^{18}F-NaF-PET/CT. This cortical shell was then unwrapped (**Fig. 8**B) into a flat projection for analysis using curved planar reformation; this method was applied in an identical manner to both ^{18}F-NaF-PET and CT. Fitting the cortical shell CT Hounsfield unit (HU) and PET standard uptake value (SUV) as 2 different channels in the AlexNet RGB input, the authors extracted features of interest. The CNN detected osteophytes with a sensitivity of 85% with 2 false positives per patient. This methodology may be useful in the detection of other bone pathologies.[18]

The authors of this study used the topological conversion of three-dimensional space to two-dimensional space. This idea can be applied in the realm of DL-based ^{18}F-NaF-PET/CT analysis rather robustly due to the currently superior ability of DL image processors to process two-dimensional data over three-dimensional data. For example, a similar cortical shell unwrapping procedure could be used in the case of diseases that cause pathology in the cortex of long bones. The cortex of the femur, for example, can be segmented using a similar method as the vertebral method described by Wang and colleagues and then HU and SUV shells can be fed to a DL algorithm for downstream analysis.

Another area in which AI can significantly impact ^{18}F-NaF-PET/CT imaging in patient care is the automated classification of lesions as benign or malignant. Perk and colleagues discuss a methodology of extracting radiomic features from PET, and then comparing various machine learning methods to analyze the features for benign versus malignant lesion classification.[19] This method was highly accurate in classifying

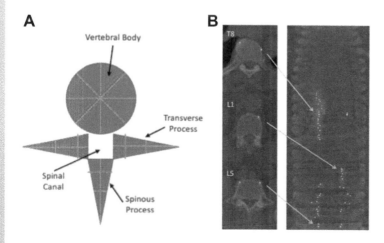

Fig. 8. (A) Simplified vertebral model based on the four-part vertebral model described by Yao and colleagues[17] (B) Axial (left) and curved planar reformed (right) views.[18] (*From* Yao J, O'Connor SD, Summers RM. Automated spinal column extraction and partitioning. In: *3rd IEEE International Symposium on Biomedical Imaging: Nano to Macro, 2006.*; 2006:390-393 and Wang Y, Yao J, Burns JE, Liu J, Summers RM. Detection of degenerative osteophytes of the spine on PET/CT using region-based convolutional neural networks. In: Vrtovec T., Zheng G., Yao J., Li S., Frangi A., Glocker B., eds. 4th International Workshop and Challenge on Computational Methods and Clinical Applications for Spine Imaging, CSI 2016 Held in Conjunction on 19th International Conference on Medical Image Computing and Computer-Assisted Intervention, MICCAI 2016. Vol 10182 LNCS. Springer Verlag; 2016:116-124.)

lesions similarly to physicians. This paper, however, uses machine learning methods on features extracted from the original ^{18}F-NaF-PET/CT images, and not a DL image processing methodology. We propose that further DL methodologies be developed for the direct analysis of ^{18}F-NaF-PET/CT images.

Deep Learning Analysis of ^{18}F-Sodium Fluoride Positron Emission Tomography/ Computed Tomography Images Using Initial ^{18}F-Sodium Fluoride Positron Emission Tomography Segmentation

The use of AI in the segmentation of bone using the ^{18}F-NaF-PET portion of ^{18}F-NaF-PET/CT has so far been limited in the literature. To our knowledge, there are no studies that have used DL methodology to segment bone on ^{18}F-NaF-PET images.

Although slightly out of the scope of this paper, methods have been previously implemented without the use of DL to segment ^{18}F-NaF-PET/CT; we have included those in **Table 2**. Most of these methods have used SUV-based simple thresholding as a way to segment lesions. In this approach, an SUV threshold is selected for exclusion of normal bone and inclusion of all the lesions of interest. One paper in the table used an adaptive thresholding method, described previously by Torigian and colleagues[20]

Perk and colleagues introduced a bone region-specific SUV thresholding method.[21] To do this,

19 bone regions were determined on the ^{18}F-NaF-PET. Then, local maxima were recovered for both healthy and pathologic region(s) of interest (ROI) after a ROI was generated for each disease site. After the identification of abnormal local maxima, a second physician evaluation was conducted. SUV thresholds for each region were set using receiver operating characteristic (ROC) analysis, which was optimized for the identification of malignant illness (**Table 3**). This method was superior in performance to the global simple thresholding methods which used an SUV threshold of 10 or 15 to differentiate normal bone uptake from diseased uptake.

Deep Learning Analysis of ^{18}F-Sodium Fluoride Positron Emission Tomography/ Computed Tomography Images Using an End-to-End Approach

End-to-end learning is an approach to solving complex tasks using a single DL model instead of using a pipeline of different image analysis methods. The end-to-end approach mimics the way experienced radiologists interpret PET/CT studies. They use all available data as input simultaneously and recognize potentially abnormal findings, streamlining the process of image analysis as well as potentially cutting down on the risk of errors along the length of an image analysis pipeline confounding the results. Despite the advantages of end-to-end DL

Table 2
Survey of various PET threshold-based bone segmentation methods in the literature

Thresholding Method	Number of Studies	Diseases Studied
≥7–8 SUV, depending on patient	1[22]	Fibrous dysplasia
≥7.7 SUV	1[23]	Fibrous dysplasia
≥8.4 SUV	1[24]	Fibrodysplasia ossificans progressiva
≥8.5 SUV	1[23]	Fibrous dysplasia
≥10 SUV	9[25–33]	Prostate carcinoma, breast carcinoma, osteosarcoma, medullary thyroid carcinoma, various urologic malignancies, and multiple myeloma metastatic to bone
≥15 SUV	5[16,34–37]	Prostate carcinoma bone mets
Statistically Optimized Regional Thresholding (SORT)	1[21]	Prostate carcinoma bone mets
Adaptive thresholding[20]	1[38]	Multiple Myeloma

Table 3
Regional SUV thresholds determined by Perk et al.'s SORT method[21]

Region	Optimal Proposed SUV Threshold Based on Empirical Data	Most *Specific* SUV Threshold Based on Empirical Data (ie, Threshold with No False Positives)	Most *Sensitive* SUV Threshold Based on Empirical Data (ie, Threshold with No False Negatives)
Skull	6.5	14.4	5.7
Mandible	8.1	12.9	8.1
Ribs	7.3	12	4.4
Cervical spine	11.8	15.4	6.5
Thoracic spine	11.8	17.3	6.3
Lumbar spine	12.9	19.2	6.7
Sacrum	10	16	7.1
Shoulders	8.1	12.2	6.1
Sternum	9.1	12.6	9.2
Humeri	6.7	12.6	6.7
Radii/ulnae	5.6	8.8	5.6
Hands	3.2	5.3	3.1
Ilium	10.9	17.5	9.1
Pubis	10.2	15	6.4
Ischium	11	15.5	5.4
Femurs	6.3	11.5	3.9
Tibias/fibulas	5.9	9.6	4.1
Feet	5.4	7.3	5.4
Patellae	5.2	6.1	5.2

algorithms, this methodology has not yet been used in the literature.

One reason why the end-to-end approach has not been widely used in the field of medical imaging is the lack of large training data sets. The DL model needs to be trained with as many or even more cases as the experienced radiologist has seen. As with ^{18}F-NaF-PET/CT databases in general, the large-scale databases required for end-to-end learning are currently not publicly available today.

THE FUTURE OF ARTIFICIAL INTELLIGENCE IN ^{18}F-SODIUM FLUORIDE POSITRON EMISSION TOMOGRAPHY/COMPUTED TOMOGRAPHY IMAGING

In this section, we discuss the ideal application of AI in ^{18}F-NaF-PET/CT bone imaging. We begin by explaining how AI-based CT bone segmentation may be made more applicable to ^{18}F-NaF-PET/CT, and then look at how AI analysis of ^{18}F-NaF-PET/CT can be used in the clinical environment to enhance bone disease diagnosis and prognosis, as well as patient care.

Future of Artificial Intelligence Bone Segmentation on Computed Tomography: Improved Utility for ^{18}F-Sodium Fluoride Positron Emission Tomography Analysis

To characterize bone diseases more effectively and objectively using ^{18}F-NaF-PET/CT, detection, segmentation, and labeling of both pathologic and healthy bone on CT scans should be more comprehensive than it currently is.

Difficulties in and potential solutions for deep learning-based computed tomography bone segmentation

Segmentation and labeling of each individual bone on CT are crucial to easily pinpoint and characterize bone disease on the fused PET. Effective segmentation of bone can allow more accurate measurement and diagnosis of processes occurring outside of the bone. The aim should be to integrate the various methods discussed in the section

'Skeletal segmentation on CT studies' to create a workflow capable of segmenting and labeling all the bones with high accuracy and precision.

The lacking accuracy of rib segmentation discussed in the section 'Skeletal segmentation on 18F-NaF-PET/CT studies' brings forward the idea of differences in the conceptualization of the bone as an organ. Clinically, the bones may all exist in a common ecosystem, but radiographically, each bone is segmented and analyzed as a separate ecosystem. If certain bones are less accurately segmented than others, there will be a downstream automation bias that may alert physicians to pathologies of certain bones more frequently than others when the difference in frequency may not be as large. To achieve more awareness of this and avoid automation bias, researchers should be transparent and deliberate about stating the uncertainty in the segmentation of each bone, and physicians should be aware of these limitations of the AI tools they use. Below, we discuss different possibilities for improving the technical robustness of CT bone segmentation.

A potential step in improving the technical robustness can be to curate and develop more comprehensive publicly available and annotated CT databases for the purpose of bone segmentation. Currently, there are 2 large-scale publicly available databases for this purpose. The CT-ORG database was introduced in 2020 due to the publishers' observation that the then available databases did not have skeletal annotations. This database consists of 140 thoracoabdominopelvic CT studies with 6 annotated organ classes: liver, lungs, bladder, kidney, brain, and bone.[39] The VerSe '20 challenge is another bone-specific dataset that consists of 374 CT studies with all of the vertebrae annotated and labeled.[14] More databases like these are necessary to advance the CT-based DL bone segmentation.

There might be a multitude of reasons for the absence of CT segmentation of deformed bone. The paucity of research on the application of DL to the segmentation of deformed bone is one of the primary causes; additionally, large-scale datasets of deformed bone are not freely available for the training and implementation of a DL algorithm. Despite this, a concerted effort can still be made to address this issue at institutions with access to these types of datasets. A proposed method to address the segmentation of deformed bone is the combination of landmark digitization with bone segmentation via CNNs. Landmark digitization traditionally involves marking common landmarks on bone to plan treatments and surgical approaches to correct deformity.[40] This combination method has previously been implemented in the context of cone-beam CT segmentation of craniomaxillofacial deformity.[40] It was also used by Lindgren-Belal and colleagues to segment similarly shaped bones adjacent to each other such as the ribs (**Fig. 5**).[9] Finding common and conserved landmarks in bone and using those as references to identify, segment, and label the bones can aid in the segmentation of deformed bone.

Future of Artificial Intelligence in ^{18}F-Sodium Fluoride Positron Emission Tomography/ Computed Tomography Imaging

^{18}F-NaF-PET/CT currently stands as the next frontier of AI application to bone disease diagnosis and prognostication. As with DL-based segmentation of bone on CT, DL-based automation of whole-body ^{18}F-NaF-PET/CT segmentation is highly beneficial for the nuclear medicine physician's workflow. In addition, interpretation of ^{18}F-NaF-PET/CT studies is currently subjective, and we discuss possibilities to make this process more objective using AI.

Proposed deep learning approaches to ^{18}F-sodium fluoride positron emission tomography/computed tomography segmentation

To automate ^{18}F-NaF-PET/CT bone scan analysis, clinicians can either use a CT-based or a PET-based approach implementing DL techniques. In the CT-based approach (**Fig. 9**A), CT is used to (1) delineate the outer border of each individual bone and classify them each into discrete objects, (2) determine the relationships of the delineated objects to each other, and (3) derive the CT HU and the PET SUV. By considering the location of the lesions within the objects, the relational properties of these objects with each other, and the HU and SUV values in the lesion, the AI will alert the radiologist to the patterns of bone disease.

In the PET-based approach (**Fig. 9**B), a CNN is trained to recognize normal patterns of ^{18}F-NaF uptake across the body. These pattern recognition algorithms should be age-aware. For example, in an older patient population, there may be a pattern of focal ^{18}F-NaF uptake in arthritic areas whereby there is greater bone turnover. Then, areas of abnormal metabolic activity on PET will be highlighted for the radiologist. Alternatively, the AI can first localize ROIs of interest based on the ^{18}F-NaF-PET SUV values. Then, the algorithm, using a combination of PET and CT phenotype

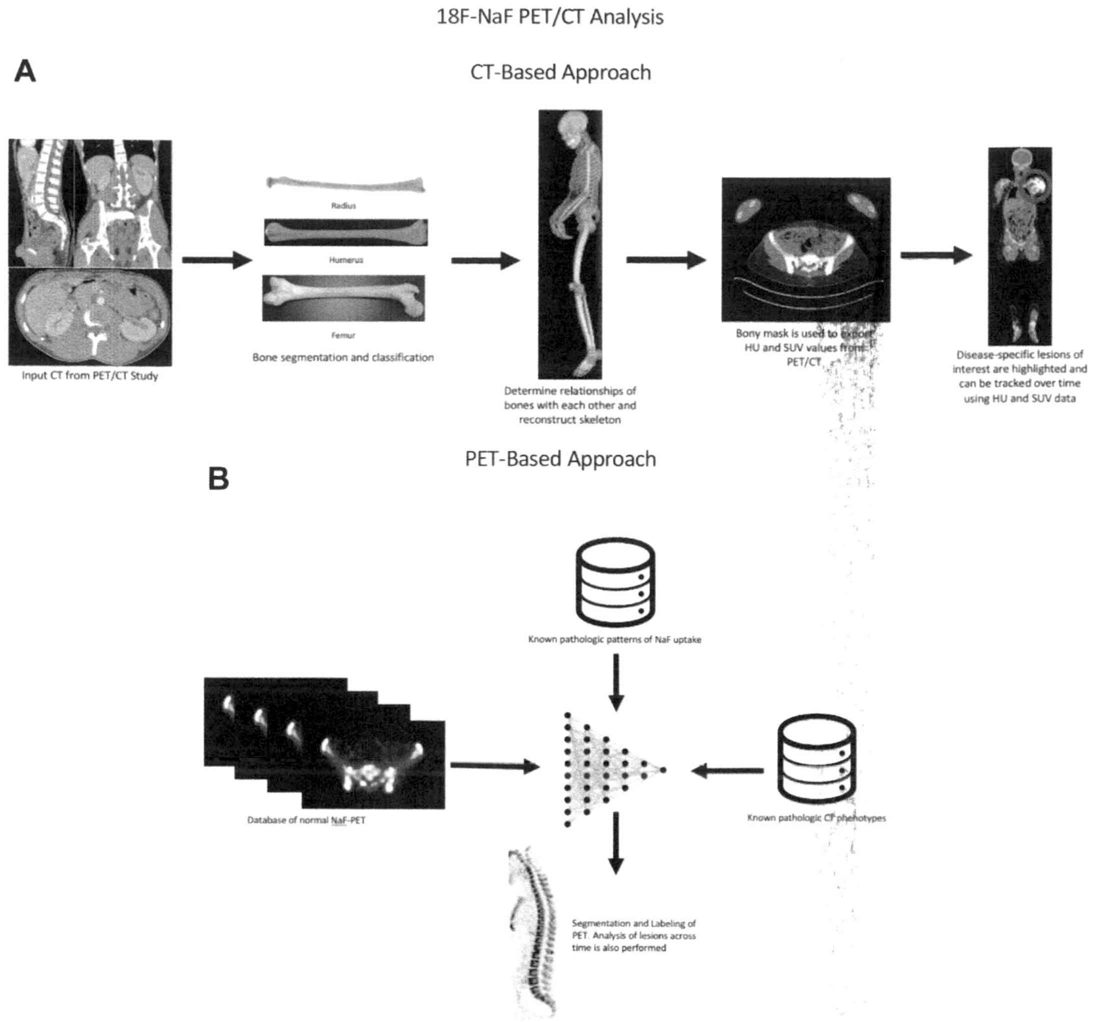

Fig. 9. Describing CT-based and PET-based approaches to ^{18}F-NaF-PET/CT automation. Part (A) describes the CT-based approach of individual bone segmentation, skeleton creation, location-based HU/SUV export, and finally lesion of interest highlighting. Part (B) describes the PET-based approach; characterization of normal ^{18}F-NaF uptake, pattern recognition of abnormal uptake, and automatic highlighting, diagnosis, or disease burden calculation.

analysis, will alert the radiologist to possible pathology. An advantage to this method is that lesions of interest in a particular disease can be tracked on PET, whereas regions of uptake that are less important to the disease process can be deprioritized for analysis. A disadvantage of simple rule-based methods, for example defining abnormal SUV uptake as "more than two standard deviations greater than the normal SUV uptake based on a reference database", is that these methods usually achieve only suboptimal performance. Therefore, it is preferable to allow the DL algorithm to analyze the complexity in SUV regional differences and use a variety of factors

in the segmentation of abnormal uptake, rather than simple rules.

To implement the CT-based and PET-based AI approaches suggested in this paper, a standardized method to localize the potential lesion and then query a database to perform pattern recognition should exist. To that end, creating a common bone atlas that is generalizable across patients and over multiple scans in the same patient is crucial. A methodology for this has been discussed previously in the literature.[41] The authors showcase a great workflow for atlas creation (Fig. 10). We can augment atlas creation by registering landmarks on bones on a query CT with the

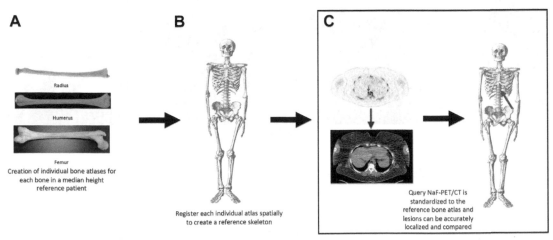

Fig. 10. Bone atlas concept for comparison on ^{18}F-NaF-PET/CT scans. Individual bone atlases are created for each bone in a median height reference patient (*A*). These individual bone atlases are then registered spatially to create a reference skeleton (*B*). Then, the query ^{18}F-NaF-PET/CT is standardized to the reference bone atlas and lesions can be accurately localized and compared (*C*).

landmarks on the reference atlas to more easily create a common bone space that can be compared. This atlas creation will enable the use of an efficient workflow to easily compare ^{18}F-NaF-PET/CT scans quantitatively.

A CNN that is objective and standardized in detecting bone pathologies on ^{18}F-NaF PET/CT must use some of the same principles that are second nature to a radiologist. For instance, while the most essential element is the region of increased uptake, the CT phenotypic information is also extremely relevant. The ^{18}F-NaF-PET scan serves as a saliency map for the CNN to look at ROIs for the disease. Using either the CT-based or PET-based localization frameworks described above, the AI must pinpoint the coordinates within the ROI on both PET and CT and delineate the ROI. Then the CNN will compare the query to a database of ^{18}F-NaF-PET/CT images to help characterize the disease of interest.

We briefly discussed the integration of various DL models into a single pipeline. In the pipeline approach, the diagnostic problem is divided into several subproblems using a step-by-step approach. For example, the pipeline can identify the location of individual bones on the CT, or what is the normal SUV in a particular bone. The subproblems can usually be solved using currently available data sets. A disadvantage of this method is that if one step in a chain of steps is inaccurate, the results are usually inaccurate. End-to-end DL approaches can be an ideal solution to this issue, once we overcome the scarcity of large-scale datasets to train DL algorithms in end-to-end ^{18}F-NaF-PET/CT processing.

Special cases High-density structures lying near bone, such as ectopic calcifications in familial tumoral calcinosis (FTC), myositis ossificans, or fibrodysplasia ossificans progressiva (FOP), should be easily segmented as distinct objects from the bone. Comparison of the number, shape, and density of the objects to databases and serial scans can be performed to predict disease progression or evaluate response to treatment. Once the bones are delineated, the AI will ignore those voxels, and then delineate the high-density structures and proceed to characterize the patient's disease. The densities can be mapped in three-dimensional space to the closest bone on a standardized atlas for easier comparison of lesion burden and size between patients and between different timepoints within the same patient.

Sometimes, the resolution of ^{18}F-NaF-PET may not allow for the clear delineation of structures near the bone. Super-resolution improves the spatial resolution of low-resolution images that suffer from low-quality imaging tools, patient movements, or long acquisition time. Generative adversarial network (GAN)-based super-resolution (SRGAN) techniques have shown remarkable performance compared to conventional algorithms.[42] A three-dimensional SRGAN system able to create thin-interval CT images from thick-interval images was developed that was able to better clarify the boundaries between bone and surrounding tissue.[43] This system can be applied in segmenting high-density structures lying in close proximity to bone; better perceptual quality of bone boundaries on ^{18}F-NaF-PET would

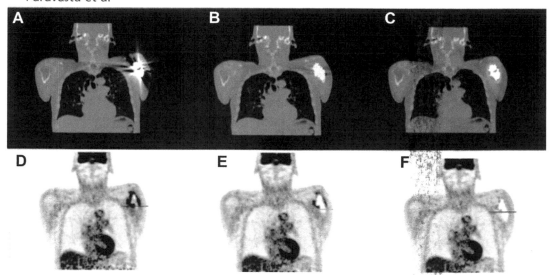

Fig. 11. Metal artefact reduction can be very useful in sharpening the hardware silhouette.[46] The CT metal arte-fact from shoulder joint hardware is reduced from panel a to c using Arabi and Zaidi's approach. This is also seen with ^{18}F-FDG-PET from panel d to f. (*From* Arabi H, Zaidi H. Deep learning-based metal artefact reduction in PET/CT imaging. Eur Radiol. 2021;31(8):6384-6396 used under an open access Creative Commons license http://creativecommons.org/licenses/by/4.0/)

simplify the delineation of the bones and high-density structures as separate objects.

Most methods reviewed in this article do not segment surgical hardware accurately. About 7 million adults in the US are living with total hip and knee prostheses.[44] This number is not comprehensive of all patients with orthopedic implants. These patients may have implants to correct complex pathologies that can be analyzed with DL. For example, an orthopedic surgeon may want to identify the degree of osseointegration of an implant based on the surrounding bone metabolism.[45] Delineation of the bones of interest, delineation of the implants, and analysis of the ^{18}F-NaF-PET/CT to determine the bone turnover surrounding the bone to assess osseointegration can be automated using DL. Metal artefact poses difficulty in identifying the boundaries of an implant. To counter this, Arabi and Zaidi published a DL-based metal artefact reduction approach for whole-body PET/CT (**Fig. 11**).[46] SRGAN can further help clearly define the region of the implant versus normal bone to assess the pathologies and metabolism of the bone surrounding the implant.

Potential applications of ^{18}F-sodium fluoride positron emission tomography/computed tomography deep learning analysis

The development of DL methodology for analysis of dynamic ^{18}F-NaF-PET/CT is very important in the context of metabolic bone disease. ^{18}F-NaF plasma clearance has been demonstrated to decrease in patients with osteoporosis compared to healthy and osteopenic patients.[47] Similarly, bone turnover at the lumbar spine as assessed by ^{18}F-NaF uptake was decreased in osteoporotic patients.[48] This presents a striking opportunity for DL applications in the diagnosis and treatment monitoring of osteoporosis using both static and dynamic ^{18}F-NaF-PET/CT. Using the PET-based automation approach mentioned above, DL-based examination of normal patterns of ^{18}F-NaF uptake can help us establish biomarkers of treatment efficacy and bone disease.

An example of automated ^{18}F-NaF-PET/CT biomarker analysis is the application of AI to determining a bone metabolism score (BMS) for patients on treatment for osteoporosis. BMS is calculated as the ratio of SUV in the volume occupied by bone tissue to the total volume contained within the neck of the femur.[49] When the BMS is calculated for the hip, the ^{18}F-NaF activity can serve as a biomarker for risk of hip fracture as well as bone quality in osteoporosis.[49] Segmenting the hip ^{18}F-NaF-PET/CT from the whole-body CT can be automated using a CT bone segmentation process, and then standardizing the patient data to the common bone atlas. Afterward, the SUV values for the bone region and the total region can be extracted easily using either a PET-based or CT-based automation scheme described above, then BMS is calculated and given to the radiologist/clinician. This can help the physician monitor response to osteoporosis therapy or predict fracture risk in an objective, standardized, automatic manner.

Outside the scope of this article but very important to ^{18}F-NaF-PET/CT analysis, is the proper registration of the ^{18}F-NaF-PET to its corresponding CT. Improper registration can have profound consequences on the downstream analysis and therefore registration practices should be reviewed and assessed.

SUMMARY

The use of DL to automate ^{18}F-NaF-PET/CT analysis is a relatively recent venture, with just a few studies in the literature. Efforts to increase the size and quality of training data sets are needed to expand the literature and clinical use. All clinical situations in which a DL model would be useful need to be represented in the training data. For example, CT with and without contrast, different image resolutions, slice thicknesses, cases with metal artefacts, different genders, ages, and normal and abnormal findings, among other factors. We have much work ahead of us, but the reward will most likely be AI models performing as extremely competent assistants to enhance the workflow of radiologists. DL technologies are generating a great deal of interest due to their enormous potential to help uncover novel bone disease biomarkers and allow radiologists and clinicians to track response to therapy more efficiently. More quantitative ^{18}F-NaF-PET/CT analysis technologies may one day allow for an elegant metric to assess medication treatment efficacy in bone for diverse illnesses. We anticipate significant advancements in this rapidly evolving field soon.

CLINICS CARE POINTS

- AI models will perform as extremely competent assistants to enhance the workflow of radiologists.
- Deep learning-based bone segmentation approaches may be valuable in improving the clinical workflow when analyzing ^{18}F-NaF-PET/CT scans.
- The RECOMIA platform provides DL-based tools that can perform basic organ segmentation on CT, including 77 bones and 23 soft tissue organs. This is currently available for research applications.
- Physicians should be aware of the limitations of any artificial intelligence tool they are using to avoid automation bias in clinical practice.

DISCLOSURE

This research was supported by the Intramural Research Program of the NIH Clinical Center and National Institute of Dental and Craniofacial Research. The opinions expressed in this publication are the author's own and do not reflect the views of the National Institutes of Health, the Department of Health and Human Services, or the United States government.

REFERENCES

1. Campanini PDP, La Rosa F. A deep learning approach to bone segmentation in CT scans. Available at: https://amslaurea.unibo.it/14561/1/A%20deep%20learning%20approach%20to%20bone%20segmentation%20in%20CT%20scans.pdf. Accessed July 8, 2021.
2. Liu P, Han H, Du Y, et al. Deep learning to segment pelvic bones: large-scale CT datasets and baseline models. Int J Comput Assist Radiol Surg 2021;16(5):749–56.
3. Moreau N, Rousseau C, Fourcade C, et al. Comparison between threshold-based and deep learning-based bone segmentation on whole-body CT images. In: Medical Imaging 2021: Computer-Aided Diagnosis. Vol 11597. SPIE; 2021:661–667.
4. Weston AD, Korfiatis P, Kline TL, et al. Automated abdominal segmentation of CT scans for body composition analysis using deep learning. Radiology 2019;290(3):669–79.
5. Klein A, Warszawski J, Hillengaß J, et al. Automatic bone segmentation in whole-body CT images. Int J Comput Assist Radiol Surg 2019;14(1):21–9.
6. Janssens R, Zeng G, Zheng G. Fully automatic segmentation of lumbar vertebrae from CT images using cascaded 3D fully convolutional networks. In: 2018 IEEE 15th international symposium on biomedical imaging (ISBI 2018). Washngton, DC, USA April 4-7 2018:893-897. https://doi.org/10.1109/ISBI.2018.8363715.
7. Lessmann N, van Ginneken B, de Jong PA, et al. Iterative fully convolutional neural networks for automatic vertebra segmentation and identification. Med Image Anal 2019;53:142–55.
8. Hemke R, Buckless CG, Tsao A, et al. Deep learning for automated segmentation of pelvic muscles, fat, and bone from CT studies for body composition assessment. Skeletal Radiol 2020;49(3):387–95.
9. Lindgren Belal S, Sadik M, Kaboteh R, et al. Deep learning for segmentation of 49 selected bones in CT scans: first step in automated PET/CT-based 3D quantification of skeletal metastases. Eur J Radiol 2019;113:89–95.
10. Noguchi S, Nishio M, Yakami M, et al. Bone segmentation on whole-body CT using convolutional neural network with novel data augmentation techniques. Comput Biol Med 2020;121:103767.

11. Trägårdh E, Borrelli P, Kaboteh R, et al. RECOMIA-a cloud-based platform for artificial intelligence research in nuclear medicine and radiology. EJNMMI Phys 2020;7(1):51.

12. Borrelli P, Kaboteh R, Enqvist O, et al. Artificial intelligence-aided CT segmentation for body composition analysis: a validation study. Eur Radiol Exp 2021;5(1):11.

13. Löffler MT, Sekuboyina A, Jacob A, et al. A vertebral segmentation dataset with fracture Grading. Radiol Artif Intell 2020;2(4):e190138.

14. Sekuboyina A, Husseini ME, Bayat A, et al. VerSe: a vertebrae labelling and segmentation benchmark for multi-detector CT images. Med Image Anal 2021;73: 102166.

15. Sekuboyina A, Rempfler M, Kukačka J, et al. Btrfly Net: Vertebrae Labelling with Energy-Based Adversarial Learning of Local Spine Prior. In: Medical Image Computing and Computer Assisted Intervention – MICCAI 2018. Springer International Publishing; 2018:649–657.

16. Lindgren Belal S, Sadik M, Kaboteh R, et al. 3D skeletal uptake of ^{18}F sodium fluoride in PET/CT images is associated with overall survival in patients with prostate cancer. EJNMMI Res 2017;7(1):15.

17. Yao J, O'Connor SD, Summers RM. Automated spinal column extraction and partitioning. In: 3rd IEEE international Symposium on biomedical imaging: Nano to Macro, 2006. 2006:390-393. DOI:10.1109/ISBI.2006.1624935.

18. Wang Y, Yao J, Burns JE, et al. Detection of degenerative osteophytes of the spine on PET/CT using region-based convolutional neural networks. In: Vrtovec T, Zheng G, Yao J, et al, editors. 4th international Workshop and challenge on computational methods and clinical applications for spine imaging, CSI 2016 Held in conjunction on 19th international conference on medical image computing and computer assisted intervention, MICCAI 2016. Vol 10182 LNCS. Springer International Publishing AG (outside the US); 2016. p. 116–24.

19. Perk T, Bradshaw T, Chen S, et al. Automated classification of benign and malignant lesions in ^{18}F-NaF PET/CT images using machine learning. Phys Med Biol 2018;63(22):225019.

20. Torigian DA, Lopez RF, Alapati S, et al. Feasibility and performance of novel software to quantify metabolically active volumes and 3D partial volume corrected SUV and metabolic volumetric products of spinal bone marrow metastases on ^{18}F-FDG-PET/CT. Hell J Nucl Med 2011;14(1): 8–14.

21. Perk T, Chen S, Harmon S, et al. A statistically optimized regional thresholding method (SORT) for bone lesion detection in ^{18}F-NaF PET/CT imaging. Phys Med Biol 2018;63(22):225018.

22. Papadakis GZ, Manikis GC, Karantanas AH, et al. F-18-NaF PET/CT imaging in fibrous dysplasia of bone. J Bone Miner Res 2019;34(9):1619–31.

23. van der Bruggen W, Vriens D, Meier ME, et al. Denosumab reduces lesional fluoride skeletal burden on Na[^{18}F]F PET-CT in patients with fibrous dysplasia/McCune–albright syndrome. J Clin Endocrinol Metab 2021;106(8):e2980–94.

24. Botman E, Raijmakers PGH, Yaqub M, et al. Evolution of heterotopic bone in fibrodysplasia ossificans progressiva: an [^{18}F]NaF PET/CT study. Bone 2019; 124:1–6.

25. Kairemo K, Kappadath SC, Joensuu T, et al. A retrospective comparative study of sodium fluoride (NaF-18)-PET/CT and fluorocholine (F-18-CH) PET/CT in the evaluation of skeletal metastases in metastatic prostate cancer using a volumetric 3-D radiomics analysis. Diagnostics (Basel) 2020;11(1):17.

26. Lim I, Lindenberg ML, Mena E, et al. ^{18}F-Sodium fluoride PET/CT predicts overall survival in patients with advanced genitourinary malignancies treated with cabozantinib and nivolumab with or without ipilimumab. Eur J Nucl Med Mol Imaging 2020;47(1): 178–84.

27. Azad GK, Siddique M, Taylor B, et al. Is response assessment of Breast cancer bone metastases better with measurement of F-18-Fluoride metabolic flux than with measurement of F-18-Fluoride PET/CT SUV? J Nucl Med 2019;60(3):322–7.

28. Etchebehere EC, Araujo JC, Fox PS, et al. Prognostic factors in patients treated with Ra-223: the role of skeletal tumor burden on baseline F-18-Fluoride PET/CT in predicting overall survival. J Nucl Med 2015;56(8):1177–84.

29. Brito AE, Mourato F, Santos A, et al. Validation of the semiautomatic quantification of ^{18}F-fluoride PET/CT whole-body skeletal tumor burden. J Nucl Med Technol 2018;46(4):378–83.

30. Letellier A, Johnson AC, Kit NH, et al. Uptake of radium-223 dichloride and early [^{18}F]NaF PET response are driven by baseline [^{18}F]NaF parameters: a pilot study in castration-resistant prostate cancer patients. Mol Imaging Biol 2018;20(3): 482–91.

31. Lapa P, Marques M, Costa G, et al. Assessment of skeletal tumour burden on ^{18}F-NaF PET/CT using a new quantitative method. Nucl Med Commun 2017;38(4):325–32.

32. Rohren EM, Etchebehere EC, Araujo JC, et al. Determination of skeletal tumor burden on ^{18}F-fluoride PET/CT. J Nucl Med 2015;56(10):1507–12.

33. Kurdziel KA, Shih JH, Apolo AB, et al. The kinetics and reproducibility of ^{18}F-sodium fluoride for oncology using current PET camera technology. J Nucl Med 2012;53(8):1175–84.

34. Muzi M, O'Sullivan F, Perk TG, et al. Whole-body [^{18}F]-fluoride PET SUV imaging to monitor response

to dasatinib therapy in castration-resistant prostate cancer bone metastases: secondary results from ACRIN 6687. Tomography 2021;7(2):139–53.

35. Weisman AJ, Harmon SA, Perk TG, et al. Quantification of bone flare on ^{18}F-NaF PET/CT in metastatic castration-resistant prostate cancer. Prostate Cancer Prostatic Dis 2019;22(2):324–30.

36. Harmon SA, Perk T, Lin C, et al. Quantitative assessment of early [F-18]Sodium fluoride positron emission tomography/computed tomography response to treatment in men with metastatic prostate cancer to bone. J Clin Oncol 2017;35(24):2829.

37. Lin C, Bradshaw T, Perk T, et al. Repeatability of quantitative ^{18}F-NaF PET: a multicenter study. J Nucl Med 2016;57(12):1872–9.

38. Zadeh MZ, Seraj SM, Østergaard B, et al. Prognostic significance of ^{18}F-sodium fluoride in newly diagnosed multiple myeloma patients. Am J Nucl Med Mol Imaging 2020;10(4):151–60.

39. Rister B, Yi D, Shivakumar K, et al. CT-ORG, a new dataset for multiple organ segmentation in computed tomography. Sci Data 2020;7(1):381.

40. Zhang J, Liu M, Wang L, et al. Context-guided fully convolutional networks for joint craniomaxillofacial bone segmentation and landmark digitization. Med Image Anal 2020;60:101621.

41. Yip S, Perk T, Jeraj R. Development and evaluation of an articulated registration algorithm for human skeleton registration. Phys Med Biol 2014;59(6):1485–99.

42. Shin Y, Yang J, Lee YH. Deep generative adversarial networks: applications in musculoskeletal imaging. Radiol Artif Intell 2021;3(3):e200157.

43. Kudo A, Kitamura Y, Li Y, et al. Virtual Thin Slice: 3D Conditional GAN-based Super-Resolution for CT Slice Interval. In: Machine Learning for Medical Image Reconstruction. Springer International Publishing; 2019:91–100.

44. Maradit Kremers H, Larson DR, Crowson CS, et al. Prevalence of total hip and knee replacement in the United States. J Bone Joint Surg Am 2015; 97(17):1386–97.

45. Jeuken RM, Roth AK, Peters MJM, et al. In vitro and in vivo study on the osseointegration of BCP-coated versus uncoated nondegradable thermoplastic polyurethane focal knee resurfacing implants. J Biomed Mater Res B Appl Biomater 2020;108(8): 3370–82.

46. Arabi H, Zaidi H. Deep learning-based metal artefact reduction in PET/CT imaging. Eur Radiol 2021; 31(8):6384–96.

47. Frost ML, Fogelman I, Blake GM, et al. Dissociation between global markers of bone formation and direct measurement of spinal bone formation in osteoporosis. J Bone Miner Res 2004;19(11):1797–804.

48. Uchida K, Nakajima H, Miyazaki T, et al. Effects of alendronate on bone metabolism in glucocorticoid-induced osteoporosis measured by ^{18}F-fluoride PET: a prospective study. J Nucl Med 2009;50(11): 1808–14.

49. Rhodes S, Batzdorf A, Sorci O, et al. Assessment of femoral neck bone metabolism using ^{18}F-sodium fluoride PET/CT imaging. Bone 2020;136:115351.

Clinical Application of Artificial Intelligence in Positron Emission Tomography: Imaging of Prostate Cancer

Kevin Ma, PhD[a], Stephanie A. Harmon, PhD[a], Ivan S. Klyuzhin, PhD[b],
Arman Rahmim, PhD, DABSNM[b,c,d], Baris Turkbey, MD[a,*]

KEYWORDS

• PET • Prostate cancer • Artificial intelligence

KEY POINTS

- Novel targeted tracers (eg, PSMA, FACBC, choline) have a big impact on the clinical management of prostate cancer.
- Artificial intelligence (AI) has been more commonly used in medical imaging
- Research in AI for prostate cancer in PET/CT is relatively new but current evidence in the literature is promising.

Artificial intelligence (AI) algorithms, particularly those based on convolutional neural networks, have shown promise for organ and lesion segmentation, patient-level and region-level classification of pathological findings, and outcome predictions in cancer imaging. Advantages of automated, AI-based image segmentation, and classification include higher annotation and processing speed than manual annotation, repeatable segmentation results, and the ability to identify and capture complex patterns or features in the images.

In PET/CT imaging of prostate cancer, however, unique challenges exist for AI-based image analysis. Manual segmentations of prostate based on CT data can often include bladder tissues, and coupled with higher radiation uptake of bladder, can result in inaccurate segmentations. Additional challenges include (a) small lesion sizes that and the resulting strong voxel-wise class imbalance, (b) wide variation in the number of lesions per patient, (c) physiologic tracer accumulation in the organs such as ureters, ganglia, and bladder, (d)

uptake overlap due to proximity of cancer lesions to surrounding organs with high tracer uptake such as bladder and bowel, (e) and finally faint uptake (SUVmax < 3) in some cancer lesions.

Several PET tracers have been developed for clinical workup of prostate cancer, such as ^{68}Ga-PSMA-11,[1] ^{18}F-DCFPyL,[2] Choline,[3] ^{18}NaF,[4] although their potential as quantitative imaging biomarkers are still being investigated.[5] Meanwhile, the usage of whole-body PET in detecting and measuring global tumor presence enables clinicians and researchers to characterize the burden of metastatic disease and its relationship with other disease characteristics, such as treatment outcome and patient survival rate.[1]

Despite the aforementioned challenges, there are several ongoing research efforts that use AI for various diagnostic tasks in molecular imaging of prostate cancer with established and novel tracers. In this work, we review the current trends and categorize the currently available research into the quantification of total tumor burden, or

[a] Artificial Intelligence Resource, Molecular Imaging Branch, NCI, NIH, Bethesda, MD, USA; [b] Department of Integrative Oncology, BC Cancer Research Institute, Vancouver, British Columbia, Canada; [c] Department of Radiology, University of British Columbia, Vancouver, British Columbia, Canada; [d] Department of Physics, University of British Columbia, Vancouver, British Columbia, Canada
* Corresponding author. 10 Center Drive, Room B3B85, Bethesda, MD 20892.
E-mail address: turkbeyi@mail.nih.gov

PET Clin 17 (2022) 137–143
https://doi.org/10.1016/j.cpet.2021.09.002
1556-8598/22/Published by Elsevier Inc.

tumor burden within a particular organ, metastasis detection and quantification, and development of AI-based clinical and research tools.

CURRENT ARTIFICIAL INTELLIGENCE RESEARCH IN PROSTATE CANCER POSITRON EMISSION TOMOGRAPHY IMAGING
Artificial Intelligence-Based Primary Tumor Segmentation

Current AI research in PET imaging for prostate cancer is in relatively early stages. A group in Sweden and Denmark has been conducting pioneering research on AI methods for predicting prostate cancer outcome, as well as evaluating AI algorithms for the segmentation and quantification of disease burden for correlation to patient outcomes. According to Mortensen and colleagues,[6] the first step was to develop a CNN segmentation algorithm for prostate on PET/CT. The model first calculates the transform between PET and CT scans for spatial alignment, then uses information from both scans for prostate segmentation. For model training, both prostate and bladder were manually annotated, with bladder assigned a negative value. The resultant segmentation and standard uptake values (SUVs) from trained CNN matched with manual-segmentation SUVmax, SUVmean, and volume of abnormal voxels with mean differences of 0.37, −0.08, and 1.4 mL, respectively.[6] They have also shown that quantitative biomarkers such as tumor volume and uptake were significantly associated with overall patient survival.[7] The same group has similarly investigated the segmentation of lymph nodes and bone metastases and found segmentation results to relate to overall patient survival.[8,9]

Artificial Intelligence-Based Primary Tumor Burden Quantification

Quantifiable tumor uptake, or SUV, in PET can be a promising biomarker in predicting treatment outcome and prognosis.[10] SUVmax measurement of primary prostate cancer depends on accurate 3D organ and tumor segmentations in the prostate. Polymeri and colleagues[7] have proposed a deep-learning model to quantify primary tumor burden in PET/CT images. A CNN model was developed for the segmentation of prostate in CT images based on individual voxel grey-scale values. The network used multi-resolution processing to evaluate the probabilities of individual voxels belonging to the prostate gland. "Abnormal" voxels within the prostate gland were defined as those with SUV greater than 2.65, and total tumor uptake in the prostate region was calculated from co-registered ^{18}F-choline PET

images. The results were validated using 2 metrics: prostate volume and abnormal PET uptake. The validation results from 43-patient cohort showed that the deep-learning-based prostate segmentation was similar to manual segmentations with a dice similarity coefficient of 0.78. Univariate survival analysis found that CNN-produced lesion volume and lesion uptake relate significantly to overall survival, prostate-specific antigen (PSA), and Gleason score. Volumetric analysis of PET/CT images is not currently in the standard clinical practice, and an automated tool may allow such analysis results to be included to increase the diagnostic value of PET/CT imaging.

Another research effort aimed to extract PET/CT voxel features and match them with ground truth obtained from histopathology slices. Rubenstein and colleagues[11] proposed an unsupervised feature detection method to improve feature detection and voxel classification in dynamic ^{11}C-choline-PET/CT, aiming to combine manual perfusion-based features with deep features. PET/CT images were matched with histopathology images, which served as a standard of reference. Deep features, extracted via an autoencoder, were analyzed along with statistics-based features (such as SUVmax (SUVs), TAC (time activity curves) and SUVmean) and kinetic modeling features. The resultant feature matrix improved tumor detection rates from AUC = 0.812 with SUVmean only to AUC = 0.899 for big tumors, which are greater than 36 mm^2 at 2D pathology slides.

Artificial Intelligence-Based Predictive Modeling

In addition to volumetric analysis, radiomics (including tumor texture, shape, or statistical features) have been explored as a potential indicator for disease staging and predictor of survival and treatment outcome. For prostate cancer, predicting biochemical reoccurrence (BCR) is very important because of the high morbidity rate associated with BCR identified during the primary treatment follow-up. Alongi and colleagues[12] aimed to develop machine learning models to discover prognostic biomarkers from choline PET/CT images in patients with high-risk prostate cancer, particularly texture analysis. Each tumor from the study cohort (n = 94) was manually segmented, and 53 features of each tumor were extracted via LIFEx toolbox,[13] plus PSA, and Gleason scores. Machine learning-based feature reduction and selection were performed, and then a predictive model was trained from features most associated with patient risks. Depending on disease types, the patient cohort was split into 3 groups: local relapse, lymph-nodal disease, and bone metastasis, and the overall predictive model has an AUROC of 67.24 for TNM prediction.

Cysouw and colleagues[14] explored machine learning-based analysis of quantitative ^{18}F-DCFPyL PET to predict metastasis and high-risk pathologic tumor features in prostate cancer. Primary tumors were manually segmented and 480 radiomic features were extracted per tumor. Standard PET metrics (SUV, PSMA + volume, lesion uptake) were also extracted for comparison. AUCs for radiomics-based lymph node involvement (LNI) prediction was slightly higher (P = .25–.29) than AUCs for traditional PET features: 0.86 versus 0.81 for patients with LNI, 0.86 versus 0.81 for the presence of metastasis, 0.81 versus 0.76 for GS greater than 8 patients, and 0.76 versus 0.67 for the presence of extracapsular extension (ECE). The results of this early study indicate that machine learning-based ^{18}F-DCFPyL PET metrics can be helpful for the prediction of LNI and high risk at pathology.

Artificial Intelligence-Based Lesion Delineation

Prostate cancer lesion segmentation in PET images can be difficult due to low resolution and suffers from inter- and intra-observer variability. A group at Johns Hopkins has begun using deep-learning methods for lesion delineation in ^{18}F-DCFPyL PET images.[15] A CNN-based method was used to segment 207 PET studies, with approximately 6 lesions per study. The results were compared with manual segmentations from 4 nuclear medicine physicians, with a DICE coefficient of 0.71, than 0.66 from a semiautomated thresholding-based technique. Deep learning (DL)-based method was significantly (P < .05) better at lesion segmentation than threshold-based methods. In another effort, a 3-D CNN method was developed for PET lesion segmentation and 9-label classification according to PSMA-RADS.[16] Prediction results on the test set (overall n = 3724 lesions, n ~ 559 for testing) showed AUC of 0.88 to 0.98 among the 9 labels, and an overall accuracy of 67.4%. These results demonstrate the potential of using DL for prostate cancer lesion segmentation and classification from PET images.

Artificial Intelligence-Based Metastasis Detection and Quantification

Identification of lymph node metastasis is key in staging patients with newly diagnosed prostate cancer and for managing patients with biochemically recurrent prostate cancer. Borrelli and colleagues[9] proposed an AI-based method for the detection and quantitative assessment of imaging biomarkers for lymph nodes on ^{18}F-choline PET/CT. An organ CNN was trained to segment organs from CT, and a detection CNN was trained for lymph node lesions based on manual annotations from a reader. Segmentation and annotation from the AI model were compared with 2 experienced readers and showed comparable sensitivity while overestimating the number of lymph node lesions. The number of detected lymph node lesions was related significantly to overall prostate cancer-specific survival. This retrospective study demonstrated that it is possible to use AI not only for the evaluation of objective PET imaging metrics, but also for prognosis estimation. In a study by Hartenstein and colleagues, CNNs were trained to determine ^{68}Ga-PSMA-PET/CT-lymph node status from CT images in 549 patients with a total of 2616 lymph nodes. ^{68}Ga-PSMA-PET was used as a reference and CNNs performed with AUC of 0.95 (nodal status based) and 0.86 (location based), whereas the AUC of experienced radiologists was 0.8.[17] This showed the AI performance in predicting lymph node metastasis on CT images was comparable to expert radiologists.

Detection and segmentation of individual metastatic lesions in ^{68}Ga-PSMA PET/CT images using DL were also recently proposed by Zhao and colleagues.[18] The group trained a CNN to detect lesions in the axial, coronal, and sagittal planes of the pelvic area. The data from 193 patients were combined from 3 different centers. The authors report 99% precision and 99% recall in bone lesion detection, and 94% precision and 89% recall in lymph node lesion detection.

In another study, Lee and colleagues aimed to evaluate the performance of DL classifiers in discriminating normal and abnormal ^{18}F-FACBC (fluciclovine) PET scans based on the presence of tumor recurrence and/or metastases in patients with prostate cancer. The study included 251 patients and CNN models were trained using 2 different architectures, a 2D-CNN (ResNet-50) using single slices (slice-based approach) and the same 2D-CNN and a 3D-CNN (ResNet-14) using a hundred slices per PET image taken from the pelvic region (case-based approach). For the 2D-CNN slice-based approach, sensitivity and specificity were 90.7% and 95.1%, and AUC was 0.971. For the case-based approaches using both 2D-CNN and 3D-CNN architectures, sensitivity, specificity, and AUC were 85.7%, 71.4%, and 0.75% and 71.4%, 71.4%, and 0.699, respectively.[19] These studies indicate that AI can assist in identifying abnormal uptake based on tumor presence or recurrence in PET images of prostate cancer.

Most of the published works on lesion detection in PSMA-PET images have leveraged supervised machine learning methods. However, the collection of training data, that is, manual delineation of primary lesions and metastases, is a difficult and time-consuming process. Moreover, as metastases can occur in semirandom locations, large quantities of lesion segmentations may be required. This problem may be alleviated by using unsupervised and self-supervised learning techniques, whereby no manually annotated training data are required. It was recently demonstrated that lesion detectability can be enhanced by training a CNN to generate a lesion-free (healthy) PET image, in a self-supervised manner.[20,21] More specifically, the CNN was trained to predict a full-resolution PET image from a pair of CT and highly blurred PET image (this is unsupervised learning in the sense that no tumors were manually segmented for the training of the network, and manual segmentations were only used for the evaluation of the network); in the predicted image, the healthy tracer uptake patterns are reproduced accurately, whereas the lesions are missing (**Fig. 1A**). In the difference (original-predicted) images, lesions then become more prominent (**Fig. 1B**): background noise (measured as spatial standard deviation) around lesion was reduced on average by 40.3% (median: 47.1%) than original images, and lesion-contrast to-background-noise ratio increased on average by 79.0% (median 47.9%). These initial findings demonstrate the promise of unsupervised machine learning techniques in prostate cancer lesion detection (see **Fig. 1**).

In addition to classic PET features and radiomics, other features such as bone scan index (BSI) and changes in bone scan index (ΔBSI) can be potentially strong quantitative biomarkers for metastatic prostate cancer prognosis.[22] BSI, defined as the percentage of bone weight affected by tumor to the entire skeleton mass, can act as a quantifiable measure of metastatic disease burden or treatment effects. BSI calculation depends on accurate bone segmentation, and the current standard of BSI calculation is based on the 2D projection of skeletal images. Lindgren and colleagues[8] explored a CNN-based 3D bone segmentation method for bone volume calculation in PET/CT scans to increase the speed of BSI calculation. The CT portion was used for anatomic bone segmentation, whereas PET tracers were used to detect tumor activity in segmented bone. The CNN segmentation method focused on 49 bone regions including rib cage, spine, and pelvis. The presented methodology focused on the segmentation speed and serves as the very first step in the creation of an automated PET/CT-based method for quantifying skeletal tumor burden. The dice similarity coefficient for CNN based versus manual segmentations ranged between 0.83 and 0.88. Although the initial results are promising, more work is needed to include all skeletal bones and a larger patient cohort to improve BSI calculation accuracy.

Artificial Intelligence-Based Clinical and Research Tools in Current Use

For AI-related clinical research, manual annotations and data preparation can be very time-consuming and remain to be a bottleneck in the research workflow. Hence, there is an incentive to develop tools that simplify and speed up the processing of PET/CT images. Tragardh and colleagues[23] proposed a cloud-based platform, RECOMIA (Research Consortium for Medical Image Analysis), that provided AI research functionalities including deidentification, web-based image viewing and tools, manual annotation, and AI-based tools for quantification and segmentation. The platform has been used in several AI research papers in PET/CT for prostate cancer due to its ability to perform multi-organ segmentation and compute PET metrics.[7,9]

Quantifying the PSMA tracer uptake in healthy organs can be used to estimate the radiation burden in targeted radionuclide therapy for prostate cancer, and to optimize the drug dose and effectiveness on a personalized level. Indeed, significant correlations were found between pretherapy PSMA-PET standardized uptake values (SUVs) in healthy organs and absorbed dose during therapy.[24] However, manual segmentation of organs is very labor-intensive, subject to operator variability, and often not feasible in the clinic or large research trials. Recently, the feasibility of fully automated, high-quality segmentation of 14 organs with high [^{18}F]DCFPyL uptake was demonstrated using a multi-target neural network.[25] An example is shown in **Fig. 2**. The overall measured Dice coefficient between manual and automatic segmentation was 0.8 or above for all organs. This demonstrates that AI algorithms can produce high-quality organ segmentations without human intervention, and potentially lead to a wide clinical adoption of personalized and precise dosimetry in prostate cancer treatment. In fact, there is increasing evidence that AI-based frameworks, due to their higher repeatability (than humans), once trained sufficiently, can point out

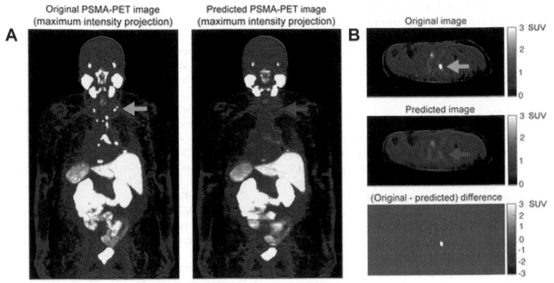

Fig. 1. (*A*) Examples of original and neural-net predicted [^{18}F]DCFPyL PSMA-PET images for a subject with metastatic prostate cancer (using unsupervised learning). The cancer lesions are not reproduced in the predicted image (*red arrow*), and lacrimal glands and other organ shapes are accurately reproduced. (*B*) Examples of original, neural-net predicted, and difference images of a single slice. The lesion (indicated by *arrow*) becomes pronounced in the difference image.

inconsistencies in manual 'reference truth' delineations, and further improve on those.[26,27]

For PET/MR scans, accurate attenuation and scatter correction can be a challenge to accurately estimate tumor uptakes. For prostate cancer PET/MR, the complex pelvic bone structure presents a unique problem in calculating attenuation maps. Pozaruk and colleagues[28] developed a DL model, based on the generative-adversarial network (GAN), to calculate PET attenuation and scatter maps (μ-map) in ^{68}Ga-PSMA PET/MR scans. PET/CT and PET/MR images of the same subjects were taken, CT and MR-Dixon images were coregistered, and normalized MR images and μ-map from CT were used to train the GAN model to estimate μ-map for PET/MR. The result was

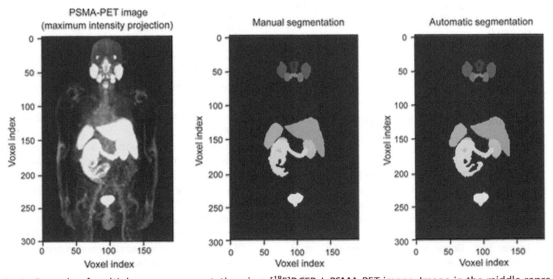

Fig. 2. Example of multiple organ segmentations in a [^{18}F]DCFPyL PSMA-PET image. Image in the middle represents manual organ delineations, and image on the right represents segmentations generated automatically by a neural network.

compared with atlas-based PET/MR μ-map, and it was observed to have lower overall relative errors. This AI method to automated PET attenuation correction has the potential to aid in other quantitative PET research in predicting outcome and classification.

SUMMARY

PET imaging of primary and metastatic prostate cancer holds significant potential for quantitative biomarker discovery and treatment planning. AI-based image analysis techniques can accelerate biomarker research, but also contribute to the clinical adoption of PET/CT in prostate cancer management. At present, there is only a limited number of applications of AI in PET imaging of prostate cancer, and most of the proposed methods are not aimed at clinical adoption. However, this is expected to change, as novel prostate-targeting tracers are developed, and data for training AI models become more readily available. Clinical patient care will benefit from these research outcomes in the future.

CLINICS CARE POINTS

- PET imaging has significant benefits for clinical prostate -cancer management.
- PET imaging offers important opportunities for quantitative imaging biomarkers for diagnosis and prognosis estimation.
- AI has the potential to accelerate and to further expand PET based imaging biomarker research.

DISCLOSURE

The authors have nothing to disclose.

REFERENCES

1. Schmidkonz C, Cordes M, Schmidt D, et al. 68)Ga-PSMA-11 PET/CT-derived metabolic parameters for determination of whole-body tumor burden and treatment response in prostate cancer. Eur J Nucl Med Mol Imaging 2018;45(11):1862–72.
2. Jansen BHE, Bodar YJL, Zwezerijnen GJC, et al. Pelvic lymph-node staging with (18)F-DCFPyL PET/CT prior to extended pelvic lymph-node dissection in primary prostate cancer - the SALT trial. Eur J Nucl Med Mol Imaging 2021;48(2):509–20.
3. Cimitan M, Evangelista L, Hodolič M, et al. Gleason score at diagnosis predicts the rate of detection of 18F-choline PET/CT performed when biochemical evidence indicates recurrence of prostate cancer: experience with 1,000 patients. J Nucl Med 2015; 56(2):209–15.
4. Harmon SA, Perk T, Lin C, et al. Quantitative assessment of early [(18)F]Sodium Fluoride positron emission tomography/Computed tomography response to treatment in men with metastatic prostate cancer to bone. J Clin Oncol 2017;35(24):2829–37.
5. Fraum TJ, Ludwig DR, Kim EH, et al. Prostate cancer PET tracers: essentials for the urologist. Can J Urol 2018;25(4):9371–83.
6. Mortensen MA, Borrelli P, Poulsen MH, et al. Artificial intelligence-based versus manual assessment of prostate cancer in the prostate gland: a method comparison study. Clin Physiol Funct Imaging 2019;39(6):399–406.
7. Polymeri E, Sadik M, Kaboteh R, et al. Deep learning-based quantification of PET/CT prostate gland uptake: association with overall survival. Clin Physiol Funct Imaging 2020;40(2):106–13.
8. Lindgren Belal S, Sadik M, Kaboteh R, et al. Deep learning for segmentation of 49 selected bones in CT scans: first step in automated PET/CT-based 3D quantification of skeletal metastases. Eur J Radiol 2019;113:89–95.
9. Borrelli P, Larsson M, Ulén J, et al. Artificial intelligence-based detection of lymph node metastases by PET/CT predicts prostate cancer-specific survival. Clin Physiol Funct Imaging 2021;41(1):62–7.
10. Naqa IE. The role of quantitative PET in predicting cancer treatment outcomes. Clin Translational Imaging 2014;2(4):305–20.
11. Rubinstein E, Salhov M, Nidam-Leshem M, et al. Unsupervised tumor detection in Dynamic PET/CT imaging of the prostate. Med image Anal 2019;55: 27–40.
12. Alongi P, Stefano A, Comelli A, et al. Radiomics analysis of 18F-Choline PET/CT in the prediction of disease outcome in high-risk prostate cancer: an explorative study on machine learning feature classification in 94 patients. Eur Radiol 2021;31(7): 4595–605.
13. Nioche C, Orlhac F, Boughdad S, et al. LIFEx: a freeware for radiomic feature calculation in multimodality imaging to accelerate advances in the characterization of tumor heterogeneity. Cancer Res 2018; 78(16):4786–9.
14. Cysouw MCF, Jansen BHE, van de Brug T, et al. Machine learning-based analysis of [(18)F]DCFPyL PET radiomics for risk stratification in primary prostate cancer. Eur J Nucl Med Mol Imaging 2021, 48(2):340–9.
15. Leung K, Ashrafinia S, Salehi Sadaghiani M, et al. A fully automated deep-learning based method for

lesion segmentation in ^{18}F-DCFPyL PSMA PET images of patients with prostate cancer. J Nucl Med 2019;60(supplement 1):399.

16. Leung MSS K, Dalaie P, Tulbah R, et al. A deep learning-based approach for lesion classification in 3D 18F-DCFPyL PSMA PET images of patients with prostate cancer. J Nucl Med 2020;61:527.

17. Hartenstein A, Lübbe F, Baur ADJ, et al. Prostate cancer nodal staging: using deep learning to predict (68)Ga-PSMA-Positivity from CT imaging Alone. Scientific Rep 2020;10(1):3398.

18. Zhao Y, Gafita A, Vollnberg B, et al. Deep neural network for automatic characterization of lesions on (68)Ga-PSMA-11 PET/CT. Eur J Nucl Med Mol Imaging 2020;47(3):603–13.

19. Lee JJ, Yang H, Franc BL, et al. Deep learning detection of prostate cancer recurrence with (18)F-FACBC (fluciclovine, Axumin®) positron emission tomography. Eur J Nucl Med Mol Imaging 2020; 47(13):2992–7.

20. I. Klyuzhin YX, S. Harsini, A. Ortiz, et al, editor Unsupervised image background removal by multimodality guidance: application to PSMA PET/CT imaging of metastases2021.

21. Klyuzhin I, Xu Y, Harsini S, et al. Unsupervised background removal by dual-modality PET/CT guidance: application to PSMA imaging of metastases 2021; 62(supplement 1):36.

22. Li D, Lv H, Hao X, et al. Prognostic value of bone scan index as an imaging biomarker in metastatic prostate cancer: a meta-analysis. Oncotarget 2017;8(48):84449–58.

23. Trägårdh E, Borrelli P, Kaboteh R, et al. RECOMIA-a cloud-based platform for artificial intelligence research in nuclear medicine and radiology. EJNMMI Phys 2020;7(1):51.

24. Violet J, Jackson P, Ferdinandus J, et al. Dosimetry of ^{177}Lu-PSMA-617 in metastatic castration-resistant prostate cancer: correlations between pretherapeutic imaging and whole-body tumor dosimetry with treatment outcomes. J Nucl Med 2019; 60(4):517–23.

25. Klyuzhin I, Chausse G, Bloise I, et al. Automated deep segmentation of healthy organs in PSMA PET/CT images 2021;62(supplement 1):1410.

26. Kirubarajan A, Taher A, Khan S, et al. Artificial intelligence in emergency medicine: a scoping review. J Am Coll Emerg Physicians Open 2020;1(6): 1691–702.

27. Lebovitz S, Levina, N., Lifshitz-Assaf, H. Is AI Ground Truth Really 'True'? The Dangers of Training and Evaluating AI Tools Based on Experts' Know-What. Management Information Systems Quarterly Forthcoming Special Issue on "Managing AI". 2021.

28. Pozaruk A, Pawar K, Li S, et al. Augmented deep learning model for improved quantitative accuracy of MR-based PET attenuation correction in PSMA PET-MRI prostate imaging. Eur J Nucl Med Mol Imaging 2021;48(1):9–20.

Artificial Intelligence in Lymphoma PET Imaging:
A Scoping Review (Current Trends and Future Directions)

Navid Hasani, BS[a,b], Sriram S. Paravastu, BA[a], Faraz Farhadi, BS[a],
Fereshteh Yousefirizi, PhD[c], Michael A. Morris, MD, MS, DABR, DABNM[a,d],
Arman Rahmim, PhD, DABSNM[c,e], Mark Roschewski, MD[f],
Ronald M. Summers, MD, PhD[a,*],
Babak Saboury, MD, MPH, DABR, DABNM[a,d,g,*]

KEYWORDS

- Artificial intelligence • Deep learning • Positron emission tomography (PET) • Lymphoma
- Radiomics • Radiophenomics • Segmentation • Detection

KEY POINTS

- One of the most serious issues in the management of lymphoma patients is treatment failure.
- Accurate quantification of tumor burden using ^{18}F-FDG-PET is an important method for therapy response assessment and prediction.
- Artificial Intelligence (AI)-based PET approaches could make this process more efficient, precise, and pave the way for future PET-based imaging biomarker applications.
- In addition to streamlining the workflow, AI can enable segmentation and radiomic analysis to acquire prognostic information regarding therapy augmentation, remission planning, and recurrence prediction.

INTRODUCTION

Lymphomas are a diverse group of hematologic malignancies, which can be broadly categorized into Hodgkin (HL) and non-Hodgkin diseases (NHL) and have a wide range of clinical presentations.[1] 2-deoxy-2-[Fluorine-18]fluoro-D-glucose (^{18}F-FDG) positron emission tomography/computed tomography (PET/CT) is extensively used for staging and response assessment in HL and NHL.[2–5] The accurate and precise quantification of tumor burden in lymphoma is critical for prognosis and treatment response evaluation and prediction. ^{18}F-FDG PET scans provide valuable information about the metabolism of lesions. This functional information combined with structural (CT or MRI) data can be used to assess the *global disease burden* in Alzheimer's disease,[6] Crohn's disease,[7] knee inflammation[8] as

[a] Department of Radiology and Imaging Sciences, Clinical Center, National Institutes of Health, 9000 Rockville Pike, Building 10, Room 1C455, Bethesda, MD 20892, USA; [b] University of Queensland Faculty of Medicine, Ochsner Clinical School, New Orleans, LA 70121, USA; [c] Department of Integrative Oncology, BC Cancer Research Institute, Vancouver, BC, Canada; [d] Department of Computer Science and Electrical Engineering, University of Maryland-Baltimore Country, Baltimore, MD, USA; [e] Department of Radiology, BC Cancer Research Institute, University of British Columbia, 675 West 10th Avenue, Vancouver, British Columbia, V5Z 1L3, Canada; [f] Lymphoid Malignancies Branch, Center for Cancer Research, National Institutes of Health, Bethesda, MD, USA; [g] Department of Radiology, Perelman School of Medicine, University of Pennsylvania, Philadelphia, PA, USA
* Corresponding authors. Department of Radiology and Imaging Sciences, Clinical Center, National Institutes of Health, 10 Center Drive, Building 10, Room 1C224D, Bethesda, MD 20892, USA (R.M.S); Department of Radiology and Imaging Sciences, Clinical Center, National Institutes of Health, 9000 Rockville Pike, Building 10, Room 1C455, Bethesda, MD 20892, USA (B.S).
E-mail addresses: rsummers@mail.cc.nih.gov (R.M.S.); babak.saboury@nih.gov (B.S.)

PET Clin 17 (2022) 145–174
https://doi.org/10.1016/j.cpet.2021.09.006
1556-8598/22/Published by Elsevier Inc.

well as lymphoma.[9] Therefore, ^{18}F-FDG PET/CT is extremely valuable in the noninvasive assessment of disease burden.[10]

To determine global disease burden, segmentation of all tumor lesions is a vital step that allows the measurement of metabolically active tumor volumes (*MTV*), mean activity of the lesion (*SUV_mean*), lesion partial volume corrected metabolic volume product (*PVC-MVP*: calculated as the product of *lesion MTV* and *lesion PVC-SUV_mean*), total metabolic tumor volume (*TMTV*: calculated as the sum of MTV of all lesions), total lesion glycolysis (*TLG*),[11] whole-body metabolic burden (*WBMB*: calculated as the sum of *lesion PVC-MVP* of all lesions),[10,12] metabolic heterogeneity (*MH*)[13,14] and lesion dissemination (*D_max*).[15,16] There are, however, *various methods for* the *segmentation* of tumor lesions (e.g. manual, thresholding-based, region-based, or boundary-based)[17,18] each with high *inter-observer variability* depending on the operator and segmentation method.[19,20] Furthermore, even for an expert, manual segmentation takes time (30–45 minutes per patient depending on tumor burden) as summary measurements of each lesion must be aggregated.[19] Lymphoma lesion segmentation is a challenging task due to the large variability in number, size, distribution, uptake, the shape of lesions, and different degrees of glucose metabolism (**Fig. 1**)[21–23] Normal biodistribution of ^{18}F-FDG creates physiologic intense activity either due to high metabolic rate (such as brain) or high concentration of excreted radiotracer (such as renal collecting ducts and bladder). This normal pattern significantly deteriorates the performance of the crude intensity-based detection and segmentation methods.[24,25] Automated segmentation and feature extraction approaches may be an exciting avenue to limit measurement discrepancies and cut image analysis to a fraction of the current required time.[19]

In general, the most critical aspects that should be evaluated during lymphoma PET are as follows: (1) quantification of disease burden,[26,27] (2) evaluation of therapy response,[28] and (3) extraction of additional image information used for prognosis and diagnosis of lymphoma.[29,30] Artificial Intelligence (AI) has ample potential to achieve the aforementioned goals by first performing automatic quantification, which entails (1) automatically identifying the location of the abnormality,[31] (2) automatically segmenting the lesion,[32,33] (3) summarizing each lesion to other dimensions (SUV_mean, SUV_max).[10,34] Finally, AI can enable registration at multiple points in time,[35,36] scaling from one space to another. This allows evaluation of lymphoma before and after diagnosis or therapy.[37,38] Given such significant promise that AI has in other fields of medical imaging and sporadic relevant evidence specific to lymphoma PET, it is important to scope and map current applications of AI in lymphoma PET imaging. However, at the time of this publication, there has not been a review of various applications of AI as it pertains to lymphoma.

Thus, in this article, we first aim to scope the breadth of evidence and systematically map literature on the topic of AI applications in lymphoma PET to identify key concepts and disseminate research evidence on various AI models. We then depict the potential clinical utility of AI in PET imaging and anticipate future directions that can be expected for AI applications in lymphoma.

A list of abbreviations used in this article are shown in **Box 1**.

METHODS

This scoping review was conducted following the preferred reporting items for systematic reviews and meta-analysis extension for scoping reviews (PRISMA-ScR) guidelines.[39]

Search Strategies

Bibliographic searches were performed in PubMed, EMBASE, Cochrane Library, and Google Scholar for articles published before September 1st, 2021. In PubMed/Medline, Medical Subject

---

Box 1
Abbreviations

AI	Artificial Intelligence	ML	Metabolic Heterogeneity
CNN	Convolutional Neural Network	MTV	Metabolic Tumor Volume
DL	Deep Learning	NHL	Non-Hodgkin Lymphoma
DLBCL	Diffuse Large B-cell Lymphoma	NM	Nuclear Medicine
FP	False Positive	OS	Overall Survival
FN	False Negative	PFS	Progression-Free Survival
^{18}F-FDG	^{18}F-fluorodeoxyglucose	RF	Random Forest
HL	Hodgkin Lymphoma	SVM	Support Vector Machine
HiNA	High Normal Activity	TLG	Total Lesion Glycolysis
ML	Machine Learning	TMTV	Total Metabolic Tumor Volume

Headings (MESH) in all fields were searched for "Artificial Intelligence" (or Deep Learning or Machine Learning or Support Vector Machine (SVM) or Convolutional Neural Network (CNN) or Artificial Neural Network (ANN)) and "Positron Emission Tomography" (PET or PET-CT or PET-MR) and "lymphoma." The remainder of the studies were identified through manual searches of bibliographies and citations until no further relevant studies were found. One investigator (N.H) independently screened titles and abstracts and selected relevant citations for full-text review.

Eligibility and Exclusion Criteria

Studies that reported the diagnostic measurement of an AI/ML/DL algorithm to investigate any type of lymphoma using PET were sought. Articles were excluded if the study was not written in English. All the nonpeer-reviewed material such as nonpeer-reviewed conference articles and archives as well as studies irrelevant to applications of AI in lymphoma PET imaging were excluded. Studies that comprised a development or assessment of an AI algorithm on PET imaging in human populations diagnosed with lymphoma or any subtypes were eligible. The search included all primary articles since the beginning of 2009.

Data Extraction and Analysis

Key study characteristics (such as tasks/models, methods, results) for selected papers are summarized. According to the specification of the task— segmentation, classification, prognostication— the articles were categorized (**Table 1**). The details of methods and the AI architecture proposed were recorded. Study characteristics extracted were the purpose of the article, authors, year of publication, AI model design, proposed AI application, and ground truth (GT). Also extracted were information regarding sample size, training sample, testing, and validation samples as well as figures

of merit (FoM) such as specificity, sensitivity, dice similarity coefficient (DSC), and Hausdorff distance (HD) (**Table 2**) depending on the proposed application of the algorithm (see **Table 1**).

RESULTS
Search Results

We retrieved 1122 documents from initial searches; 1089 met the eligibility criteria for the title and abstract review and 75 met the final criteria for full-text review as shown in **Fig. 2**. After the screening process, 20 articles were included; these covered both the AI development and clinical assessment fields (see **Fig. 2**). All 20 papers examined AI applications in lymphoma PET imaging. These studies either developed an original model or evaluated a previously proposed AI model to perform detection, classification, segmentation, characterization, prediction/prognosis, or a combination of these tasks on PET/CT or PET images. The definition of the aforementioned tasks is provided in "Terminology for Elucidating Algorithm Aim" under the Results section.

Overview: Key Literature Characteristics

In this section, we will systematically examine how each study performed these tasks assigned to AI. We first identify the reported AI task (detection, segmentation, classification, radiophenomics), then determine the model's input and output for that specific task. For instance, regarding the detection task, we identify the AI's input, which is frequently in the form of pixels, and the output would be detecting areas suspicious for cancer (high FDG uptake). **Table 1** summarized the results of each study as it pertains to the proposed model (such as CNN, ANN, and so forth), task (classification, detection, segmentation, prediction, prognosis, and so forth), FoM provided specific to each task (see **Table 2**), and the GT definition for evaluating the results. Based on the current

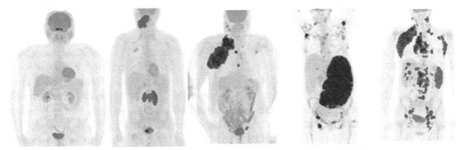

Fig. 1. Examples of different sizes and distributions of tumor in 5 patients with diffuse large B-cell lymphoma[25]. (*From* Barrington SF, Meignan M. Time to Prepare for Risk Adaptation in Lymphoma by Standardizing Measurement of Metabolic Tumor Burden. *J Nucl Med.* 2019;60(8):1096-1102: under Open Access Creative Commons License https://creativecommons.org/licenses/by/4.0/)

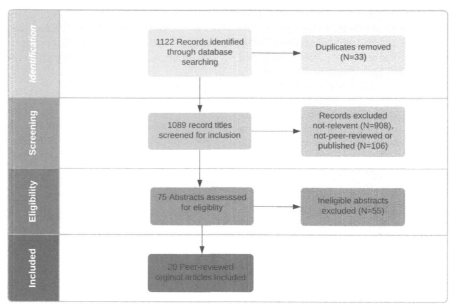

Fig. 2. Demonstrates the summary of the literature search strategies and the results at each stage.

literature, the 2 main applications for radiomics in lymphoma: distinguishing lymphomas as separate form other tumors, and prediction or prognostication of lymphomas.[40]

Appropriate GT and label for an imaging AI application are highly related to AI objectivity. PET images are often visually analyzed, and this may often lead to high inter-and intraoperator variability. Thus, it is a challenge to define optimal GT for datasets to be used for AI training, and a suboptimal GT will hamper the predictive accuracy of the model.[41,42] For these reasons, here, we present a definition of GT specific to the AI objective as provided by each of the studies (see **Table 1**).

Terminology for Elucidating Algorithm Aim

Detection

Detection as a task refers to locating an area within an image that contains an object of interest with a stated level of certainty. This task often involves a combination of localization and some level of classification, finding a nodule in the lung is an example of a detection task. As referred to in **Table 1**, the input to an AI algorithm that performs detection should be a type of image (pixel/voxel), and the output should also be a location containing the object of desire.[24] For example, Bi and colleagues use 3D WB, coronal ^{18}F-FDG PET with CT slices (2 channels) as an input to detect individual regions of High Normal Activity (HiNA) (also referred to as sites of FDG excretion and physiologic FDG uptake (sFEPU) by Bi and colleagues)

using their multi-scale superpixel encoding CNN model.[24] In addition, Sibille and colleagues proposed a model that automatically detects HiNA and lesions suspicious of lung cancer and lymphoma lesions[50] (**Fig. 3**). Similarly, Wiseman and colleagues proposed a 3D DeepMedic model that implicitly learned information about the HiNA regions during model training achieving 85% detection TPR on average.[49] Due to the increased heterogeneity of HiNA regions below the diaphragm (for example in bladder, kidney, and ureter) this model performed better above the diaphragm than the below.[49]

In this scoping review, we found 7 studies for lymphoma lesion detection in PET/CT imaging (see **Table 1** - Yuan and colleagues (2021),[46] Zhou and colleagues (2021)[38] Weisman and colleagues (2021),[61] Sibille and colleagues (2020),[50] Hu and colleagues (2019),[56] Yu and colleagues (2018),[57] Bi and colleagues (2017)[24]).

Segmentation

Delineation of the boundary of an *object of interest* given its location is referred to as segmentation.[62] Accurate segmentation of lymphoma is an important task as it permits the extraction of both lesion-level (such as SUV_{max} and SUV_{mean}) and whole-body quantitative metrics (such as TMTV) which provide important predictive and prognostic information.[63,64] The image input data for the segmentation task can be as large as a 3D WB PET image or as small as a group of pixels.

Table 1
Summary of characteristics of selected literature

Author (Year)	Tasks Performed	Task Specific Input/Out	FoM	Details (Model-Related)	Details (Ground Truth, Sample Size)
CNN Models					
Pinochet et al,[43] 2021	Classification (Radiophenomics)	Input: 2D; WB; axial/sagittal/coronal 18F-FDG PET slice Output: slice-level 3-category classification (Benign, Malignant, Equivocal lymph nodes)	AUC = 0.62	Evaluate PET Assisted Reporting System (PARS-PET) by Siemens on DLBCL patients CNN model: PET Assisted Reporting System (PARS)	GT: 2 NM physicians segmented DLBCL lesions Testing: 119 patients (research cohort) + 430 patients (routine cohort)
	Segmentation	Input 1: 2D; WB; axial/sagittal/coronal 18F-FDG PET slices Input 2: detection map provided by PARS prototype software Output: 2D; segmented lesions with borders masked on PET slice	DSC = 0.65 (research cohort) DSC = 0.48 (routine cohort) TMTV ICC = 0.68 (research cohort) TMTV ICC = 0.61 (routine cohort)		
	Statistical Classification (Prediction/Prognosis)	Input: TMTV value from WB PET Image (Method: TMTV thresholding) Output: Prognostication (PFS, OS)	OS Hazard ratio = 2.4 PFS Hazard ratio = 2.1		
Sadik et al,[44] 2021	Classification (Radiophenomics)	Input: 2D; WB; sagittal/coronal/axial; 18F-FDG PET slice and CT slice (2 channel input) Output: Pt-level 4-class classification [high vs low diffuse bone marrow uptake] x [presence vs absence of focal lesion])	PA = 0.85 Kappa = 0.41	Highlight foci of skeletal and bone marrow uptake in Hodgkin's Lymphoma patients CNN model: based on RECOMIA prototype	GT: 10 independent experienced NM clinicians classified lesions Training: 156 patients Testing: 49 patients

(continued on next page)

Table 1
(continued)

Author (Year)	Tasks Performed	Task Specific Input/Out	FoM	Details (Model-Related)	Details (Ground Truth, Sample Size)
Guo et al,[45] 2021	Characterization (deepRadiomics)	Input: Manually segmented lesions (3D; axial; 1 channel; Rank 3 Tensor [combined ^{18}F-FDG PET and CT]) Output: 16 x 8 feature maps, total of 128 features	AUC = 0.88 (for PSI) PSI-based PFS prediction: Spec = 0.80, Sens = 0.83, Accuracy = 0.85	Extraction of feature maps surrogates for prognosis prediction in nasal ENKTL. Proposes PSI be a predictor of PFS; PSI is the ratio of the PPV to NPV Model: Weakly supervised deep learning (WSDL) based on Residual Network-18 (ResNet-18) and PNU classifier.	GT: 1 NM physician (15 y experience) segmented nasal ENKTL lesions Training sample: 64 patients Testing: 20 patients
	Statistical Classification (Radiophenomics)	Input: Prediction similarity index (PSI) derived from image features Output: Relapsed vs nonrelapsed classes for ENKTL			
Yuan et al,[46] 2021	Detection	Input: 2D; axial; neck/chest/abdomen; ^{18}F-FDG PET slice and CT slices (2 channel input) Output: 2D; axial; detection map with lesions in rectangular boxes	Sens (chest) = 83.2%, Spec (chest) = 99.75%, Accuracy = 99.5%	Hybrid Learning for feature fusion of DLBCL Segmentation Hybrid CNN models can create feature fusion maps and quantify the spatial contributions of each modality. PET and CT image feature-based hybrid learning CNN model architecture	GT: 1 physician manually segmented DLBCL lesions Training and Validation: Cross-validation using a dataset with total of 1242 PET-CT slice pairs from 45 PET-CT samples
	Segmentation	Input 1: 2D; axial; neck/chest/abdomen; ^{18}F-FDG PET slice and CT slices (2 channel input) Input 2: Detection map results Output: lesions border segmentation map	DSC = 0.73, MHD = 4.38 mm		

Zhou et al,[38] 2021	Detection	Input: 2D; axial/coronal; WB ^{18}F-FDG PET/CT (1 channel) or ^{18}F-FDG PET alone Output: Map of detected mantle cell lymphoma	Sens = 0.88 FP/patient = 15 For outside-institute patients Sens = 0.84 FP/patient = 14	Xception-based U-Net Localized lesions on PET/CT and labeled each pixel as MCL or not MCL. High FPs/patient needs to be corrected through physicians' inspection	GT: 3 NM physicians each with more than 10 y of experience identified and contoured MCL lesions Training: 110 patients Validation: 5-fold cross-validation Testing: 32 outside-institute patients
	End-to-end Segmentation	Input: 3D; coronal; WB; ^{18}F-FDG PET and 3D CT 2 separate channels Output: Mask of segmented lesions with calculated TMTV on 18F-FDG PET/CT	JSC = 0.60, DSC = 0.73 Predicted TMTV R = 0.88, 0.82 in first cohort, second cohort, respectively	Fully automatic segmentation of DLBCL lesions for total MTV prediction – 3D [18]FDG-PET/CT	GT: masks were manually obtained with 41% SUV_{max} adaptive thresholding. TMTV protocol from LIFEx used for VOI semiautomatically segmented. 2 experienced physicians reviewed clustering results and remove physiologic uptakes Training: 639 patients Validation: 5-fold cross-validation Testing: 94 patients

(continued on next page)

Table 1
(continued)

Author (Year)	Tasks Performed	Task Specific Input/Out	FoM	Details (Model-Related)	Details (Ground Truth, Sample Size)
Weisman et al,[48] 2020	End-to-end Segmentation	Input: 3D; coronal; WB; ^{18}F-FDG PET and CT image (2 channels) (Hidden input 2: integrated detection of lymph node map by DeepMedic) Output: Map of masked segmented lesions	DSC = 0.86	Measures PET imaging features in pediatric lymphoma PET/CT scans in a fully-automated fashion. Model: an ensemble of 3 DeepMedic	GT: 1 NM physician with 11 yrs of experience segmented and determined malignancy status at lymph nodes Training/validation: 80 patients Testing: 20 patients
	Characterization (Radiomics)	Input: 3D; coronal; WB; PET-CT slices with segmented lesions Output: SUV_{max}, MTV, TLG, SA/MTV, measure of disease spread ($Dmax_{patient}$)	R = 0.95		
Weisman et al[49] (with Kieler) 2020	Detection	Input: 2D; coronal; WB; ^{18}F-FDG PET slice (from PET/CT) Output: Lymph nodes probability map contoured	TPR = 0.85 4 FP/patient	Automated detection of diseased lymph node Burden in lymphoma patients – PET/CT Model: an ensemble of 3 DeepMedics	GT: 1 NM physician with 11 yrs of experience segmented and determined malignancy status at lymph nodes Training: 58 patients Testing: 90 patients
Sibille et al,[50] 2020	Detection (localization + 4-category classification suspicious vs nonsuspicious for lung cancer or lymphoma)	Input: 2D; coronal; WB; ^{18}F-FDG PET slice fused with CT, MIP, anatomic atlas Output: Map of detected lesions classified under [suspicious or nonsuspicious] x [lung cancer or lymphoma]	For Localization: Sens = 0.81, Spec = 0.97, accuracy = 0.96 (for body parts), 0.87 (for region), 0.81 (for subregion) For Classification: FP = 1.47 (96 of 65), FN = 1.76 (of 65), AUC = 0.98	^{18}F-FDG Uptake Classification in Lymphoma and Lung Cancer – using CT, PET, MIP, and atlas information	GT: 2 NM physicians annotated and segmented foci with increased ^{18}F-FDG uptake specified the anatomic location and classified. Training: 380 patients Validation:126 patients Testing: 123 patients

Study	Task	Input/Output	Metrics	Purpose/Model details	Ground truth/Validation
Li et al,[51] 2019	End-to-end Segmentation	Input 1: 2D; axial; WB; ^{18}F-FDG PET and CT slices (6 channels) (Hidden input: single pixel probability map of lesions) Output: segmentation map of lymphoma	DSC = 0.73, Precision = 0.70, Recall = 0.81	End-to-end lymphoma segmentation – WB PET/CT Model details: DenseX-Net	GT: 3 clinicians delineated images, then verified and revised by 1 nuclear medicine expert Validation: 5-fold cross-validation Testing: 80 patients
Sadik,[52] 2019	Segmentation	Input 1: 2D axial/ sagittal, coronal CT (3 channels) Input 2: manually detected liver and aorta Output: Segmentation of liver and aorta	DSC = 0.95	Automated calculation of liver and aortic ^{18}F-FDG uptake levels to serve as a reference for therapy response classification in HL and NHL CT segmentation maps were resampled to fit the ^{18}F-FDG-PET image in order to calculate SUVmedian Model details: CNN adopted from Goodfellow et al,[53] 2016	GT: 2 radiologists segmented images Training: 80 patients Validation: 6 patients
Bi et al,[24] 2017	Detection	Input: 3D; WB; coronal; ^{18}F-FDG PET with CT slices (2 channels) Output: 3D; WB; coronal; map of sFEPU regions (ie, Left, and right kidneys, bladder, brain, heart)	DSC: 0.92	Automatic detection of superpixel regions of FDG uptake of lymphoma regions Model details: MSE + CFSC	GT: 1 experienced operator manually identified ROI using PERCIST thresholding and the diagnostic report of PET-CT scan Training: 1.5 million nonmedical images, validated: 50,000 nonmedical images Testing: 11 patients

(continued on next page)

Table 1
(continued)

Author (Year)	Tasks Performed	Task Specific Input/Out	FoM	Details (Model-Related)	Details (Ground Truth, Sample Size)
Classic Machine Learning Models					
Annunziata et al,[22] 2021	Statistical Classification (Prediction/Prognosis)	Input: Deauville Score, qPET, MTV_0, slope (slope of a linear function of MTV) features from 3D; axial/coronal end-of-treatment than beginning-of-treatment ^{18}F-FDG PET and CT slices Output: Patient-level 2-class prediction (relapse vs progression)	PPV = 0.55, NPV = 0.83 (for DS 4–5) PPV = 0.89, NPV = 0.82 (for positive qPET) R = 0.63 (for ANN)	Assess the prognostic capacity of post-treatment ^{18}F-FDG-PET/CT in DLBCL patients Model details: multi-regression model, ANN	GT: 2 NM physicians independently evaluated using a dedicated fusion and display software Training: 26 patients Testing: 11 patients K-fold cross-validation
Lippi et al,[54] 2020	Classification (Radiophenomic)	Input: 3D; WB; coronal ^{18}F-FDG PET slices Output: Patient-level 4-class classification of malignant lymphoma (DLBCL, HL, follicular and mantle cell lymphoma)	Sens = 0.97, PPV = 0.94	Texture analysis and classification of malignant lymphoma Model details: SVM + RF	GT: 1 NM physician with 5 y of experience extracted VOIs using a 40%-threshold of SUV_{max} Evaluation: leave-one-out procedure, whereby each patient was used, in turn, as the test set, and all the other patients constituted the training set.

Mayerhoefer et al,[55] 2019	Statistical Classification (Prediction/Prognosis)	Input: TMTVs, SUV_mean, TLG, entropy, and 15 other textural radiomic features Output: Patient-level 3-category metabolic risk (low, intermediate, high) of progression	AUC = 0.72	Radiomic features for prediction of outcome in mantle cell lymphoma International prognostic indices for MCL = MIPI and MIPI-b Model details: Multilayer perceptron feed-forward ANN	GT: TMTV protocol used to semiautomatically construct with 41% SUV_max threshold Training: 75 patients Testing: 32 patients
Hu et al,[56] 2019	Detection	Input: 3D; WB; coronal/axial/sagittal ^{18}F-FDG PET slices and CT slices (2 Channels) Output: 3D probability map of the segmented lesion (normal organ and tumors)	Sens = 0.80, DSC = 0.59	Physical spatial characteristics of the lesions along with prior knowledge were used to optimize the technique. Density-based spatial clustering of applications with noise (DBSCAN)	GT: Segmentation ground truth obtained by 41% SUV max thresholding, no information on the physicians Testing: 48 patients
	Segmentation	Input1: 3D; WB; coronal/axial/sagittal ^{18}F-FDG PET slices and CT slices (2 Channels) Input2: Detection results Output: 3D, coronal/axial/sagittal slice with segmented normal organ and tumor lesions.	D_{ref} (DSC) = 0.74, D_{global} = 0.50, Volume_sup = .39		

(continued on next page)

Table 1
(continued)

Author (Year)	Tasks Performed	Task Specific Input/Out	FoM	Details (Model-Related)	Details (Ground Truth, Sample Size)
Yu et al,[57] 2018	Detection	Input: 2D; WB; coronal/axial/sagittal ^{18}F-FDG PET slices and CT slices (2 Channels) Output: probability map of detected lymphoma lesions	Sens = 1.0	Semiautomatic lymphoma detection and segmentation	GT: 1 physician contoured images Training/validation: 11 patients
	Segmentation	Input1: PET/CT images with physiologic hypermetabolic organs removed. Input2: Detection results Output: Border mask segmentation visualized on software on axial, sagittal, and coronal	DSC = 0.84	Model details: FC-CRF	
Grossiord et al,[58] 2017	Classification (Radiophenomics)	Input: 2D; coronal; ^{18}F-FDG PET and CT slices (2 channel) Output: slice-level 3-class classification (Organ, tumor, nonrelevant)	Sens = 0.65, Spec = 0.92, Accuracy = 0.86	Automated 3D lymphoma lesion segmentation - PET/CT Model details: PET/CT feature extraction, random forest classification, mixed spatial-spectral space of component-trees	GT: 1 expert manually expert segmentation at 41% SUV_{max} Training/validation : 43 patients Leave-one patient-out cross-validation for classification task
	Segmentation	Input 1: 2D; WB; coronal ^{18}F-FDG PET and CT slices (2 channel) Input 2: single cluster representative of each lesion Output: 2D, WB, coronal segmentation map	DSC = 0.75		

Desbordes et al,[59] 2016	End-to-end Segmentation	Input: 2D; WB; coronal/ axial/sagittal PET slices and CT slices (2 Channels) (Hidden input: single pixel representative each lesion (based on automatic seed definition)) Output: 2D, WB, lesion segmentation map	DSC = 0.80	Cellular automata define tumor seed within ROI to obtain final segmentation by iterative growth. Model details: auto-initialization cellular automata	GT: 1 NM physician manually selected and segmented the ROI Testing: 12 patients
Lartizien et al,[60] 2014	Classification (Radiophenomics)	Input: 3D; supraclavicular; axial ^{18}F-FDG PET slices and CT slice images Output: 2-class classification (benign vs cancer)	AUC = 0.91	SVM classifier applied on 12 most discriminant 1st and 2nd order textural features derived from the registered PET and contrast CT images	Evaluation set: 156 lymphomatous and 32 suspicious 25 (11 males and 14 females) baselines with B-cell lymphoma or HL.

Abbreviations: ^{18}F-FDG, ^{18}F-fluorodeoxyglucose; ANN, artificial neural network; AUC, area under curve; CFSC, class-driven feature-selection & classification; DLBCL, diffuse large B-cell lymphoma; DSC, dice similarity coefficient; ENKTL, extranodal NK/T cell lymphoma; nasal type; FC-CRF, fully connected conditional random fields; FCN, fully convolutional network; FoM, figures of merit; FROC, free-response receiver operating characteristic; ICC, intraclass correlation coefficient; JSC, Jaccard similarity coefficient; MH, metabolic hetero-geneity; MHD, modified Hausdorff distance; MIP, maximum intensity projection; MLP, multilayer perception; MM, multi-regression model, MSE, multi-scale super pixel-based encod-ing; MTV, metabolic tumor volume; NHL, non-Hodgkin lymphoma; NM, nuclear medicine; NPV, negative predictive value; OS, overall survival; PA, percentage agreement; PERCIST, PET response criteria in solid tumors; PFS, progression-free survival; PPV, positive predictive value, PSI, prediction similarity index; R, Pearson correlation coefficient; RF, random forest; ROI, region of interest; Sens, sensitivity, sFEPU, sites of FDG excretion and physiologic FDG uptake; Spec, Specificity; SVM, Support Vector Machine, TLG, Tumor lesion glycolysis; TMTV, total Metabolic Tumor volume.

Table 2
The mathematical definitions for the evaluation metrics used in the reviewed articles

Evaluation Measure	Mathematical Definition
Sensitivity	$\dfrac{TP}{TP+FN}$
Specificity	$\dfrac{TN}{TN+FP}$
PPV or Precision	$\dfrac{TP}{TP+FP}$
Dice similarity coefficient (DSC) (Synonyms: Dice similarity index, Sorensen–Dice coefficient, F1-Score, Sorensen–Dice index, Dice's Coefficient)	$\dfrac{2TP}{2TP+FP+FN}$
Dice $_{Ref}$ (equivalent to Dice) F(M) is defined as the number of elements in set M. G = ground truth regions composed of g_i voxels. B = set of detected lymphoma regions consisting of b_i voxels.[56]	$\dfrac{2F(B\cap G)}{F(G)+F(B)}$
Dice $_{Global}$[56] Same as the Dice$_{Ref}$ reference but includes false-positive regions. S is the set of all detected false regions.	$\dfrac{2F(B\cap G)}{F(G)+F(B)+F(S)}$
Volume $_{sup}$[56] For evaluating the volume of the false-positive region.	$\dfrac{F(S)}{F(B\cup S)}$
Jaccard similarity coefficient (JSC)	$\dfrac{TP}{TP+FP+FN}$

The segmentation task which is the combination of localization and pixel/voxel level classification often has two inputs (1) the image that contains an *object of interest* (input 1) (2) the location of that *object of interest* with a certain level of certainty (input 2). Input 2 can either be a probability map of coarse region of the lesions, or single-pixel locations representative of the lesion locations which can be derived from a localization or a detection task. The *output* of segmentation is an image that encodes the membership of each voxel to the *object of interest* (this output can be referred to as a segmentation map).

The second input for the tumor segmentor can be entered manually (eg, Sadik (2019)[52]) or automatically (eg, Yuan and colleagues)[46] into the system. In case of automatic input, the detection probability map results can be fed into the algorithm. This can be called a *cascaded approach* whereby all of the steps are performed separately and sequentially by one or several neural networks (**Fig. 4**). These techniques often divide the segmentation process into detection, and segmentation phases and provide specific evaluation metrics for each step along the way.

In this scoping review, six studies performed the segmentation task (see **Table 1** - Pinochet and colleagues (2021)[43] Yuan and colleagues (2021)[46] Sadik (2019)[52] Hu and colleagues (2019)[56] Yu and colleagues (2018)[57] Grossiord and colleagues (2017).[58])

End-to-end segmentation
When the segmentation task is done in one step, we use the term end-to-end segmentation in which case the only input is the image data. These approaches optimize for efficiency and performance in terms of memory consumption and in case of limited access to well-annotated training data.[65] An example, Weisman and colleagues proposed an end-to-end segmentation model that receives WB ^{18}F-FDG PET and CT image through 2 channels and without an additional detection step, the CNN is able to provide a map of masked segmented lymphoma lesions with DSC of 0.86 (**Fig. 5**).[48]

In this review, there were 4 studies that performed the end-to-end lesion segmentation task (see **Table 1** - Blanc-Durand and colleagues (2020),[47] Weisman and colleagues (2020),[48] Li and colleagues (2019),[51] and Desbordes and colleagues (2016)[59]).

Classification
Through reviewing the literature, we recognized 2 distinct usages of the word classification. To avoid ambiguity, we have to clarify these terms here: in a mathematical and statistical context, categorization of members of a set to various classes is defined as "classification." This is a broad meaning of this term, and we refer to this as "statistical classification." However, in computer vision, classification has a narrower meaning. It refers to the categorization of an image. We refer to this meaning as "image classification." For example, we refer to the process of using radiomic feature inputs to assign patients to different diagnostic or prognostic groups by the term "statistical classification" (Refer to Section "Prediction and Prognosis" under Results

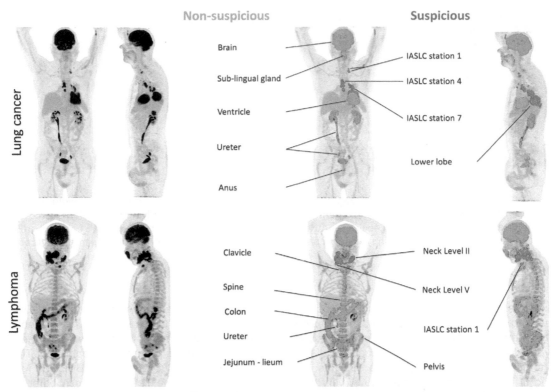

Fig. 3. Maximum intensity projection ^{18}F-FDG PET/CT images were processed in 2 patients using the constructed CNN. The test data consists of patients with both lung cancer and lymphoma; the detected lesions are color coded accordingly. IASLC is the abbreviation for the International Association for the Study of Lung Cancer. (*From* Sibille L, Seifert R, Avramovic N, et al. 18F-FDG PET/CT Uptake Classification in Lymphoma and Lung Cancer by Using Deep Convolutional Neural Networks. Radiology. 2020;294(2):445-452; with permission.)

section). For example, Annunziata and colleagues[22] used image features such as Deauville Score, qPET, MTV_0 from end-of-treatment ^{18}F-FDG PET, and CT to classify the prognosis of patients into "relapse" or "progression" classes. In contrast, the process of categorizing an image input (such as the axial slice of the PET) to normal versus abnormal is "image classification." For

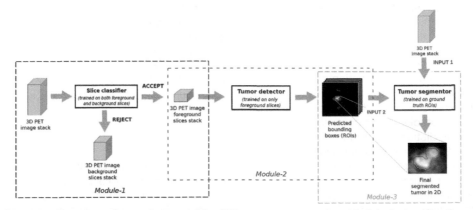

Fig. 4. Schematic of a proposed cascaded model for PET tumor segmentation; Module 1, classifies the axial slices to suspicious and non-suspicious ones; Module 2, detects the lymphoma lesions in axial slices that are a candidate by Module 1. In Module 3, the 3D PET image and detection results are given to the tumor segmentation algorithm to segment the lesions inside the bounding boxes provided by Module 2.

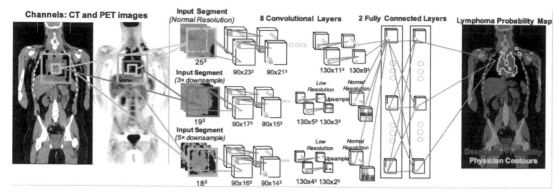

Fig. 5. CT and coronal PET multicenter images are input to 3 segment layers, there are then 8 convolution layers and two fully connected layers that subsequently generate a probability map for lymphoma lesions as shown in purple. (*From* Weisman AJ, Kim J, Lee I, et al. Automated quantification of baseline imaging PET metrics on FDG PET/CT images of pediatric Hodgkin lymphoma patients. *EJNMMI Phys.* 2020;7(1):76: under Open Access Creative Commons License http://creativecommons.org/licenses/by/4.0/.)

example, Lippi and colleagues used a machine-learning algorithm that classified the lesions within the image into 4 malignant lymphoma subtypes: DLBCL, HL, follicular and mantle cell lymphomas.[54] Radiomics signatures such as PET and CT textural features have shown very good performance to classify the disease sites from physiologic uptake sites and inflammatory non-lymphomatous sites. For instance, to classify an ^{18}F-FDG avid lesion (benign vs malignant), Lartizien and colleagues developed an SVM and Random Forest (RF) model based on 12 different radiomic features extracted from PET and CT scans achieving Area Under the Curve (AUC) of 0.91[60].

In this scoping review, there were 5 studies that performed image classification (see **Table 1.**— Pinochet and colleagues (2021),[43] Sadik and colleagues (2021),[44] Guo and colleagues (2021),[45] Lippi and colleagues (2019),[54] Grossiord and colleagues (2017),[58] and Lartizien and colleagues (2014).[60]

Prediction and prognosis

Recurrence is common in patients with HL and NHL, emphasizing the importance of risk stratification, prognostication, and relapse prediction based on PET studies. In the context of this paper, the task of prediction and prognosis of lymphoma based on PET imaging is performed by *statistical classification*. The inputs in statistical classification are radiomic features (eg, SUV, TMTV, TLG, entropy among others). These inputs are used to inform the output in the form of a prognostic or predictive classification.[65]

Baseline TMTV can be used for risk stratification and be a prognostic factor in a range of

lymphomas (DLBCL, primary mediastinal B-cell lymphoma (PMBCL) and HL).[11,66] This is exemplified by Vercellino and colleagues, whereby the authors analyzed the prognostic capability of TMTV in patients aged 60 to 80 with DLBCL and found that a high baseline TMTV indicates poorer PFS and OS.[66]

In addition to the usage of a singular radiomic feature to predict and prognose lymphoma, some studies may combine various radiomic features to perform the same task. Mayerhoefer and colleagues used both the maximal standardized uptake value (SUV$_{max}$) and entropy to predict survival in mantle cell lymphoma (MCL).[22,43,55] Entropy is a measure of glucose metabolism heterogeneity within the TMTV.[55] Demonstrating the concept of combination of radiomic features to predict and prognose, Mayerhoefer and colleagues, used entropy (heterogeneity of glucose metabolism) as well as TMTV and SUV$_{max}$ for the prediction and prognosis of PFS in mantle cell lymphoma patients with 0.72 AUC.[55]

In this scoping review, we found 3 studies that performed the statistical classification of lymphoma (see **Table 1.** Pinochet and colleagues, Annunziata and colleagues, Mayerhoefer and colleagues[22,43,55])

DISCUSSION

The major objective of this study is to review recent papers in the field of artificial intelligence-based PET medical imaging in lymphoma. According to our findings, the most prevalent uses of artificial intelligence in lymphoma PET imaging are presently focused on tumor burden evaluation (detection, segmentation, and advanced quantification of lesions). In our discussion, we focus on two key themes derived from our research findings. First, we review the implications for the clinical transition of AI-based applications in lymphoma patient care. Next, we cover some critical concepts that clinicians should consider when evaluating and validating AI algorithms. In addition, we offer our thoughts on the field's future directions.

Clinical Implementation of Artificial Intelligence in the Management of Lymphoma

Currently, a prominent objective in lymphoma PET image quantification is the evaluation of disease burden by TLG and TMTV, which requires the detection and segmentation of all lesions.[67,68] In this workflow, a major bottleneck toward improved prognostic pipelines and treatment planning is the segmentation.[51,69] This is in part due to the time-consuming task of manual segmentation and a high degree of intra- and interobserver variability.[70,71]

AI approaches can help by: (1) Automated detection and segmentation (fully-automated) and [32,58,72] (2) user detection/selection of the lesion followed by AI-based segmentation (semi-automated). A clear advantage of a fully automated AI model is that it can further enhance the workflow without requiring the nuclear radiologist to identify each lesion separately. Given the extent of lymphomatous involvement, individual identification of each lesion could be time-consuming, and unlikely feasible in the routine workflow given clinical demands and traditionally available resources. A few studies carried out a fully automatic disease burden assessment of lymphoma on PET images (see **Table 1**- Pinochet and colleagues,[43] Bi and colleagues,[24] Li and colleagues,[51] Blanc-Durand and colleagues[47]). For example, Grossiord and colleagues used RF classifier and morphologic hierarchy to first extract PET and CT image features to classify lesions into 3 categories: organ, tumor, and nonrelevant. Then, they automatically segment lesions into the tumor category.[58] Although fully automated models can remove a layer of physician lesion identification from the workflow, semiautomated models may provide other benefits in terms of accuracy or precision. Human involvement in semiautomatic methods manifests in 2 ways: (1) Presegmentation human-based lesion detection and identification + automatic segmentation of the identified lesion (2) Automatic detection and segmentation of lesions with high false-positive rate and reliance on human

agents to select the real lesions and discard the false-positives. As an example of the human selection of real lesions and deletion of false-positives, Yu and colleagues[57] manually identified lesions of true lymphoma after all possible detected lesions were automatically segmented.[57]

The biodistribution of ^{18}F-FDG creates regions with HiNA (for example in kidneys, bladder, brain, and heart) which can cause inaccurate AI-based identification and segmentation of lymphoma lesions. However, to improve the performance of a model one may attempt to exclude HiNA regions from the scene before the process of lesion detection. This may be conducted manually or automatically as a pre or postprocessing step.[51,73] By removing the HiNA regions from the training data, the performance of automated AI techniques for lesion detection and segmentation can be improved. For example, Yu and colleagues used a semiautomatic approach to identify and remove HiNA regions followed by an AI algorithm to automatically detect lymphoma lesions in patients.[57] For the purpose of improving workflow and integration into clinical practice, an end-to-end lymphoma detection AI algorithm can be trained to combine the task of HiNA region identification and detection of lymphoma regions.

We previously discussed methods of lymphoma segmentation on ^{18}F-FDG PET/CT studies. Along with simplifying the clinician's workflow, automatic segmentation of lymphoma lesions can enable end-to-end prognostication and radiomic analysis of the studies to gain valuable insight into therapy augmentation, remission planning, and recurrence prediction. There are 2 avenues for downstream prediction and prognosis of lymphoma: (1) an end-to-end prognostication/prediction task (whereby the image input is processed to output a prognostication/risk stratification category directly, with no reporting of the intermediate steps; for example Sadik and colleagues),[44] or (2) a radiomic analysis based prognostication, which is carried out as a secondary step after explicit segmentation. For example, Guo and colleagues[11] employ deep radiomics by using a neural network to derive deep features. Deep features, in contrast to handcrafted features of classical radiomics, are not predefined; a CNN learns features of interest depending on the task at hand and the input images. Automatically segmented lesions can also be entered into a classic radiomics pipeline to derive handcrafted features such as SUV, volume, or entropy. These features are predefined by formulas and can be statistically analyzed to derive prognoses or a risk stratification schema. A range of studies showcasing classification, prognostication, and prediction based on ^{18}F-FDG-PET radiomic features is presented in **Table 3**.

Important Considerations for Evaluating and Validating Artificial Intelligence in Lymphoma Positron Emission Tomography

The transition of AI-based technologies to patient care requires important considerations that are both general for any AI algorithm and specific to lymphoma. In addition to the accuracy of the lesion detection and segmentation, it is very important to report the amount of time clinicians should dedicate to verify and correct model outcomes. Lumped sensitivity and specificity for lesion detection are not reflective of clinical significance as some lesions are much more important than others and "critical misses" are not tolerable. In both detection and segmentation tasks, missed lesions occur particularly for the interim scans with shrunk tumors or patients with smaller lesions. TMTV, as the only figure of merit for the assessment of detection/segmentation, may undermine the smaller missed lesions. To address this shortcoming, additional performance evaluation measures such as the D_{max} and MH should be used to define a task-specific composite FoM. Weisman and colleagues characterized the results of their end-to-end segmentation using SUVmax, MTV, TLG, SA/MTV, D_{max} to depict a well-rounded assessment of the CNN performance.[48]

As demonstrated in **Table 1**, the studies use a range of different methods to determine their GT based on which the AI algorithm is tested. Therefore, a degree of uncertainty is expected due to this nonuniformity.[92] A standardized approach for GT determination must be sought as it can be less user-dependent and capable of constructing generalizable algorithms.[49]

Future Directions

After a review of current trends in AI applications in the PET imaging of lymphoma, we aim to place a special focus on describing likely future directions in this field. The discussion related to the future directions is primarily aimed at depicting the potential clinical utility of AI in the management of lymphoma with ^{18}F-FDG-PET imaging.

From spatial domain to spatiotemporal realm
Current AI-based methods rarely use prior images in their models. This is counterintuitive for clinicians who consider prior images as one of the most important sources of information.[93–95] In clinical practice, temporal changes in a lesion may provide much more useful information than

imaging features of a lesion in one study. As an example, conventional PET radiomics methods usually use a single-time-point for analysis, which does not take into account the interim change of the lesions throughout the treatment process.[96] However, "Delta-radiomics"[95] appraise the change in radiomic features during or after treatment to enhance information extraction.[95,97] Several studies have shown that CT-based Delta-radiomics can be used for the prediction of lung cancer, gastric cancer, and also the detection of side effects to radiation therapy.[94,98–100] Therefore, this method will be better suited to evaluate tumor response of treatment.[56] Creation of the Delta image permits identifying any posttreatment tumor transformations.[94,101] The difference between the baseline and interim parameters may be measured (ΔSUV, ΔMTV, ΔTLG, and ΔADC) for this purpose.[102] Delta radiomics as a quantitative assessment can be used for the evaluation of the changes over time and for the prediction of treatment response earlier in the treatment course.[101] Time-interval changes in the features such as SUV_{max}, TMTV, MH, and D_{max} and the other features can be considered as the complementary important features that have not been considered before, especially for analysis of lymphoma data.

Using AI capabilities to generate and visualize Delta images will provide insight into the intralesional tumor heterogeneity, such as when a piece of a bulky tumor shrinks/improves while the other portion of the lesion grows. This capacity will be revolutionary for the detection and evaluation of tumor heterogeneity and heterogeneous response of tumor colonies to therapies. Future studies should also determine how to appropriately visualize the Delta image for better interpretability. Furthermore, the quantification of Delta images and identification of nonresponders at an earlier stage is a key direction AI-based algorithms can move toward.[103] This utility allows the optimization of treatment or biopsy of the non-responding lesion (or portion of a lesion) for new mutations. By identifying the nonresponder region of the tumor clinicians will also be able to use external beam radiation or percutaneous ablation sooner during lymphoma treatment. Recommendations for posttreatment lymphoma recurrence surveillance using AI-based PET imaging can be included in guidelines. Particularly in those with cancer remission, the Delta image could allow important insights on early and accurate detection of potential recurrence.

From data silos to large shared databases
Accessible, high-quality, and diverse imaging datasets are essential for accelerating the development

Table 3
Survey of classification, prognostication, and prediction methods based on ^{18}F-FDG-PET radiomics

Authors (Year)	Lymphoma Subtypes	Aim of Study Input	Goal	Extraction Method	Features Used	Notable Radiomic Features	Discriminator Used	Figures of Merit
Studies in which radiomic features were utilized for the classification of lymphoma								
Ou et al,[74] 2020	Breast lymphoma	Segmented breast tumor VOIs on ^{18}F-FDG-PET/CT	Differentiation (breast lymphoma vs breast carcinoma)	LifeX	First and second-order radiomic features	PETa and CTa models demonstrated great potential to differentiate in training and validation group	LDA	Not given for testing datasets
Xu et al,[75] 2019	Hepatic lymphoma	Segmented hepatic tumor VOIs on ^{18}F-FDG-PET	Differentiation (hepatic lymphoma vs HCC)	LifeX	6 image-based parameters and 39 texture features	Combination model of texture and image features had greater diagnostic capability	ROC analysis	AUC = 0.898
Ou et al,[76] 2019	Breast lymphoma	Segmented breast tumor VOIs on ^{18}F-FDG-PET/CT	Differentiation (breast lymphoma vs breast carcinoma)	LifeX	First and second-order radiomic features	Combination model of PET and CT features had greater diagnostic capability	Binary logistic regression	PET: AUC = 0.751. CT: AUC = 0.729; PET + CT: AUC = 0.771
Aide et al,[77] 2018	DLBCL	Axial skeleton segmented on ^{18}F-FDG-PET	Identify bone marrow involvement in DLBCL based on radiomic features from ^{18}F-FDG-PET	LifeX	4 first-order, 6 second-order and 11 third-order texture features	SkewnessH was most predictive of lymphoma	Linear regression, ROC analysis	AUC = 0.820
Lartizien et al,[60] 2014	All types	Segmented suspicious regions of interest on ^{18}F-FDG-PET/CT	Lymphoma vs HINA	Not reported	105 features (GLDM, GLCM, GLISZ, GLRLM, and first order)	Combination model of PET and CT features had greater diagnostic capability	SVM	Combination of CT and PET: AUC = 0.910
Studies in which radiomic features were used for the prognosis/prediction of lymphoma								
Rodriguez Taroco et al,[78] 2021	HL	Segmented tumor VOIs on ^{18}F-FDG-PET	Prediction of PFS from 18F-FDG-PET radiomic features in HL and DLBCL	Not specified	8 first-order features, 23 features from GLCM, 11 features from GLRLM, 5	PFS in patients with Deauville scores of 1, 2, 3, and X at initial PET was higher than that in patients with	Univariate and multivariate Cox regression analysis	Average PFS, for patients with Deauville 4 score, of 1120 d

(continued on next page)

Table 3
(continued)

Authors (Year)	Lymphoma Subtypes	Aim of Study		Radiomic Feature Information			Discriminator Used	Figures of Merit
		Input	Goal	Extraction Method	Features Used	Notable Radiomic Features		
					features from NGLM, 3 features from the neighborhood grey-tone difference	a Deauville score of 4		(95% CI, 229–672)
Eertink et al,[79] 2021	DLBCL	Segmented tumor VOIs on 18F-FDG-PET	Prediction of treatment outcome with first-line treatment of DLBCL from baseline 18F-FDG-PET radiomic features	RaCat	Large number of morphologic and texture features were extracted	Five models were created based on radiomic features as well as clinical predictors; combination of clinical and radiomics predictors was best	ROC analysis	Combined model: HR = 4.6 (95% CI, 2.6–7.9)
Wang et al,[80] 2020	ENKTL	Segmented tumor VOIs on 18F-FDG-PET	Identify a 18F-FDG-PET radiomics-based model for predicting PFS and OS in ENKTL	LifeX	41 features	Radiomics and metabolism-based models were combined to predict both PFS and OS	Univariate and multivariate Cox regression analysis	PFS: 0.788 (95% CI = 0.682–0.895) and 0.473 (P = .803) OS: 0.637 (95% CI = 0.488–0.786) and 0.730 (95% CI = 0.548–0.912)
Sun et al,[81] 2020	Primary gastric DLBCL	Segmented tumor VOIs on 18F-FDG-PET	Texture analysis of 18F-PET-CT scans to predict interim response after 3–4 rounds of chemotherapy in primary gastric DLBCL	In-house software	First and second-order features	Combination of SUV_{max}, volume, and entropy in one model best predicted treatment response	Mann-Whitney U	AUC = 0.915
Aide et al,[82] 2020	DLBCL	Segmented tumor VOIs on 18F-FDG-PET	Prognosticate DLBCL treated with first-line immunotherapy using radiomic features from baseline 18F-FDG-PET	LifeX	19 features	18F-FDG-PET heterogeneity of the largest lymphoma lesion is associated with 2y-event free survival (EFS)	Univariate and multivariate Cox regression analysis	EFS: HR = 7.47 (95% CI = 0.83–66.99)
Wu et al,[83] 2019	DLBCL	18F-FDG-PET/CT pre and posttreatment	Radiomics-based treatment	MATLAB	GLCM, GLRLM, GLSZM	Belief-function theory-based outcome	EK-NN and SVM	Therapy response: NS

		outcome prediction model						
Tatsumi et al,[84] 2019	FL	Segmented tumor VOIs on 18F-FDG-PET	Predict response and recurrence after therapy in FL	PETSTAT	6 texture features	low gray-level zone emphasis (LGZE) in texture features predicted complete response	Logistic regression	Therapy response: AUC = 0.720; PFS: NS
Lue et al,[85] 2019	HL	Segmented tumor VOIs on 18F-FDG-PET	18F-FDG-PET was analyzed using radiomics to predict/prognose HL	OsiriX, CGITA MATLAB	11 first-order, 39 higher-order, 400 wavelet features	Ann Arbor stage, GLRLM and SUV kurtosis were associated with PFS	Univariate and multivariate Cox regression analysis	PFS: HR = 6.640 (95% CI, 1.261–34.96; P = .026); OS: HR = 14.54 (95% CI, 1.808–117.0; P = .012)
Lue et al,[86] 2019	HL	Segmented tumor VOIs on 18F-FDG-PET	Radiomic intratumor heterogeneity in 18F-FDG-PET to predict treatment response and survival outcomes in patients with HL	OsiriX, CGITA MATLAB	7 SUV and HU, 78 second- and higher-order, 624 wavelet features	Treatment response was associated with high-intensity run emphasis (HIR) was performed on PET images and run-length nonuniformity (RLNU) of CT extracted from gray-level run-length matrix (GLRM) in high-frequency wavelets. PFS was independently associate with intensity nonuniformity (INU) of PET and wavelet short-run emphasis (SRE) of CT from GLRM and Ann Arbor stage. OS was associated with zone-size nonuniformity (ZSNU) of PET from gray-level size zone matrix (GLSZM)	Cox proportional hazards model, ROC curve, logistic regression	PET: Therapy response: OR = 36.4 (95% CI, 2.060–642.0, P = .014); PFS: HR = 9.286 (95% CI, 1.341–66.28; P = .023); OS: HR = 41.02 (95% CI, 4.206–400.1; P = .001) CT:Therapy response: OR = 30.4 (95% CI, 1.700–545.0; P = .014); PFS: HR = 18.480 (95% CI, 1.918–178.1; P = .012); OS: NS

(continued on next page)

Table 3
(continued)

Authors (Year)	Lymphoma Subtypes	Aim of Study		Radiomic Feature Information				Figures of Merit
		Input	Goal	Extraction Method	Features Used	Notable Radiomic Features	Discriminator Used	
Zhou et al,[87] 2019	Primary gastric DLBC-	Segmented tumor VOIs on ^{18}F-FDG-PET	Prediction of OS and PFS from ^{18}F-FDG-PET radiomic features in primary gastric DLBCL	LifeX	44 texture features	Kurtosis, TMTV, GLNU, and HGZE were identified as independent prognostic factors	Univariate and multivariate Cox regression analysis	PET: PFS: HR = 14.642 (95% CI, 2.661–80.549; P = .002); OS: HR = 28.685 (95% CI, 2.067–398.152; P = .012) CT: PFS: HR = 11.504 (95% CI, 1.921–68.888; P = .007); OS: HR = 11.791 (95% CI, 1.583–87.808; P = .016)
Milgrom et al,[88] 2019	Mediastinal HL	Segmented nodal disease on ^{18}F-FDG-PET/CT	Predict response to therapy in mediastinal HL	MIM, IBEX	GLCM, intensity histogram, shape	A combination model of 5 most predictive features accomplished the highest AUC (SUV$_{max}$, TMTV, inverse variance, and 2 measures of tumor heterogeneity)	ROC analysis	AUC = 0.952
Wang et al,[89] 2019	Renal/adrenal lymphoma	Segmented tumor VOIs on ^{18}F-FDG-PET	Prognose patients with primary renal lymphoma and primary adrenal lymphoma using texture features	LifeX	37 texture features	GLRLM_RLNU (gray-level co-occurrence matrix run-length nonuniformity) was most predictive of OS.	Univariate and multivariate Cox regression analysis	OS: HR = 9.016 (95% CI, 1.041–78.112; P = .046)
Parvez et al,[90] 2018	NHL	TMTV using thresholding and radiomic features	Predict response to therapy and outcome in NHL using radiomic features extracted from ^{18}F-FDG-PET/CT	LifeX	GLCM, NGLDM, GLRLM, GLZLM, indices from sphericity and histogram	GLNU correlated to DFS, and kurtosis correlated with OS	Univariate Cox regression analysis	Therapy response: NS; DFS: P = .013; OS: P = .035

Aide et al,[77] 2018	DLBCL	Axial skeleton segmented on ^{18}F-FDG-PET	Determine prognostic value of skeletal textural features in DLBCL	LifeX	4 first-order, 6 second-order and 11 third-order texture features	The only independent predictor of PFS was SkewnessH	ROC analysis	PFS: HR = 3.17 (95% CI, 1.00–10.04; P = .032)
Ben Bouallègue et al,[91] 2017	Bulky HL and NHL	Segmented tumor VOIs on ^{18}F-FDG-PET	Predict response to therapy in bulky HL and NHL	In-house software	Shape, texture features	SVM accounting for both texture and shape features achieved the highest ROC AUC	ROC analysis	AUC = 0.820

Abbreviations: ^{18}F-FDG-PET, ^{18}F-fluorodeoxyglucose-positron emission tomography; ACC, accuracy; AUC, area under the curve; DFS, disease-free survival; DLBCL, diffuse large B cell lymphoma; EFS, event-free survival; EK-NN, evidential k-NN; FL, follicular lymphoma; GLCM, grey-level co-occurrence matrix; GLRLM, grey-level run-length matrix; GLSZM, grey-level size-zone matrix; GLZLM, grey-level zone length matrix; HL, Hodgkin's lymphomas; HR, hazard ratio; LDA, linear discriminant analysis; MCL, mantle cell lymphoma; NGLDM, neighborhood grey-level different matrix; NHL, non-Hodgkin's lymphomas; NS, not significant; OR, odds ratio; OS, overall survival; PFS, progression-free survival; ROC, receiver operating characteristic; RUN, run-length matrix; SEN, sensitivity; SPE, specificity; SVM, support vector machine; TF, texture features; VOI, volume of interest.

of AI algorithms in lymphoma and successful transition of these technologies into routine clinical practice.[104] These repositories can bypass many barriers for researchers and diversify the patient population and their lymphoma subtypes, therefore, improving the generalizability of the algorithms. Especially when these datasets include multi-centric GT data and were generated by expert with varying levels of experience to recreate the heterogeneities that exist in real clinical practice rather than a controlled setting for biomedical research.

Currently, there is no centralized publicly available medical imaging data repository for lymphoma. There have, however, been minor initiatives to establish open access data sets. The Cancer Imaging Archive (TCIA) contains almost 31 million de-identified cancer medical images that are accessible to the public[105] which includes CT and ^{18}F-FDG PET studies of 155 DLBCL patients.[106] Additionally, the National Institutes of Health (NIH) has made available over 10,500 labeled CT imaging studies of 4400 different patients (DeepLesion dataset) with lung nodules, liver tumors, enlarged lymph nodes, and other critical findings throughout the body.[107] With the rapid growth of AI algorithms in lymphoma PET imaging, there is an increasing demand for institutional collaboration to enable the gathering and curation of both large data sets and labeled images necessary for the establishment of centralized yet diverse open access data repositories.

SUMMARY

Almost 35 years after the first utilization of ^{18}F-FDG PET in lymphoma,[108,109] this modality has proven its value in a wide spectrum of management from diagnosis and staging to treatment response assessment and prognostication. Alongside the significant improvement in treatment measures, from biological agents[110] to CAR-T cell therapy,[111] there have been substantial efforts to improve the quantitative aspect of ^{18}F-FDG PET to produce robust, reliable, and feasible metabolic imaging biomarkers. Establishment of PERCIST was a monumental event,[112] 2 years after universal acceptance of PET imaging for lymphoma response assessment by International Working Group (IWG).[113] ^{18}F-FDG PET was extremely successful in the elimination of "complete remission unconfirmed" (CRu) category in treatment response assessment. CRu was assigned to patients with a residual mass detected by CT after treatment that was unlikely to be malignant. Lugano classification,[1] a consensus document of the 11th International Conference on Malignant Lymphoma, reemphasized the role of ^{18}F-FDG-

PET. Advancement of biological agents underscored the importance of the "tumor flare" phenomenon (pseudo-progression) and resulted in the refinement of Lugano classification by the introduction of immune-related criteria (IRC)[114] emphasizing the importance of clinical context in the process of image interpretation and quantification.

Treatment failure is the major problem in the management of patients with lymphoma and ^{18}F-FDG-PET has been providing valuable information to predict this event[115,116] and guide the treatment (response-adapted therapy).[117,118] Furthermore, the importance of biologic heterogeneity in treatment failure[119] motivated the molecular imaging community to detect and quantify this heterogeneity using Radiomics.[119]

In spite of all these achievements, the clinical adaptation of quantitative PET-based imaging biomarkers has been limited so far. Workflow integration barriers are one of the major contributing factors. Deep learning has the potential to make this process more efficient and more precise at the same time and this will open the door for all the subsequent utilization of PET-based imaging biomarkers. But the utility of AI is not limited to lesion detection and segmentation. Almost 20 years after wide utilization of ^{18}F-FDG-PET in lymphoma, we are experiencing a major transformation powered by AI affecting the entire imaging lifecycle: from scheduling and operational tasks [Beegle and colleagues' article "Artificial Intelligence and Positron Emission Tomography Imaging Workflow: Technologists' Perspective," in this issue], to image acquisition optimization [Muhammad Nasir Ullah and Craig S. Levin's article, "Application of Artificial Intelligence (AI) in Positron Tomography (PET) instrumentation," in this issue], enhancement of image reconstruction[120] and harmonization of the images[121] toward high-throughput imaging biomarkers[122] and multi-omics data integration for prediction and prognosis [Yousefirizi and colleagues' article, "Artificial Intelligence-Based Detection, Classification and Prediction/Prognosis in PET Imaging: Towards Radiophenomics," in this issue].[123]

CLINICS CARE POINTS

- In order to efficiently extract valuable information about tumor biology from ^{18}F-FDG-PET, we need to move beyond SUV measurement. The first step in this path is detection and delineation of hypermetabolic lesions.

- AI based methods have the potential to provide clinicians with a high throughput platform to perform these steps efficiently and accurately.

- Clinicians should be aware of pearls and pitfalls of AI algorithms. Deep learning is very efficient when utilized in the correct setting and could be prone to bias and aberrant performance if used out of scope of training and testing. It is ultimately the responsibility of physicians and the healthcare system to verify the trustworthiness and reliability of AI as Medical Devices (AIMDs).

- Despite their significant advances, PET-based AI applications have had limited clinical implementation. Immaturity of PACS architecture is among the important reasons. AI orchestrators will play an important role in future of imaging workflow.

DISCLOSURE

This research was supported by the Intramural Research Program of the NIH, Clinical Center and NIDCR. The opinions expressed in this publication are the author's own and do not reflect the view of the National Institutes of Health, the Department of Health and Human Services, or the United States government.

REFERENCES

1. Cheson BD, Fisher RI, Barrington SF, et al. Recommendations for initial evaluation, staging, and response assessment of Hodgkin and non-Hodgkin lymphoma: the Lugano classification. J Clin Oncol 2014;32(27):3059–68.

2. El-Galaly TC, Hutchings M, Mylam KJ, et al. Impact of 18F-fluorodeoxyglucose positron emission tomography/computed tomography staging in newly diagnosed classical Hodgkin lymphoma: fewer cases with stage I disease and more with skeletal involvement. Leuk Lymphoma 2014;55(10): 2349–55.

3. Hutchings M, Barrington SF. PET/CT for therapy response assessment in lymphoma. J Nucl Med 2009;50(Suppl 1):21S–30S.

4. Baba S, Abe K, Isoda T, et al. Impact of FDG-PET/CT in the management of lymphoma. Ann Nucl Med 2011;25(10):701–16.

5. Meignan M, Itti E, Gallamini A, et al. FDG PET/CT imaging as a biomarker in lymphoma. Eur J Nucl Med Mol Imaging 2015;42(4):623–33.

6. Alavi A, Newberg AB, Souder E, et al. Quantitative analysis of PET and MRI data in normal aging and Alzheimer's disease: atrophy weighted total brain metabolism and absolute whole brain metabolism as reliable discriminators. J Nucl Med 1993; 34(10):1681–7.

7. Saboury B, Salavati A, Brothers A, et al. FDG PET/CT in Crohn's disease: correlation of quantitative FDG PET/CT parameters with clinical and endoscopic surrogate markers of disease activity. Eur J Nucl Med Mol Imaging 2014;41(4): 605–14.

8. Saboury B, Parsons MA, Moghbel M, et al. Quantification of aging effects upon global knee inflammation by 18F-FDG-PET. Nucl Med Commun 2016;37(3):254–8.

9. Basu S, Zaidi H, Salavati A, et al. FDG PET/CT methodology for evaluation of treatment response in lymphoma: from "graded visual analysis" and "semiquantitative SUVmax" to global disease burden assessment. Eur J Nucl Med Mol Imaging 2014;41(11):2158–60.

10. Basu S, Saboury B, Torigian DA, et al. Current evidence base of FDG-PET/CT imaging in the clinical management of malignant pleural mesothelioma: emerging significance of image segmentation and global disease assessment. Mol Imaging Biol 2011;13(5):801–11.

11. Guo B, Tan X, Ke Q, et al. Prognostic value of baseline metabolic tumor volume and total lesion glycolysis in patients with lymphoma: a meta-analysis. PLoS One 2019;14(1):e0210224.

12. Saboury B, Moghbel M, Basu S, et al. Modern Quantitative Techniques for PET/CT/MR Hybrid Imaging. In: Schaller B, ed. Molecular Imaging. IntechOpen; 2012.

13. Ceriani L, Milan L, Martelli M, et al. Metabolic heterogeneity on baseline 18FDG-PET/CT scan is a predictor of outcome in primary mediastinal B-cell lymphoma. Blood 2018;132(2):179–86.

14. Ceriani L, Gritti G, Cascione L, et al. SAKK38/07 study: integration of baseline metabolic heterogeneity and metabolic tumor volume in DLBCL prognostic model. Blood Adv. 2020;4(6):1082-1092. Blood Adv 2020;4(10):2135.

15. Cottereau A-S, Nioche C, Dirand A-S, et al. 18F-FDG PET dissemination features in diffuse large B-cell lymphoma are predictive of outcome. J Nucl Med 2020;61(1):40–5.

16. Cottereau A-S, Meignan M, Nioche C, et al. New approaches in characterization of lesions dissemination in DLBCL patients on baseline PET/CT. Cancers 2021;13(16). https://doi.org/10.3390/cancers13163998.

17. Foster B, Bagci U, Mansoor A, et al. A review on segmentation of positron emission tomography images. Comput Biol Med 2014;50:76–96.

18. Dewalle-Vignion A-S, Yeni N, Petyt G, et al. Evaluation of PET volume segmentation methods:

comparisons with expert manual delineations. Nucl Med Commun 2012;33(1):34–42.

19. Burggraaff CN, Rahman F, Kaßner I, et al. Optimizing workflows for fast and reliable metabolic tumor volume measurements in diffuse large B cell lymphoma. Mol Imaging Biol 2020;22(4):1102–10.

20. Zijlstra JM, Comans EF, van Lingen A, et al. FDG PET in lymphoma: the need for standardization of interpretation. An observer variation study. Nucl Med Commun 2007;28(10):798–803.

21. Frood R, Burton C, Tsoumpas C, et al. Baseline PET/CT imaging parameters for prediction of treatment outcome in Hodgkin and diffuse large B cell lymphoma: a systematic review. Eur J Nucl Med Mol Imaging 2021. https://doi.org/10.1007/s00259-021-05233-2.

22. Annunziata S, Pelliccioni A, Hohaus S, et al. The prognostic role of end-of-treatment FDG-PET/CT in diffuse large B cell lymphoma: a pilot study application of neural networks to predict time-to-event. Ann Nucl Med 2021;35(1):102–10.

23. Whiting PF, Rutjes AWS, Westwood ME, et al. QUADAS-2: a revised tool for the quality assessment of diagnostic accuracy studies. Ann Intern Med 2011; 155(8):529–36.

24. Bi L, Kim J, Kumar A, et al. Automatic detection and classification of regions of FDG uptake in whole-body PET-CT lymphoma studies. Comput Med Imaging Graph 2017;60:3–10.

25. Barrington SF, Meignan M. Time to prepare for risk adaptation in lymphoma by standardizing measurement of metabolic tumor burden. J Nucl Med 2019;60(8):1096–102.

26. Berkowitz A, Basu S, Srinivas S, et al. Determination of whole-body metabolic burden as a quantitative measure of disease activity in lymphoma: a novel approach with fluorodeoxyglucose-PET. Nucl Med Commun 2008;29(6):521–6.

27. Akhtari M, Milgrom SA, Pinnix CC, et al. Reclassifying patients with early-stage Hodgkin lymphoma based on functional radiographic markers at presentation. Blood 2018;131(1):84–94.

28. Kostakoglu L, Goldsmith SJ. 18F-FDG PET evaluation of the response to therapy for lymphoma and for breast, lung, and colorectal carcinoma. J Nucl Med 2003;44(2):224–39.

29. Gallamini A. PET scan in Hodgkin lymphoma: role in diagnosis, prognosis, and treatment. New York City, NY, USA: Springer; 2016.

30. Punwani S, Taylor SA, Saad ZZ, et al. Diffusion-weighted MRI of lymphoma: prognostic utility and implications for PET/MRI? Eur J Nucl Med Mol Imaging 2013;40(3):373–85.

31. Gull S, Akbar S. Artificial intelligence in brain tumor detection through MRI Scans. Artif Intelligence Internet Things 2021;241–76. https://doi.org/10.1201/9781003097204-10.

32. Yousefirizi F, Jha AK, Brosch-Lenz J, et al. Towards high-throughput AI-based segmentation in oncological PET imaging. arXiv [physics.med-ph]. 2021. Available at: http://arxiv.org/abs/2107.13661. Accessed September 10, 2021.

33. Taghanaki SA, Abhishek K, Cohen JP, et al. Deep semantic segmentation of natural and medical images: a review. Artif Intelligence Rev 2021;54(1):137–78.

34. Hirata K, Manabe O, Magota K, et al. A preliminary study to use SUVmax of FDG PET-CT as an identifier of lesion for artificial intelligence. Front Med 2021;8:647562.

35. Spatial and temporal image registration. In: Yankeelov TE, Pickens DR, Price RR, editors. Quantitative MRI in cancer. Boca Raton, FL: CRC Press; 2011. p. 256–69.

36. Jiao J, Searle GE, Tziortzi AC, et al. Spatio-temporal pharmacokinetic model based registration of 4D PET neuroimaging data. Neuroimage. 2014;84: 225-235.

37. Pereira G. Deep Learning techniques for the evaluation of response to treatment in Hogdkin Lymphoma. 2018. Available at: https://estudogeral.uc.pt/handle/10316/86276. Accessed September 10, 2021.

38. Zhou Z, Jain P, Lu Y, et al. Computer-aided detection of mantle cell lymphoma on 18F-FDG PET/CT using a deep learning convolutional neural network. Am J Nucl Med Mol Imaging 2021;11(4):260.

39. Tricco AC, Lillie E, Zarin W, et al. PRISMA extension for scoping reviews (PRISMA-ScR): checklist and explanation. Ann Intern Med 2018;169(7): 467–73.

40. Mayerhoefer ME, Umutlu L, Schöder H. Functional imaging using radiomic features in assessment of lymphoma. Methods 2021;188:105–11.

41. Sheng VS, Provost F, Ipeirotis PG. Get another label? improving data quality and data mining using multiple, noisy labelers. In: Proceedings of the 14th ACM SIGKDD International Conference on Knowledge Discovery and Data Mining. KDD '08. Association for Computing Machinery; Las Vegas, Nevada, USA: August 24–27, 2008:614-622.

42. Park SH, Han K. Methodologic guide for evaluating clinical performance and effect of artificial intelligence technology for medical diagnosis and prediction. Radiology 2018;286(3):800–9.

43. Pinochet P, Eude F, Becker S, et al. Evaluation of an automatic classification algorithm using convolutional neural networks in oncological positron emission tomography. Front Med 2021;8:628179.

44. Sadik M, López-Urdaneta J, Ulén J, et al. Artificial intelligence could alert for focal skeleton/bone marrow uptake in Hodgkin's lymphoma patients staged with FDG-PET/CT. Sci Rep 2021;11(1): 10382.

45. Guo R, Hu X, Song H, et al. Weakly supervised deep learning for determining the prognostic value of 18F-FDG PET/CT in extranodal natural killer/T cell lymphoma, nasal type. Eur J Nucl Med Mol Imaging 2021. https://doi.org/10.1007/s00259-021-05232-3.

46. Yuan C, Zhang M, Huang X, et al. Diffuse large B-cell lymphoma segmentation in PET-CT images via hybrid learning for feature fusion. Med Phys 2021. https://doi.org/10.1002/mp.14847. mp.14847.

47. Blanc-Durand P, Jégou S, Kanoun S, et al. Fully automatic segmentation of diffuse large B cell lymphoma lesions on 3D FDG-PET/CT for total metabolic tumour volume prediction using a convolutional neural network. Eur J Nucl Med Mol Imaging 2021;48(5):1362–70.

48. Weisman AJ, Kim J, Lee I, et al. Automated quantification of baseline imaging PET metrics on FDG PET/CT images of pediatric Hodgkin lymphoma patients. EJNMMI Phys 2020;7(1):76.

49. Weisman AJ, Kieler MW, Perlman SB, et al. Convolutional neural networks for automated PET/CT detection of diseased lymph node burden in patients with lymphoma. Radiol Artif Intell 2020;2(5): e200016.

50. Sibille L, Seifert R, Avramovic N, et al. 18F-FDG PET/CT uptake classification in lymphoma and lung cancer by using deep convolutional neural networks. Radiology 2020;294(2):445–52.

51. Li H, Jiang H, Li S, et al. DenseX-Net: an end-to-end model for lymphoma segmentation in whole-body PET/CT Images. IEEE Access 2020;8:8004–18.

52. Sadik M, Lind E, Polymeri E, et al. Automated quantification of reference levels in liver and mediastinal blood pool for the Deauville therapy response classification using FDG-PET/CT in Hodgkin and non-Hodgkin lymphomas. Clin Physiol Funct Imaging 2019;39(1):78–84.

53. Goodfellow I, Bengio Y, Courville A. Deep learning. Cambridge, MA, USA: MIT Press; 2016.

54. Lippi M, Gianotti S, Fama A, et al. Texture analysis and multiple-instance learning for the classification of malignant lymphomas. Comput Methods Programs Biomed 2020;185:105153.

55. Mayerhoefer ME, Riedl CC, Kumar A, et al. Radiomic features of glucose metabolism enable prediction of outcome in mantle cell lymphoma. Eur J Nucl Med Mol Imaging 2019;46(13): 2760–9.

56. Hu H, Decazes P, Vera P, et al. Detection and segmentation of lymphomas in 3D PET images via clustering with entropy-based optimization strategy. Int J Comput Assist Radiol Surg 2019;14(10):1715–24.

57. Yu Y, Decazes P, Lapuyade-Lahorgue J, et al. Semi-automatic lymphoma detection and segmentation using fully conditional random fields. Comput Med Imaging Graph 2018;70:1–7.

58. Grossiord É, Talbot H, Passat N, Meignan M, Najman L. Automated 3D lymphoma lesion segmentation from PET/CT characteristics. In: 2017 IEEE 14th International Symposium on Biomedical Imaging (ISBI 2017). Melbourne, VIC, Australia; 18-21 April 2017:174-178.

59. Desbordes P, Petitjean C, Ruan S. Segmentation of lymphoma tumor in PET images using cellular automata: a preliminary study. IRBM 2016;37(1): 3–10.

60. Lartizien C, Rogez M, Niaf E, et al. Computer-aided staging of lymphoma patients with FDG PET/CT imaging based on textural information. IEEE J Biomed Health Inform 2014;18(3):946–55.

61. Weisman A, Kim J, Lee I, et al. Automated deep learning-based quantification of baseline imaging PET metrics on FDG PET/CT images of pediatric lymphoma patients. J Nucl Med 2020;61(Suppl 1):506.

62. Puttagunta M, Ravi S. Medical image analysis based on deep learning approach. Multimed Tools Appl 2021;1–34.

63. Kostakoglu L, Chauvie S. PET-derived quantitative metrics for response and prognosis in lymphoma. PET Clin 2019;14(3):317–29.

64. Lucignani G. SUV and segmentation: pressing challenges in tumour assessment and treatment. Eur J Nucl Med Mol Imaging 2009;36(4):715–20.

65. Yousefirizi F, Jha AK, Brosch-Lenz J, et al. Toward high-throughput artificial intelligence-based segmentation in oncological PET imaging. PET Clin 2021;16(4):577–96.

66. Vercellino L, Cottereau A-S, Casasnovas O, et al. High total metabolic tumor volume at baseline predicts survival independent of response to therapy. Blood 2020;135(16):1396–405.

67. Weisman AJ, Kieler MW, Perlman S, et al. Comparison of 11 automated PET segmentation methods in lymphoma. Phys Med Biol 2020; 65(23):235019.

68. Rahim MK, Kim SE, So H, et al. Recent trends in PET image interpretations using volumetric and texture-based quantification methods in nuclear oncology. Nucl Med Mol Imaging 2014;48(1):1–15.

69. Rizzo A, Triumbari EKA, Gatta R, et al. The role of 18F-FDG PET/CT radiomics in lymphoma. Clin Translational Imaging 2021. https://doi.org/10.1007/s40336-021-00451-y.

70. Starmans MPA, van der Voort SR, Castillo Tovar JM, et al. Chapter 18 - radiomics: Data mining using quantitative medical image features. In: Zhou SK, Rueckert D, Fichtinger G, editors. Handbook of medical image computing and computer assisted intervention. Cambridge, MA, US: Academic Press; 2020. p. 429–56.

71. Hatt M, Le Rest CC, Tixier F, et al. Radiomics: data are also images. J Nucl Med 2019;60(Suppl 2): 38S–44S.

72. Blanc-Durand P, Van Der Gucht A, Schaefer N, et al. Automatic lesion detection and segmentation of 18FET PET in gliomas : a full 3D U-Net convolutional neural network study. J Nucl Med 2018; 59(Suppl 1):330.

73. Klyuzhin I, Xu Y, Harsini S, et al. Unsupervised background removal by dual-modality PET/CT guidance: application to PSMA imaging of metastases. J Nucl Med 2021;62(Suppl 1):36.

74. Ou X, Zhang J, Wang J, et al. Radiomics based on 18 F-FDG PET/CT could differentiate breast carcinoma from breast lymphoma using machine-learning approach: a preliminary study. Cancer Med 2020;9(2):496–506.

75. Xu H, Guo W, Cui X, et al. Three-dimensional texture analysis based on PET/CT images to distinguish hepatocellular carcinoma and hepatic lymphoma. Front Oncol 2019;9:844.

76. Ou X, Wang J, Zhou R, et al. Ability of 18F-FDG PET/CT radiomic features to distinguish breast carcinoma from breast lymphoma. Contrast Media Mol Imaging 2019;2019:4507694.

77. Aide N, Talbot M, Fruchart C, et al. Diagnostic and prognostic value of baseline FDG PET/CT skeletal textural features in diffuse large B cell lymphoma. Eur J Nucl Med Mol Imaging 2018; 45(5):699–711.

78. Rodríguez Taroco MG, Cuña EG, Pages C, et al. Prognostic value of imaging markers from 18FDG-PET/CT in paediatric patients with Hodgkin lymphoma. Nucl Med Commun 2021;42(3):306–14.

79. Eertink JJ, van de Brug T, Wiegers SE, et al. 18F-FDG PET baseline radiomics features improve the prediction of treatment outcome in diffuse large B-cell lymphoma. Eur J Nucl Med Mol Imaging 2021. https://doi.org/10.1007/s00259-021-05480-3.

80. Wang H, Zhao S, Li L, et al. Development and validation of an 18F-FDG PET radiomic model for prognosis prediction in patients with nasal-type extranodal natural killer/T cell lymphoma. Eur Radiol 2020;30(10):5578–87.

81. Sun Y, Qiao X, Jiang C, et al. Texture analysis improves the value of pretreatment 18F-FDG PET/CT in predicting interim response of primary gastrointestinal diffuse large B-cell lymphoma. Contrast Media Mol Imaging 2020;2020:2981585.

82. Aide N, Fruchart C, Nganoa C, et al. Baseline 18F-FDG PET radiomic features as predictors of 2-year event-free survival in diffuse large B cell lymphomas treated with immunochemotherapy. Eur Radiol 2020;30(8):4623–32.

83. Wu J, Lian C, Ruan S, et al. Treatment outcome prediction for cancer patients based on radiomics and belief function theory. IEEE Trans Radiat Plasma Med Sci 2019;3(2):216–24.

84. Tatsumi M, Isohashi K, Matsunaga K, et al. Volumetric and texture analysis on FDG PET in evaluating and predicting treatment response and recurrence after chemotherapy in follicular lymphoma. Int J Clin Oncol 2019;24(10):1292–300.

85. Lue K-H, Wu Y-F, Liu S-H, et al. Prognostic value of pretreatment radiomic features of 18F-FDG PET in patients with Hodgkin lymphoma. Clin Nucl Med 2019;44(10):e559–65.

86. Lue K-H, Wu Y-F, Liu S-H, et al. Intratumor heterogeneity assessed by 18F-FDG PET/CT predicts treatment response and survival outcomes in patients with Hodgkin lymphoma. Acad Radiol 2020; 27(8):e183–92.

87. Zhou Y, Ma X-L, Pu L-T, et al. Prediction of Overall survival and progression-free survival by the 18F-FDG PET/CT radiomic features in patients with primary gastric diffuse large B-cell lymphoma. Contrast Media Mol Imaging 2019; 2019:5963607.

88. Milgrom SA, Elhalawani H, Lee J, et al. A PET radiomics model to predict refractory mediastinal Hodgkin lymphoma. Sci Rep 2019;9(1). https://doi.org/10.1038/s41598-018-37197-z.

89. Wang M, Xu H, Xiao L, et al. Prognostic value of functional parameters of 18F-FDG-PET images in patients with primary renal/adrenal lymphoma. Contrast Media Mol Imaging 2019;2019: 2641627.

90. Parvez A, Tau N, Hussey D, et al. Erratum to: 18F-FDG PET/CT metabolic tumor parameters and radiomics features in aggressive non-Hodgkin's lymphoma as predictors of treatment outcome and survival. Ann Nucl Med 2018; 32(6):410–6.

91. Ben Bouallègue F, Tabaa YA, Kafrouni M, et al. Association between textural and morphological tumor indices on baseline PET-CT and early metabolic response on interim PET-CT in bulky malignant lymphomas. Med Phys 2017;44(9): 4608–19.

92. Pfaehler E, Burggraaff C, Kramer G, et al. PET segmentation of bulky tumors: strategies and workflows to improve inter-observer variability. PLoS One 2020;15(3):e0230901.

93. Noortman WA, Vriens D, Slump CH, et al. Adding the temporal domain to PET radiomic features. PLoS One 2020;15(9):e0239438.

94. Fave X, Zhang L, Yang J, et al. Delta-radiomics features for the prediction of patient outcomes in non–small cell lung cancer. Sci Rep 2017;7(1):1–11.

95. Carvalho S, Leijenaar RTH, Troost EGC, et al. Early variation of FDG-PET radiomics features in NSCLC is related to overall survival - the "delta radiomics" concept. Radiother Oncol 2016;118(Suppl 1): S20–1.

96. Mayerhoefer ME, Materka A, Langs G, et al. Introduction to radiomics. J Nucl Med 2020;61(4): 488–95.

97. Alahmari SS, Cherezov D, Goldgof D, et al. Delta radiomics improves pulmonary nodule malignancy prediction in lung cancer screening. IEEE Access 2018;6:77796–806.

98. Wang L, Gao Z, Li C, et al. Computed tomography–based delta-radiomics analysis for discriminating radiation pneumonitis in patients with esophageal cancer after radiation therapy. Int J Radiat Oncol Biol Phys 2021. Available at: https://www.sciencedirect.com/science/article/pii/S036030162 1004752?casa_token=klpUfNmgEhEAAAAA:ZOA ShjEEgzDXK6JxuvCplWKcps-6o7x51hP4a952C9k qQMbH7zXrqgkjlhumgcLoWkrVJu8.

99. Mazzei MA, Di Giacomo L, Bagnacci G, et al. Delta-radiomics and response to neoadjuvant treatment in locally advanced gastric cancer—a multicenter study of GIRCG (Italian Research Group for Gastric Cancer). Quantitative Imaging Med Surg 2021;11(6):2376–87.

100. Liu Y, Shi H, Huang S, et al. Early prediction of acute xerostomia during radiation therapy for nasopharyngeal cancer based on delta radiomics from CT images. Quant Imaging Med Surg 2019;9(7):1288–302.

101. Nasief H, Zheng C, Schott D, et al. A machine learning based delta-radiomics process for early prediction of treatment response of pancreatic cancer. NPJ Precis Oncol 2019;3:25.

102. Fave X, Zhang L, Yang J, et al. Using pretreatment radiomics and delta-radiomics features to predict non–small cell lung cancer patient outcomes. Int J Radiat Oncol Biol Phys 2017;98(1):249.

103. Bera K, Velcheti V, Madabhushi A. Novel quantitative imaging for predicting response to therapy: techniques and clinical applications. Am Soc Clin Oncol Educ Book 2018;38:1008–18.

104. Kohli MD, Summers RM, Geis JR. Medical image data and datasets in the era of machine learning-whitepaper from the 2016 C-MIMI meeting dataset session. J Digit Imaging 2017;30(4):392–9.

105. Prior F, Smith K, Sharma A, et al. The public cancer radiology imaging collections of the cancer imaging archive. Sci Data 2017;4:170124.

106. Dose-adjusted EPOCH-R compared with R-CHOP as frontline therapy for diffuse large B-cell lymphoma (CALGB50303) - the cancer imaging archive (TCIA) public access - cancer imaging archive wiki. Available at: https://wiki.cancerim agingarchive.net/pages/viewpage.action?pageI d=70225094. Accessed October 1, 2021.

107. Yan K, Wang X, Lu L, et al. DeepLesion: automated mining of large-scale lesion annotations and universal lesion detection with deep learning. J Med Imaging (Bellingham) 2018;5(3):036501.

108. Kiyosawa M, Ohmura M, Mizuno K, et al. [18F-FDG positron emission tomography in orbital lymphoid tumor]. Nihon Ganka Gakkai Zasshi 1985;89(12):1329–33.

109. Kuwabara Y, Ichiya Y, Otsuka M, et al. High [18F]FDG uptake in primary cerebral lymphoma: a PET study. J Comput Assist Tomogr 1988;12(1):47–8.

110. Coiffier B, Lepage E, Briere J, et al. CHOP chemotherapy plus rituximab compared with CHOP alone in elderly patients with diffuse large-B-cell lymphoma. N Engl J Med 2002;346(4):235–42.

111. Schuster SJ, Bishop MR, Tam CS, et al. Tisagenlecleucel in adult relapsed or refractory diffuse large B-cell lymphoma. N Engl J Med 2019;380(1):45–56.

112. Wahl RL, Jacene H, Kasamon Y, et al. From RECIST to PERCIST: evolving Considerations for PET response criteria in solid tumors. J Nucl Med 2009;50(Suppl 1):122S–50S.

113. Cheson BD, Pfistner B, Juweid ME, et al. Revised response criteria for malignant lymphoma. J Clin Oncol 2007;25(5):579–86.

114. Cheson BD, Ansell S, Schwartz L, et al. Refinement of the Lugano Classification lymphoma response criteria in the era of immunomodulatory therapy. Blood 2016;128(21):2489–96.

115. Hutchings M, Loft A, Hansen M, et al. FDG-PET after two cycles of chemotherapy predicts treatment failure and progression-free survival in Hodgkin lymphoma. Blood 2006;107(1):52–9.

116. Burggraaff CN, de Jong A, Hoekstra OS, et al. Predictive value of interim positron emission tomography in diffuse large B-cell lymphoma: a systematic review and meta-analysis. Eur J Nucl Med Mol Imaging 2019;46(1):65–79.

117. André MPE, Girinsky T, Federico M, et al. Early positron emission tomography response-adapted treatment in stage I and II Hodgkin lymphoma: final results of the randomized EORTC/LYSA/FIL H10 trial. J Clin Oncol 2017;35(16):1786–94.

118. Borchmann P, Goergen H, Kobe C, et al. PET-guided treatment in patients with advanced-stage Hodgkin's lymphoma (HD18): final results of an open-label, international, randomised phase 3 trial by the German Hodgkin Study Group. Lancet 2017;390(10114):2790–802.

119. Sehn LH, Gascoyne RD. Diffuse large B-cell lymphoma: optimizing outcome in the context of clinical and biologic heterogeneity. Blood 2015;125(1):22–32.

120. Gong K, Kim K, Cui J, Wu D, Li Q. The Evolution of Image Reconstruction in PET: From Filtered Back-Projection to Artificial Intelligence. PET Clin 2021 Oct;16(4):533–42. https://doi.org/10.1016/j.cpet.2021.06.004.

121. Liu J, Malekzadeh M, Mirian N, Song TA, Liu C, Dutta J. Artificial Intelligence-Based Image

Enhancement in PET Imaging: Noise Reduction and Resolution Enhancement. PET Clin 2021 Oct; 16(4):553–76. https://doi.org/10.1016/j.cpet.2021. 06.005.

122. Yousefirizi F, Jha AK, Brosch-Lenz J, Saboury B, Rahmim A. Toward High-Throughput Artificial Intelligence-Based Segmentation in Oncological PET Imaging. PET Clin 2021 Oct;16(4):577–96. https://doi.org/10.1016/j.cpet.2021.06.001.

123. Jha AK, Myers KJ, Obuchowski NA, et al. Objective Task-Based Evaluation of Artificial Intelligence-Based Medical Imaging Methods: Framework, Strategies, and Role of the Physician. PET Clin. 2021;16(4):493–511.

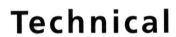

Technical

Application of Artificial Intelligence in PET Instrumentation

Muhammad Nasir Ullah, PhD[a], Craig S. Levin, PhD[a,b,c,d],*

KEYWORDS

- Artificial intelligence • Crystal • Positron Emission Tomography • Photon • Scintillator
- Time of flight • Depth of Interaction • Photodetector

KEY POINTS

- Application of AI in PET Instrumentation.
- Challenges in PET instrumentation.
- Various detector design for time of flight (ToF) PET system.
- Improving coincidence resolving timing and spatial resolution of PET detector.

INTRODUCTION

PET is a noninvasive molecular imaging modality widely used in medical imaging for characterization of various types of diseases. PET relies on the radioactive decay phenomenon known as positron emission.[1,2] The positron-emitting radionuclides are incorporated into molecular contrast agents (a.k.a. radiotracers) that are injected into patient's body and distributed based on the patient's physiology and disease biology. For each decay, the emitted positron propagates through the surrounding tissue losing its energy quickly and scattering, respectively, via interactions with atomic electrons and nuclei along its path. When the positron achieves near-zero momentum, it combines with an electron and the total rest mass energy of the electron and positron is converted into electromagnetic energy in the form of 2 simultaneously emitted (a.k.a. "coincident"), oppositely directed 511 keV photons.[3] This pair of photons can be detected by radiation detectors configured around the patient's body as illustrated in **Fig. 1**. The tracer biodistribution will produce millions of such oppositely directed 511 keV photon pair events that can be collected by a PET system. The measured events can be used to reconstruct the 3D bio-distribution of the injected tracer that created the 3-dimensional (3D) pattern of hits in the PET system detectors. This imaging process provides noninvasive information about a patient's disease.

The performance of PET systems relies on various key parameters and processes such as annihilation photon (511 keV) detection efficiency, the arrival time of coincident photons, the location of the photon interaction in the PET detector, and image reconstruction and processing methods.[4,5] The photon detection efficiency, arrival time, energy, and event position estimation are generally considered as the PET instrumentation tasks. These parameters highly influence the overall PET system performance such as system sensitivity, spatial resolution, contrast resolution, and signal-to-noise ratio performance. Artificial intelligence (AI) has gained a high level of recognition recently, especially in molecular imaging.[5] To date, time-of-flight (TOF) and 3D photon interaction localization information extraction seem to

[a] Department of Radiology, Stanford University, Stanford, CA 94305, USA; [b] Department of Bioengineering, Stanford University, Stanford, CA 94305, USA; [c] Department of Physics, Stanford University, Stanford, CA 94305, USA; [d] Department of Electrical Engineering, Stanford University, Stanford, CA 94305, USA
* Corresponding author.
E-mail address: cslevin@stanford.edu

PET Clin 17 (2022) 175–182
https://doi.org/10.1016/j.cpet.2021.09.011

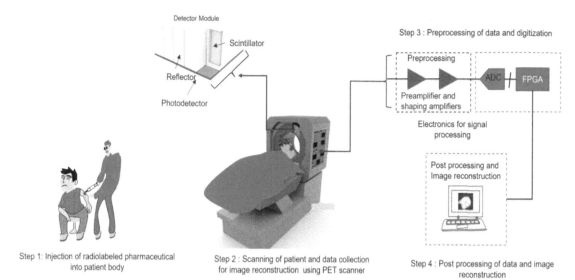

Fig. 1. PET scanning procedure, whereby millions of oppositely directed photon pairs are collected in a ring of detectors surrounding the patient. These data are used to reconstruct the 3D biodistribution of the radiotracer, giving quantitative disease information.

be the most prevalent areas in PET instrumentation where AI can play very important role.[5–9]

This article provides a brief overview of current AI research topics related to PET instrumentation and future potential applications, ranging from photon detection to system calibration and optimizing data correction methods for quantitative imaging.[10,11] This article is further divided into the following subsections: first, the fundamental physics of PET scanners and instrumentation is discussed in order to gain an understanding of the various types of detectors and the signals generated by these detectors. Following the PET physics, critical parameters such as event localization, including depth of interaction (DOI) of photon, and TOF are discussed in relation to the AI application for each of these tasks. Finally, a future prospective for AI in PET instrumentation is discussed.

BASICS OF PET INSTRUMENTATION

Conventional PET scanners consist of scintillators that convert high-energy radiation (individual 511 keV annihilation photons) to a flash of visible photons.[3] The inherent properties of scintillators such as good stopping power and timing resolution make them an attractive choice to be used as detector for PET.[12] Scintillators are coupled to photodetectors for the conversion of visible photons into the electrical signals for further processing and information extraction. Because of compact size, high gain, and sensitivity, silicon photomultipliers (SiPMs) are the most common

choice of photodetector in current PET scanner designs.[2,13] In PET, the ring of scintillation detectors usually comprises modules consisting of arrays of long and narrow crystal elements (eg, 16 x 16 array with crystal size of 3 mm × 3 mm x 20 mm) read-out by an array of photodetectors through optical multiplexing (a.k.a. light-sharing) and/or electronic multiplexing approaches to reduce the number of readout channels. Fig. 2 illustrates the basic mechanism of radiation detection in a PET detector.[1]

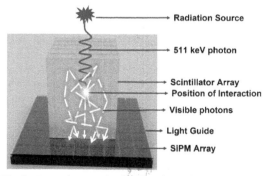

Fig. 2. Detection method of 511 keV photons in a PET detector. Each 511 keV photon is converted into a flash comprising thousands of visible light photons using a scintillator crystal. Reflectors between and on top of the crystal array direct those photons toward the photodetector plane. Photodetectors such as SiPMs are used to convert these visible light photons into electrical signals that are subsequently digitized to record parameters such as photon energy, arrival time, and interaction position.

In this particular "light sharing" detector module design depicted in **Fig.2**, localization of each detected high-energy photon (511 keV) is obtained from the scintillation light signal recorded from each crystal element, measured using the relative photodetector pulse heights and the energy sum.[3,12,14,15] The total energy of the detected high energy photon is determined from the sum of all scintillation light collected. In PET, coincident photon pair detection and TOF information is achieved by precisely measuring the arrival time of each photon interaction event using the first detected scintillation photons observed in the photodetectors.[16] A typical PET scanner has large numbers of these detectors that result in thousands of readout channels. A system design may readout each photodetector output individually, or, to reduce complexity and lower the system costs, various light or electronic signal multiplexing schemes[17–20] can used to reduce the number of readout channels, perhaps with some tradeoff of system performance such as energy, timing, and event positioning resolutions.

In case of electronic signal multiplexing, various schemes are used to minimize the number of readout channels.[17,21,22] With the reduction of readout channels, all the necessary information such as energy, timing, and position are incorporated in a fewer number of signals. For instance, in case of charge division multiplexing, an 8 x 8 photodetector array output, for example, can be multiplexed into 4 readout channels. The energy and timing information is acquired at the postprocessing stage of the signals by summing the 4 signals and picking off the leading edge, respectively, whereas the event position can be acquired using various formulas that use the amplitude of the charge at each output channel. The probability of error increases in case of event positioning from multiplexed signal, due to electronic and random noise, nonlinearity of each photodetector, and scatter events within scintillators. AI has the potential to be used for this task, which will not only improve the performance but also be helpful to multiplex a large number of photodetector outputs at once.

AI can be used for improved accuracy of the estimated parameters (ie., event localization, energy , and timing information extraction) and/or open the way for new detection methods and detector designs. At the system level, AI may be used to enable new system geometries designed to achieve specific tasks, such as sparse detector configurations, compensation for defective detectors, or to build long axial field-of-view systems with large gaps between detector rings. The remainder of this article details the developments and future directions in each of these areas.

EVENT POSITIONING AND SPATIAL RESOLUTION

Typically, a PET scanner consists of large numbers of detector modules arranged in a cylindrical geometry. Each detector module consists of a scintillator array coupled to a photodetector array as discussed above. In most of the PET scanners, the position of a photon interaction in the scintillator block is estimated using the light distribution observed at each photodetector output. However, in the case of one-to-one coupling module design where each scintillator is directly coupled to a single photodetector, the position can be directly estimated. Event positioning has a direct relation to the resulting spatial resolution of the PET scanner.

PET scanner performance characterization is based on various parameters, among which the spatial resolution is one of the most important metrics.[12,23] One of the major focuses of PET instrumentation during the past decades has been to improve the spatial resolution of PET scanners. Scintillator element size, system diameter, and the range of the positron before it annihilates mainly dictate the spatial resolution of PET scanner.[24] By using a finer scintillation crystal element width in the array, smaller system diameter, accurate methods of localization of photon interaction within the scintillator detector, and radionuclides with low positron emission energy (eg, F-18), the spatial resolution can be substantially improved. However, nonlinear distribution of light, intercrystal Compton scatter, the internal reflection of light within the scintillator detector, light sharing, electronic readout multiplexing, and electronic noise within the photodetector make the event positioning a very complex task. AI techniques require minimal human interference and can be used for accurate event positioning, especially when compared to conventional methods of crystal of interaction identification such as center-of-gravity (COG) and anger logic. AI may be tailored to augment these instrument issues and bring about further improvements in imaging spatial resolution that are necessary for the detection of smaller lesions and their improved quantification in reconstructed images.

The multiple output signals from each detector module used in conventional preclinical and clinical PET systems represent a highly suitable data input vector for several modern machine learning algorithms, including convolutional neural networks or classic machine learning algorithms such as k-nearest neighbors or k-nearest means. In practice, this implies that an AI algorithm may be trained to precisely and accurately estimate the position of interaction of the high-energy photons in the detector better than conventional classic algorithms that are most often used, for example, Anger logic[25] that correlates the fractional light collection of each photodetector to a given single position of interaction. However, these classic algorithms demonstrate rather poor statistical estimation characteristics in contrast to modern AI algorithms (reference), thus illuminating the potential of AI toward improved spatial resolution and event localization.

This aforementioned result is highlighted in monolithic scintillation crystal detector designs (references—including Andrea's recent review article on this topic), where a thick nonsegmented slab of scintillator (eg, L(Y)SO, BGO) is coupled to an array of photodetectors, such as SiPMs. These monolithic scintillators provide continuous position estimation compared with pixelated detector modules and achieve higher sensitivity owing to the absence of gaps between individual crystal elements that are normally filled with a reflective material in traditional block detector designs. In monolithic detector designs, machine learning algorithms are routinely used to estimate the position of interaction in all 3 dimensions using the set of photodetector amplitude signals as an input to either a pretrained convolutional neural network (CNN) or using a library of reference events acquired with a dedicated calibration measurement with k-nearest neighbors.[7–9,26]

Traditionally, in a pixelated scintillator array detector design, event positioning often refers to the single crystal element of interaction. However, for intercrystal Compton scatter, where the photon's energy is deposited in 2 or more crystal elements, which is more probable than a signal photoelectric interaction, the event might be more accurately positioned at the centroid of the interactions, or, for example, at the crystal element that received the smallest interaction energy.[27] These approaches provide an estimate of the 2D position for the incoming 511 keV photon interaction but do not give any information regarding the single or multiple DOIs within the crystal elements hit (the third coordinate). This missing DOI information often leads to parallax error (**Fig. 3**.), specifically in PET detectors where longer or thicker scintillators are used.[28] The perceived line of response (LOR) without DOI information does not represent the actual position of detected photons; this positioning error affects the spatial resolution both in the transverse and axial direction, as well as in the radial direction.[29]

There are several conventional methods to extract the DOI information.[30–36] The most widely used DOI encoding techniques include (1) discrete DOI measurement by implementing multilayered scintillators (phoswich design); this DOI extraction method can only provide the information regarding the layer at which the interaction happens rather than exact position of interaction; (2) direct DOI measurement using multiple detectors (scintillator + photodetector); and (3) continuous DOI measurement with either double-ended readouts of scintillation crystal elements or the light spread distribution in monolithic scintillators readout from one face only with a 2D array of photodetectors.[37] Some of the readout schemes are illustrated in **Fig. 4** as an example for DOI position estimation. Note, there are also various other methods that are not illustrated in **Fig. 4** that can be used to estimate the 3D DOI position. However, each of these methods have their own limitations,[28] which in turn can affect the key

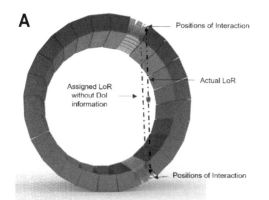 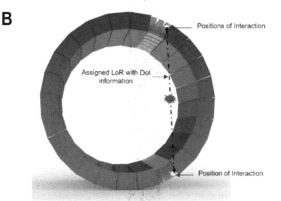

Fig. 3. Parallax error in a PET detector system. (*A*) Positioning events along a particular line of response (LOR) without and (*B*) with depth of interaction (DOI) information. The varying photon interaction depth leads to an error in LOR assignment when there is no DOI information, which blurs the radial resolution in the final reconstructed image.

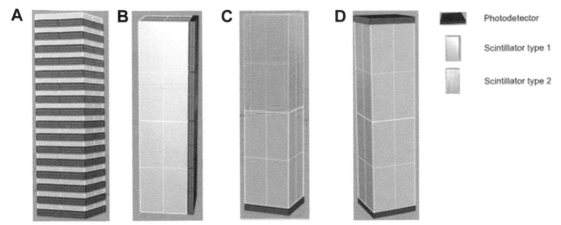

Fig. 4. Various types of readout schemes for DOI estimation. Each scintillator can be readout individually and stacked together in order to estimate the position of interaction (*A*); side readout for DOI estimation is illustrated (*B*), whereas (*C*) and (*D*) show the single and dual side readout of scintillator for DOI position estimation. Note that there are also other light sharing schemes that are also extensively studied to estimate DOI position, which are not shown here.

performance properties of the PET scanners such as timing, energy resolution, and/or detector packing fractions. AI can be advantageous for estimating DOI due to its ability to extract key information from the training data set, which can be otherwise missed by the conventional DOI positioning methods with minimal human interference.

In recent studies, several algorithms of AI are proposed to encode the DOI information in various PET detector designs.[5,7,29,38–42] For instance, Wang and colleagues presented an artificial neural network (ANN) to extract the 3D interaction position of the scintillation point within the crystal. Their results showed that the ANN was effective for plane DOI estimation.[43] Muller and colleagues proposed a method for reducing the nonlinear dimensionality and predicting detector response features.[44] They presented a gradient tree boosting (GTB) algorithm and a fast beam calibration approach with an efficacy of positioning calibration in less than an hour per detector module. However, GTB is a machine learning approach that builds a set of sequential decisions (decision trees) in a supervised manner, with the ability to handle different sets of inputs, combinations of inputs, and partially missing data. GTB models are very flexible, affecting the positioning performance as well as the memory requirements of trained positioning models.[44] There are several challenges associated to the DOI estimation in monolithic scintillators, including the computational cost and calibration complexity. The GTB method outperformed the other methods studied for retrieving the scintillation position in monolithic crystals, with a spatial resolution of 2.12 mm.[44] Similarly, Sanaat

and colleagues presented a new approach to evaluate the advantages of DOI estimation in an entire PET system geometry, specifically at the corners of the FOV.[40] Their research mainly focused on developing the 3D approximation of the scintillation position in monolithic crystals through supervised DNN and using Monte Carlo simulations.

In order to achieve high performance using AI, a highly accurate and diverse data set is required for the training of the network. In the case of event localization, generating a training data set with high accuracy is a complex task. Specifically, in the case of the detector module, due to multiple interactions owing to the higher probability of intercrystal scatter versus a single photoelectric interaction to occur, the actual position of interaction becomes uncertain and thus makes it much more difficult to accurately label the data as ground truth for the training data set.

TIME-OF-FLIGHT

Another venue for the application of AI in PET instrumentation is for signal processing tasks necessary to extract precise detection time differences of coincident 511 keV photon pairs for TOF-PET. In a TOF-PET scanner, the photon pair TOF difference information (detected time difference between the photons in each annihilation pair) is used to localize the annihilation point to a smaller region along the LOR.[13,16] The additional information provided by TOF-PET along system LORs enables much better reconstructed image signal-to-noise ratio and thus more precise measurement of the 3D activity distribution of the radiopharmaceutical.[16,45] In PET, coincidence

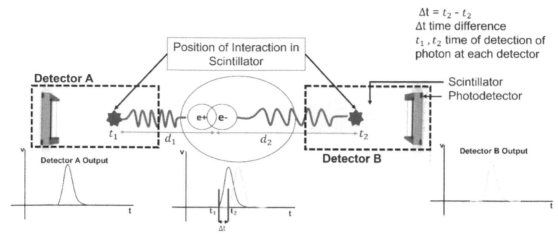

Fig. 5. Basic measurement method of photon time-of-flight (TOF) information in a PET scanner. Oppositely directed annihilation photons interact at location d_1 and d_2, from the annihilation point with arrival times t_1 and t_2, respectively.

timing resolution (CTR) refers to the variation in time difference measured for all possible pairs of opposing detector elements (**Fig. 5**), which is reported as the full width at half maximum (FWHM) of the distribution of TOF difference between all such detector pairs. The accurate measurement of coincidences not only improves the TOF capability of the scanner but may also be helpful in rejection of random coincidence events.[5] The first few visible light photons created in the scintillation crystal are normally used for the photon interaction time measurement in SiPMs.

The timing information of interacting photons are determined from the photodetector (eg, SiPMs) output signals (see **Fig. 5**). The 2 most common methods used for coincidence timing measurements are a single leading-edge threshold and constant fraction discrimination. Both of these are simple in nature, as they look for signals to cross certain threshold values for an arrival time calculation. The simplistic nature of these methods makes it easy to use the digitized output signals or readily available dedicated ASICs for arrival timing estimations.[46] However, both the leading-edge discrimination and constant fraction discrimination are susceptible to the noise at the output of photodetector and may be biased by differences in the temporal properties of the photodetector output waveforms, which limit the overall timing performance. In addition, both methods overlook many features of the signals such as shape and rising edge, which hold crucial information that can be used to improve the CTR of the system. On the other hand, AI algorithms that can be trained to learn complex features from a training data set are attractive alternatives

to be used for the estimation and calculation of CTR.[6]

AI provides several advantages for the estimation of TOF. For example, a CNN can be trained to take advantage of the various parameters of the photodetector to accurately measure the photon arrival time difference between 2 detector elements in the PET ring, which may be overlooked by using conventional methods due to the noise factor.[5,6] In particular, Berg & Cherry applied a CNN to estimate the TOF, and a significant (23%) improvement in comparison to conventional methods was observed.[6]

A necessary extension of this AI technique for its use in PET systems is to incorporate multiple photodetector waveforms into the CNN for timing estimation. The traditional algorithms rely on a summed signal owing to noise limitations that preclude the independent use of multiple photodetector signals in PET detector modules. However, the superior statistical estimation properties of CNNs compared with thresholding algorithms may enable the independent and simultaneous use of multiple input signals for timing estimation.

FUTURE PROSPECTIVE OF ARTIFICIAL INTELLIGENCE IN PET INSTRUMENTATION
Crystal Calibrations and Data Correction

Small nonuniformities in scintillator and photodetector performance due to manufacturing variations or other issues can greatly influence the image performance of the overall system. All PET detectors require a set of calibration steps before any image is reconstructed. These include the calibration of each scintillator light yield, photodetector gain, unique position of interaction within a detector module and timing offset of each detector. Precalibrated lookup-tables are used to mitigate the non-uniformity within the system. The data needed for these lookup tables need to be acquired at regular intervals due to the change in performance of detectors over a time. These routine data acquisition processes to generate lookup tables are time consuming and complex. AI algorithms may be a useful tool to ensure more accurate calibrations for both fast and slow changes in PET system calibration, for example, identifying detectors in the system with operational characteristics beyond the normal range, including normalization, TOF calibration, and energy calibration.

SUMMARY

AI is being increasingly explored in nuclear medicine, not only for postreconstructed image processing or image reconstruction tasks, but also in instrumentation and system design. Although many of these techniques are still relatively immature, there remains several potential applications of machine learning and AI aside from imagespace in the detector readout and system calibration processes that may provide more robust scanner performance and improved image quality and accuracy.

DISCLOSURE

The authors have nothing to disclose.

FUNDING

This work was supported in part by a grant awarded from the Emerson Colletive.

REFERENCES

1. Lewellen TK. Recent developments in PET detector technology. Phys Med Biol 2008;53(17):R287–317.
2. Berg E, Cherry SR. Innovations in instrumentation for positron emission tomography. Semin Nucl Med 2018;311–31.
3. Ullah MN, Pratiwi E, Cheon J, et al. Instrumentation for time-of-flight positron emission tomography. Nucl Med Mol Imaging 2010;50:112–22.
4. Gong K, Berg E, Cherry SR, et al. Machine learning in PET: from photon detection to quantitative image reconstruction. Proc IEEE IEEE 2019;108:51–68.
5. Arabi H, Zaidi H. Applications of artificial intelligence and deep learning in molecular imaging and radiotherapy. Eur J Hybrid Imaging 2020;4:1–23. Springer.
6. Berg E, Cherry SR. Using convolutional neural networks to estimate time-of-flight from PET detector waveforms. Phys Med Biol 2018;63:02LT01. IOP Publishing.
7. Bruyndonckx P, Lemaitre C, Van Der Laan DJ, et al. Evaluation of machine learning algorithms for localization of photons in undivided scintillator blocks for PET detectors. IEEE Trans Nucl Sci 2008;55:918–24.
8. Jaliparthi G, Martone PF, Stolin AV, et al. Deep residual-convolutional neural networks for event positioning in a monolithic annular PET scanner. Phys Med Biol 2021. IOP Publishing.
9. Tao L, Li X, Furenlid LR, et al. Deep learning based methods for gamma ray interaction location estimation in monolithic scintillation crystal detectors. Phys Med Biol 2020;65:115007. IOP Publishing.
10. Spencer BA, Berg E, Schmall JP, et al. Performance evaluation of the uEXPLORER total-body PET/CT scanner based on NEMA NU 2-2018 with additional Tests to characterize PET scanners with a long axial field of view. J Nucl Med Soc Nucl Med 2021;62:861–70.
11. Van Sluis J, De Jong J, Schaar J, et al. Performance characteristics of the digital biograph vision PET/CT system. J Nucl Med Soc Nucl Med 2019;60:1031–6.
12. Ullah MN, Pratiwi E, Park JH, et al. Studies on submillimeter LYSO:Ce, Ce:GAGG, and a new Ce:GFAG block detector for PET using digital silicon photomultiplier. Nucl Instr Methods Phys Res Sect A Accel Spectrometers 2018;911:115–22. Detect Assoc Equip. Elsevier B.V.
13. Slomka PJ, Pan T, Germano G. Recent Advances and future Progress in PET instrumentation. Semin Nucl Med 2016;46:5–19.
14. Karp JS, Muehllehner G, Beerbohm D, et al. Evemt localization in a continuous scintillation detector using digital processing. IEEE Trans Nucl Sci 1986;33:550–5. IEEE.
15. Tornai MP, Germano G, Hoffman EJ. Positioning and energy response of PET block detectors with different light sharing schemes. IEEE Trans Nucl Sci 1994;41:1458–63. IEEE.
16. Cates JW, Levin CS. Advances in coincidence time resolution for PET. Phys Med Biol 2016;61:2255–64. IOP Publishing.
17. Downie E, Yang X, Peng H. Investigation of analog charge multiplexing schemes for SiPM based PET block detectors. Physics in Medicine & Biology 58, no. 11 2013: 3943.
18. Park H, Ko GB, Lee JS. Hybrid charge division multiplexing method for SiPM-based high-resolution PET detectors. Volume No 57 2016;589.
19. Yang Q, Kuang Z, Sang Z, et al. Performance comparison of two signal multiplexing readouts for SiPM-based pet detector. Physics in Medicine & Biology 64, no. 23 2019;23NT02.
20. Park H, Lee JS. Highly multiplexed SiPM signal readout for brain-dedicated TOF-DOI PET detectors. Physica Medica 68 2019;117–23.

21. Yoon HS, Lee JS. Feasibility of new analog signal multiplexing techniques for SiPM PET detectors to reduce readout complexity. Volume 53 2012; 2389–489.

22. Park H, Ko GB, Lee JS. Hybrid charge division multiplexing method for silicon photomultiplier based PET detectors. Physics in Medicine & Biology 62, no. 11 2017;4390.

23. Pratiwi E, Leem HT, Park JH, et al. Performance of a 0.4 mm pixelated Ce: GAGG block detector with digital silicon photomultiplier. IEEE Trans Radiat Plasma Med Sci 2017;1:30–5. IEEE.

24. Levin CS, Hoffman EJ. Calculation of positron range and its effect on the fundamental limit of positron emission tomography system spatial resolution. Physics in Medicine & Biology 1999 Mar;44(3):781.

25. Anger HO. Scintillation camera. Review of scientific instruments. 1958 Jan;29(1):27-33.

26. Li X, Tao L, Levin CS, et al. Fast gamma-ray interaction-position estimation using kd tree search. Phys Med Biol 2019;64:155018. IOP Publishing.

27. Pratx G, Levin CS. Bayesian reconstruction of photon interaction sequences for high-resolution PET detectors. Phys Med Biol 2009;54:5073. IOP Publishing.

28. Ullah MN, Pratiwi E, Park JH, et al. Wavelength discrimination (WLD) TOF-PET detector with DOI information. Physics in Medicine & Biology 65, no. 5 2020;055003.

29. Peng P, Judenhofer MS, Jones AQ, et al. Compton PET: a simulation study for a PET module with novel geometry and machine learning for position decoding. Biomed Phys Eng Express 2018;5:15018. IOP Publishing.

30. Miyaoka RS, Lewellen TK, Yu H, et al. Design of a depth of interaction (DOI) PET detector module. IEEE Transactions on Nuclear Science 45, no. 3 1998;1069–73.

31. Ling T, Lewellen TK, Miyaoka RS. Depth of interaction decoding of a continuous crystal detector module. Physics in Medicine & Biology 52, no. 8 2007; 2213.

32. Li X, Lockhart C, Lewellen TK, et al. A high resolution, monolithic crystal, PET/MRI detector with DOI positioning capability. Eng Med Biol Soc 2008; 2287–90, 2008 EMBS 2008 30th Annu Int Conf IEEE. IEEE.

33. Maas MC, Schaart DR, Van Der Laan DJ, et al. Monolithic scintillator PET detectors with intrinsic depth-of-interaction correction. Physics in Medicine & Biology 54, no. 7 2009;1893.

34. Ullah MN, Pratiwi E, Park JH, et al. Wavelength discrimination (WLD) TOF-PET detector with DOI information. Phys Med Biol 2019. Available at: https://iopscience.iop.org/article/10.1088/1361-6560/ab6579.

35. Hyun Chung Y, Baek CH, Lee SJ, et al. Preliminary experimental results of a quasi-monolithic detector with DOI capability for a small animal PET. Nuclear Instruments and Methods in Physics Research Section A: Accelerators, Spectrometers, Detectors and Associated Equipment 621, no. 1-3 2010;590–4.

36. Tsuda T, Murayama H, Kitamura K, et al. A four-layer depth of interaction detector block for small animal PET. IEEE Transactions on Nuclear Science 51, no. 5 2004;2537–42.

37. Ito M, Hong SJ, Lee JS. Positron emission tomography (PET) detectors with depth-of-interaction (DOI) capability. Biomedical Engineering Letters 1, no. 2 2011;70.

38. Pedemonte S, Pierce L, Van Leemput K. A machine learning method for fast and accurate characterization of depth-of-interaction gamma cameras. Phys Med Biol 2017;62:8376. IOP Publishing.

39. Balibrea-Correa J, Lerendegui-Marco J, Babiano-Suárez V, et al. Machine Learning aided 3D-position reconstruction in large LaCl3 crystals. Nucl Instr Methods Phys Res Sect A Accel Spectrometers, Detect Assoc Equip. Elsevier 2021;1001:165249.

40. Sanaat A, Zaidi H. Depth of interaction estimation in a preclinical PET scanner equipped with monolithic crystals coupled to SiPMs using a deep neural network. Appl Sci 2020;10:4753. Multidisciplinary Digital Publishing Institute.

41. Zatcepin A, Pizzichemi M, Polesel A, et al. Improving depth-of-interaction resolution in pixellated PET detectors using neural networks. Phys Med Biol 2020; 65:175017. IOP Publishing.

42. Mohammadi I, Castro IFC, Correia PMM, et al. Minimization of parallax error in positron emission tomography using depth of interaction capable detectors: methods and apparatus. Biomed Phys Eng Express 2019;5:62001. IOP Publishing.

43. Wang Y, Zhu W, Cheng X, et al. 3D position estimation using an artificial neural network for a continuous scintillator PET detector. Phys Med Biol 2013; 58:1375. IOP Publishing.

44. Müller F, Schug D, Hallen P, et al. Gradient tree boosting-based positioning method for monolithic scintillator crystals in positron emission tomography. IEEE Trans Radiat Plasma Med Sci 2018;2:411–21. IEEE.

45. Ota R, Kwon S II, Berg E, et al. Direct positron emission imaging: ultra-fast timing enables reconstruction-free imaging. arXiv Prepr arXiv210505805. 2021;

46. Rolo MD, Bugalho R, Goncalves F, et al. Tofpet asic for pet applications. J Instrum 2013;8;C02050. IOP Publishing.

AI-Based Detection, Classification and Prediction/Prognosis in Medical Imaging:
Towards Radiophenomics

Fereshteh Yousefirizi, PhD[a],*, Pierre Decazes, MD[b,c], Amine Amyar, PhD[c,d],
Su Ruan, PhD[c], Babak Saboury, MD, MPH, DABR, DABNM[e,f,g],
Arman Rahmim, PhD, DABSNM[a,h,i]

KEYWORDS

- Artificial intelligence • Machine learning • Nuclear medicine • PET • Convolutional neural network
- Detection • Segmentation • Radiomics • Radiophenomics

KEY POINTS

- Artificial intelligence (AI) techniques are being increasingly explored in medical imaging. Innovations in machine learning (ML) and deep learning (DL) have helped unlock the potentials of AI for successful applications.
- Patient health information, including demographic information, electronic medical record notes, diagnostic imaging at different time-points, and radiologist reports, along with radiomic features can be used as input to AI techniques for detection, classification, and outcome prediction.
- There is a significant value for reliable and automated AI-based tools for improved clinical task performance.
- We also discuss needed efforts to enable the translation of AI techniques to routine clinical workflows, and potential improvements and complementary techniques such as the use of natural language processing on electronic health records and neuro-symbolic AI techniques.
- The phenomics approach as it is introduced for precision medicine enables the systematic discovery of structural and functional patterns associated with disease presentation or drug response, we considered the application of AI techniques for radiophenomics that is, radiomics and phenomics in this artcile.

[a] Department of Integrative Oncology, BC Cancer Research Institute, 675 West 10th Avenue, Vancouver, British Columbia V5Z 1L3, Canada; [b] Department of Nuclear Medicine, Henri Becquerel Centre, Rue d'Amiens - CS 11516 - 76038 Rouen Cedex 1, France; [c] QuantIF-LITIS, Faculty of Medicine and Pharmacy, Research Building - 1st floor, 22 boulevard Gambetta, 76183 Rouen Cedex, France; [d] General Electric Healthcare, Buc, France; [e] Department of Radiology and Imaging Sciences, Clinical Center, National Institutes of Health, Bethesda, MD, USA; [f] Department of Computer Science and Electrical Engineering, University of Maryland, Baltimore County, Baltimore, MD, USA; [g] Department of Radiology, Hospital of the University of Pennsylvania, Philadelphia, PA, USA; [h] Department of Radiology, University of British Columbia, Vancouver, British Columbia, Canada; [i] Department of Physics, University of British Columbia, Vancouver, British Columbia, Canada
* Corresponding author.
E-mail address: frizi@bccrc.ca

PET Clin 17 (2022) 183–212
https://doi.org/10.1016/j.cpet.2021.09.010
1556-8598/22/© 2021 Elsevier Inc. All rights reserved.

INTRODUCTION

The task of clinical interpretation of medical images starts with the *scanning* of the presented image to *detect* the suspicious finding ("observation" in RadLex terminology (RID5)[1] which is also used in various Reporting and Data Systems (RADS), such as LI-RADS for liver imaging[2]), with subsequent attention to details (*characterize)* in combination with clinical history (*contextualization*) to *classify* the finding/observation as "normal variant", benign, or malignant with a certain level of confidence and various amount of details (*diagnosis*). There are 2 kinds of errors in this process: "perceptual error" (not detecting the finding) and "faulty reasoning" (attributing the discovered observation to wrong cause).[3] Using Kahneman terminology,[4] these 2 categories are the errors of "system 1" thinking (automatic and intuitive) versus "system 2" thinking (logical and based on reasoning).

Analysis of medical errors in diagnostic radiology reveals that 71% of all errors are "missed findings."[5] Kim-Mansfield radiologic error classification of these "perceptual errors" demonstrates 2 subcategories: *detection error* (looking but not seeing, 60%) and *suboptimal/insufficient scanning* (40%, either due to the satisfaction of search or locations outside the intended focus of the image, such as a pulmonary nodule in CT of the abdomen). This high rate of error shows the complexity of "detection process" even for the human brain.

There are multiple sources of lexical ambiguity here. The terminology of *visual processing* in neuroscience is based on the biology of the brain and connected networks. Those terms might be used in a completely different sense in the *computer vision and image processing* field. It is important to be cognizant of this potential confusion. The brain visual processing pathways are schematically shown in **Fig. 1**(2 parallel streams of "what pathway" [involved in the recognition, identification, and categorization of visual stimuli] and "where pathway" [involved in spatial attention] make the process more complex[6]). In neuroscience, vision has 3 stages: encoding, selection, and decoding/inference. Encoding is to sample and represent the visual input. Selection or "attention selection" is to select a tiny fraction of input for further analysis; and decoding is "recognition" of the object.[6,7] Perception means "inferring or decoding the visual scene properties" from the visual input (to form *percept*). Object recognition (OR) refers to the ability to identify the object in the scene by matching the processed input (percept) with "mental representation" of the

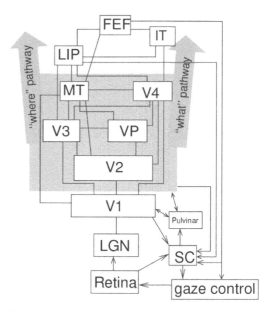

Fig. 1. Neuroscience of visual processing demonstrating the hierarchy of information processing from lower stage (retina) to higher stage (FEF). Each neuron typically responds to inputs from a limited extend of visual space called its receptive field (RF). The RF of retinal neurons is small (0.06°) and gets progressively larger (V4 neuron: 10°; IT neuron: 20–50°). In early areas such as retina RF and V1 RF are fixed and independent of "attention" while it is variable in later areas (consider a range of RF in IT). Each area has millions of neurons (about half of areas in the monkey brain are involved in vision). LGN: Lateral geniculate Nucleus (part of the thalamus). V1: visual area one in the occipital cortex; largest visual cortex in the brain. V2: visual area 2. V4: visual area4. MT: middle temporal area (terminology from macaque); neurons are sensitive to motion. LIP: lateral intraparietal area; involved in decision making for eye movement. IT: infratemporal cortex which responds to complex shapes. FEF: frontal eye field in the frontal cortex. SC: superior colliculus (part of the midbrain); both FEF and SC are involved in the control of eye movement. (*From* Zhaoping, L. and Z. Li, Understanding vision: theory, models, and data. 2014: Oxford University Press, USA.)

object. OR is hierarchical and complex.[8–11] Failure in the recognition of an object is called *visual agnosia* and has 2 subcategories: *apperceptive agnosia* (failure in recognition due to perception error; inadequate integration of simple sensory information such as color or edges to form an integrated property; eg, one cannot identify the shape) versus *associative agnosia* (perception is intact but one still cannot recognize the objects in general [*object agnosia*] or specific objects such as face [*prosopagnosia*] (face blindness), word [*agnostic alexia*], or location/environment [*topographagnosia*], and so forth).

In computer vision, object detection is defined as the combination of *localization* (identifying the object location) and some level of *classification* (identifying a broad object category; eg, when applied to medical imaging: "likely not benign", thus eliminating some normal physiologic uptake patterns). Both localization and classification tasks need robust features; however, they have different properties. The shift-variant task of localization often searches the entire image domain and is cognizant of spatial coordinates, whereas classification is a shift-invariant task that mainly requires features from the zoomed-in part of the image to determine the object category.[12]

Artificial intelligence (AI)-based detection algorithms have been used in diagnostic radiology with various intentions: to accelerate the detection of critical findings (such as the automatic detection of large vessel occlusion detection[13] for stroke management), to facilitate the processes with high cognitive burden (such as the detection of lung nodule[14]), to augment the diagnostic accuracy of radiologist (such as the detection of a suspicious lesion in mammography[15 15]), to prioritize the reading list,[16] and many more use cases. It is important to distinguish between "detection" and "diagnosis." Occlusion of large pulmonary vessel is a "detection" but identifying that finding as pulmonary thromboembolism is a "diagnosis." This difference is not merely semantic and has significant legal and regulatory consequences (c.f. Computer-Aided Detection, CADe,[17] is regulated under 21 CFR 892.2050 and 2070; however Computer Aided Diagnosis, CADx, is regulated under 21 CFR 892.2060[18]). These implications have an important role in "terminology confusion" of the scientific field. A task could be very similar to diagnosis but the claim may be merely detection and results communicated using different terms depends on the audiences, context, and intention of the writer.

There are 4 sources of "terminology confusion": 1. difference between visual neuroscience and AI-based computer vision, 2. evolving practice and developments in medical image analysis and inconsistency of usage among scientific groups, 3. borrowing terms from other fields; for example, signal detection theory or psychology, and 4. legal implications of specific terms. To make this "tower of babel" a better place, we have to redefine these words/terms in this paper in a careful way to decrease the ambiguity and increase the clarity of the language.

From an AI point of view, *detection* and *characterization* both involve classification tasks (broad definition). Here, we refer to "detection" as a task that finds a subspace in an image scene (localization) that contains a "specific object class" (classification) with a certainty level. However, we use a narrower definition of "classification" than statistical/AI terminology. Here, "classification" refers to the process of *characterization and identification* of already-detected/localized lesions. It can be an end-to-end process (input: image; output: category) or composite process (combination of *feature extraction* plus *statistical classification* of the features). However, examination (image) classification can also occur in the context of *prediction/prognosis*, enabling *risk stratification*, which we additionally review in this work. Stratification of cancer into reliably distinct risk subgroups enables the personalization of treatment. Radiomics is the large numbers of quantitative features combined with machine learning (ML) methods to determine relationships between the image and relevant clinical outcomes.[19] We can call the process of "categorization of features into clinically meaningful phenotypes" *phenomics.*[20–26] If the task of "image classification" has significant clinical value (diagnostic or prognostic), we call it *radiophenomics.* It could be either an end-to-end process (input: image; output: category/phenotype) or composite process (combination of radiomics and phenomics).

In this work, we first discuss advanced image quantification, leading to the field of radiomics in general, including *explicit* (handcrafted/engineered) radiomics versus *deep* radiomics paradigms. Next, our focus will be specifically on (i) detection, (ii) classification (characterization) of detected lesions, and (iii) prediction/prognosis tasks. Unlike (ii), (iii) usually involve the utilization of a wide search space (eg, various identified tumors and areas just outside, and distances between them, and so forth). As an example we describe the current status of different AI applications in PET imaging for detection, classification, and prognosis/prediction, and share our vista about upcoming opportunities and future directions while reminding potential hurdles in the path of translating these methods into clinical practice. The examples of PET imaging in this article are limited to cancer imaging and here we do *not* review AI techniques used in nononcological applications; for example, cardiovascular SPECT/PET and brain PET.[27]

ADVANCED IMAGE QUANTIFICATION; THE FIELD OF RADIOMICS

Medical images contain a significant minable and potentially valuable quantitative information beyond what is nowadays captured in routine clinical evaluations, motivating the field of radiomics.[28,29] An array of AI techniques in the field of medical imaging have emerged in the past decade to derive imaging biomarkers based on this information, using explicit (ie, handcrafted/engineered) radiomics features or deep radiomics features (ie, derived via deep neural networks (NNs)). These techniques have significant potential given their ability to reproducibly extract valuable information, including some that are beyond visual limits. Radiomic features are useful in numerous critical tasks from automated tumor detection in routine screening to radiogenomics including, classification of patients, and the spectrum of tumor histologies, severity scoring, prognosis, clinical outcome prediction (based on clinical and radiological features), treatment planning, and assessment and monitoring response to therapy.[30–34]

Fig. 2 shows a spectrum of AI applications (including ML and DL) in medical imaging based on varying complexity, expertise, and data. Ongoing studies (reviewed in this work) offer a glimpse into how AI can effectively support radiologists and nuclear medicine physicians by automating certain time-consuming measurements in medical imaging, consequently facilitating improved clinical tasks. Having access to appropriate labeled data with consistent labels is crucial for supervised AI techniques for classification and detection. At the same time, image labels for detection tasks including annotations of tumors location and the relevant classes are not yet extensively available in the field of medical imaging. Weakly supervised techniques have been introduced to tackle this limitation by decreasing the dependency on precise annotations for example, using image-level annotations[35,36] for detection and classification tasks. We will review these considerations.

Radiomics is an umbrella term that includes the use of single- or hybrid-imaging modalities, with the potential to identify novel imaging biomarkers for improved detection, classification, staging, prognosis, prediction, and treatment planning in different cancers.[37–43] Next, we discuss the applications of AI techniques within explicit (handcrafted) versus deep radiomics paradigms toward derivation and validation of radiomics signatures.

RADIOMICS SIGNATURES

Radiomics analyses can augment visual assessments made by radiologists.[44] AI techniques can perform quantitative high-throughput image phenotyping (extracting numerous image-based features) and identifying important discriminative features that individually or in combination form an effective radiomics signature for a given task. The field of radiomics has been introduced and elaborated in an accompanying article by Orlhac and colleagues.[29] The challenging task of detecting suspicious regions and differentiating (classifying) benign versus malignant nodules may be enhanced using AI techniques that have the potential to "see" beyond human perception using high dimensional data by radiomics, and/or enable potentially more robust clinical task performances.

Radiomics signatures have been effectively used for detection, classification, and prediction/prognosis (eg,[45,46]). As specific examples, Lartizien and colleagues[47] showed that textural features of PET and CT images have a high diagnostic ability in discriminating lymphomatous disease sites from physiologic uptake sites and inflammatory nonlymphomatous. They used ML techniques (SVM and random decision forest) for supervised classification. Nevertheless, the repeatability and reproducibility of textural features should be carefully considered in clinical settings.[48] Kebir and colleagues[49] assessed the diagnostic value of textural features of PET images for detecting true tumor progression. They found that clustering-based analysis of the heterogeneity features can be

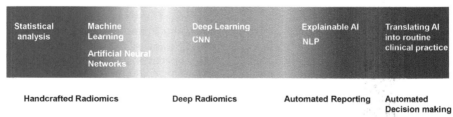

Fig. 2. Spectrum of AI applications in medical imaging based on varying complexity, expertise, and data. From the infra-zone (applications of conventional statistical analysis, artificial neural networks (ANNs), and ML to ultra-zone (AI techniques for decision-making and clinical reporting) the complexity of AI applications are amplified. CNNs for different tasks (eg, detection, classification, prediction/prognosis) are in the middle parts of the spectrum. (*Adapted from* Currie, G. and E. Rohren. *Intelligent imaging in nuclear medicine: the principles of artificial intelligence, machine learning, and deep learning.* in *Seminars in Nuclear Medicine.* 2020. Elsevier.)

used to differentiate the disease progression from pseudoprogression. The present section elaborates on some important aspects of radiomics analyses, as these issues are highly relevant and important in specific clinical tasks. **Fig. 3** depicts 2 different paradigms of AI-based analysis of medical images, namely explicit versus deep features: that is, use of ML techniques that use explicit features as extracted from segmented images versus DL techniques that use deep feature extraction or end-to-end learning from images. AI (ML and DL) techniques as mentioned previously can be supervised and weakly/semi/unsupervised, which we have discussed in the accompanying article [see Yousefirizi and colleagues' article, "Towards High-throughput AI-based Segmentation in Oncological PET Imaging," in this issue].

Next, we elaborate the explicit (handcrafted/ engineered) radiomics versus deep radiomics paradigms:

(i) Explicit (i.e. handcrafted/engineered) radiomics: This framework relies on extracting predefined with explicit mathematical definitions (eg, sphericity). Subsequently, statistical or ML-based techniques can be used to combine these features into a radiomics signature. ML-based techniques include unsupervised techniques (such as k-means clustering and hierarchical clustering) and supervised techniques (such as logistic regression, decision tree, SVM, and so forth). An explicit radiomics workflow, as shown in **Fig. 4**, typically involves the following steps[29,50]: (1) study design, (2) image acquisition and reconstruction, (3) ROI (VOI) segmentation, (4) spatial resampling and intensity discretization (except for shape features), (5) feature extraction, (6) radiomics model building (using statistical and ML methods),

followed by (7) model evaluation, and (8) sharing and reporting of findings. There are several tools to extract explicit radiomics features (intensity, shape, and texture features), for example, PyRadiomics,[51] LIFEx,[52] SERA,[53] CERR,[54] and others that have been standardized through the image biomarker standardization initiate (IBSI).[55]

Some explicit features are first-order or histogram-based features (such as standardized uptake value (SUV) maximum, mean, peak, median, first-quartile, third-quartile, standard-deviation, skewness, kurtosis, energy, and entropy) or texture features (such as gray-level co-occurrence matrix (GLCM), gray-level run length matrix (GLRLM), gray-level zone length matrix (GLZLM), and neighborhood gray-level dependence matrix (NGLDM)). Because of a potentially massive number of extracted radiomics features, radiomics model building typically involves feature selection and dimensionality reduction.[48,56] Different approaches can be used for feature selection[57] including: (1) pre-elimination of features, such as removing features known in the literature to have poor reproducibility (eg, overly sensitive to segmentation method), (2) using data-specific unsupervised methods (eg, removing features that are highly correlated, or with very low dynamic range in the data), and/or (3) supervised methods for dimensionality reduction (ie, removing features that do not add value on a separate labeled training set). Unsupervised approaches that is, principal component analysis (PCA) or cluster analysis remove redundant features without considering the class labels,[58] whereas supervised techniques consider class labels, and select the features based on their discriminative contribution in the specific tasks.[59]

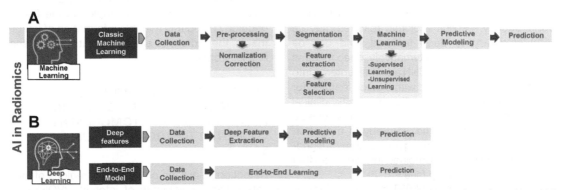

Fig. 3. Typical architecture and workflow of AI systems for predictive modeling: (*A*) classic machine learning, with the various processing steps involving handcrafted (explicit) features; (*B*) deep-learning-based techniques involving "deep features" that is, deep image feature extraction and "end-to-end learning". (*Modified from* Castiglioni, I., L. Rundo, M. Codari, et al., AI applications to medical images: From machine learning to deep learning. Physica Medica, 2021. 83: p. 9-24.)

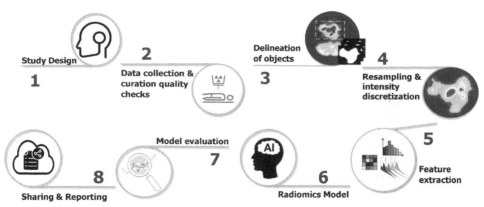

Fig. 4. The general workflow for explicit radiomics analysis by AI techniques. (1) Study design step and (2) data collection sometimes can be reversed or combined. Data quality should be checked before any further analysis. (3) The features can be directly affected by ROI/VOI delineations, so this step should be done carefully by automatic or semiautomatic techniques. (4) Spatial resampling and intensity discretization (except for shape features) are performed in this step (5) Explicit (engineered) features are extracted in step 5 and (6) radiomics model is then applied. The model is evaluated and shared in the final steps (7 and 8). (*Modified from Orlhac, F., C. Nioche, I. Klyuzhin, et al.,* Radiomics in PET imaging: a practical guide for newcomers. *PET Clinics, 2021.*)

(ii) Deep radiomics: Data-driven DL approaches are directly applied on the input image or ROI/VOI of the images, and "deep features" are learned; for example, by using convolutional neural networks (CNNs) or auto-encoder networks. DL approaches are capable of automatically identifying parts of the image most relevant to the task.[60] Auto-encoder networks, as unsupervised variant of CNNs, are able to extract compressed image content and map it onto representative features.[61] Consequently, deep features are extracted, instead of using explicit mathematical definitions of features. Despite theoretic considerations on the greater expressive power of deep features than explicit features, it has been shown that some explicit features are difficult to capture by CNNs of limited depth given limited training data.[62,63] Furthermore, CNNs can be negatively biased in capturing shape information[64,65] which can be important for a range of clinical tasks.[55] Consequently, explicit radiomic features may be complementary to deep features, and can be used as input to CNNs. Alternatively, deep features can be extracted using a CNN and then entered into a classifier,[66,67] integrated with explicit features for overall radiomics analysis. For a specific clinical task (eg, predictive modeling), **Fig. 3** shows classic ML versus DL paradigms, whereby in the latter, both steps of feature learning and radiomics signature derivation can be combined into one step that is, "end-to-end" training (see **Fig. 3**).

In the specific context of PET and PET/CT imaging, which the rest of this article focuses on, there are a number of challenges on the path to routine deployment of radiomics. There remain limited studies on multi-centric data in some cancer types

such as lymphoma to investigate the importance of radiomics analysis and avoid overfitting and degraded generalizability.[68] Overall, these issues need to be carefully considered toward appropriate radiomics frameworks including for specific detection and classification tasks. The emergence of AI techniques and incorporation of radiomics signature from anatomic information of CT images can yield better models with good performance and generalization for classification, detection, and prognosis and outcome prediction. There are some challenges in PET imaging due to the inherent image quality, standardization of imaging, and reconstruction that should be taken into consideration. The limited available data and limited interpretability of DL approaches challenge trustworthiness of AI applications in the field of medical imaging in general. In the next section, we briefly consider classification and detection techniques and provide examples in the field of oncology using this minable information of images that is, the radiomics signature that we discussed in this section.

CLINICAL UTILITY OF ARTIFICIAL INTELLIGENCE-BASED DETECTION IN POSITRON EMISSION TOMOGRAPHY/ COMPUTED TOMOGRAPHY: CURRENT STATUS

Detection of organs or lesions as regions of interests (ROIs) or volumes of interests (VOIs) is an important step toward the classification of the regions.[69] Besides, most existing segmentation approaches have an embedded detection step; we discuss segmentation methods in another work [see Yousefirizi and colleagues' article, "Towards High-throughput AI-based Segmentation in Oncological PET Imaging," in this issue]. End-to-end detection systems developed by AI techniques can effectively remove the need for further processing steps or prior knowledge about the detection task. Such networks can learn the most salient features based on various medical images in the training data such as PET, CT, or PET/CT scans. By contrast, conventional techniques for detection have the following two stages: (1) candidate generation based on specific features of the voxels in CT or PET images; that is, based on Hounsfield unit (HU) or standardized uptake value (SUV) and (2) false positive (FP) reduction.[70,71] Example attempts on the use of AI techniques for candidate generation[72] or for both steps[73] have been reported.

CNNs have opened up far-reaching opportunities in medical image analysis.[74–76] The potential of using CNNs for detection is based on their ability to extract data-driven features and relationships between adjacent pixels (voxels) in 2D (3D) schemes. These hierarchical features extracted in convolutional layers of CNNs can be highly representative if sufficient training data are available.[77] There are several studies on detection tasks in PET or CT images; meanwhile, detection based on combined PET/CT has gained more attention recently. **Table 1** lists several important studies involving the application of AI for detection. We review detection from PET, CT, and PET/CT next.

Detection of malignant lesions in fluorodeoxyglucose positron emission tomography/computed tomography imaging

Positron emission tomography -only images as input

PET imaging is used routinely and extensively for the detection and characterization of lesions in cancer examinations. Detection task in PET images is mostly degraded to high-uptake region detection using thresholding approaches. The use of physiologic uptakes to detect abnormal uptakes has been mostly used to this aim.

Some authors attempted to come up with a magical SUV threshold to detect pathologic FDG uptakes as any region with activity more than that value.[78] The threshold used can be a fixed value, for example, SUV$\geq$2.5,[79] or in reference to background uptake (eg, using liver or surrounding tissue).[80] Nonetheless, this approach is neither biologically plausible nor clinically meaningful as it ignores the normal biodistribution of a radiotracer. Each radiotracer has a specific time-dependent pattern of biodistribution in the healthy body. The concept of "sFEPU" (sites of FDG excretion and physiologic uptake) is misleading. Any uptake of FDG in normal tissue is "physiologic uptake," whether low level/background level (as in subcutaneous fat or blood pool) or high level (as in brain). However, in the literature, the term sFEPU only refers to the physiologic uptakes that are above a certain level of activity (ie, above background conceptually). The term high normal activity (HiNA) is a better term (ND = LoNA + HiNA).

The attempts to find a spatially-invariant/global threshold to detect "sFEPU" (a.k.a. HiNA) is destined to fail based on biological concepts; the poor performance of these methods has been demonstrated empirically multiple times [see Paravastu and colleagues' article, "Applications of Artificial Intelligence in 18F-NaF PET/CT: Current State and Future Directions," in this issue]. Moving beyond *spatially-invariant thresholding*, Bi and colleagues[81] proposed a multi-scale superpixel encoding approach that first groups the fragments that are obtained based on a multi-scale superpixel-based encoding method (MSE) and a class-driven feature selection and classification model for sFEPU classification in whole-body lymphoma PET-CT scans. The features are then extracted using domain-transferred CNNs to classify the regions into sFEPU and anomalies. Deng and colleagues[82] proposed a network composed of 2 parts for the detection of lymphomas and sFEPU. Their model consists of 5 fully connected convolutional neural networks (FCNs) in parallel. The input image is resized into 5 different spatial scales (100%, 95%, 90%, 85%, 80% of PET image dimensions), and each is entered as an input to the corresponding FCN model. In the second step, the detected sFEPUs in different scales are integrated to determine the exact sFEPU boundary.

Afshari and colleagues[83] and Kawakami and colleagues[84] applied the deep CNNs, You Only Look (YOLO),[85] to detect HNA on 2D PET images. YOLO detected multiple organs in 2D slices of the maximum intensity projection (MIP) images. Afshari and colleagues[83] then aggregated the detection results on 2D images to produce a 3D probability map. The size and metabolic levels of lesions impacted the performance of tumor detection techniques.

There are some attempts to augment the training data for detection tasks by generating synthetic PET. Generative adversarial networks (GANs) can use the existing CT data to synthesize PET images with high uptake region and constrain the appearance of the generated PET images.[86] This data augmentation method may help the model with FP; in other words, applying thresholding to the synthesized PET image to extract

Table 1
Selected studies on AI applications for tumor detection in CT, PET, and PET/CT images

Study	Task	Modality	Method	# Of Scans (n) # Of Cases (N)	Results
Cai et al,[180] 2020	To harvest lesions from incompletely labeled datasets. (Composed of lung nodules, liver tumors, and enlarged lymph nodes)	CT	CNN	n = 10,594 N = 4427	Precision = 90% annotating 5% of the volumes → harvest 9, 805 additional lesions: 47.9% recall at 90% precision, (s a boost of 11.2% in recall over the original RECIST marks)
Huang et al,[181] 2019	fully-automated end-to-end system to detect & segment the lung nodule	CT	CNN Nodule detection: Faster regional-CNN (R-CNN),	n = 1018	Detection Accuracy:91.4% and 94.6% with an average of 1 and 4 false positives (FPs) per scan
Zhu et al,[182] 2017	Lung nodule detection & classification benign/malignant)	CT	Detection: 3D Faster R-CNN Classification: gradient boosting machine	LIDC-IDRI dataset (n = 1018 cases)	Detection accuracy: 84.2% Classification accuracy: 92.74
Xie et al,[183] 2017	Pulmonary nodule detection	CT	ResNet for detection DenseNet for false positive reduction,	LUNA16(n = 888)	Sensitivity: 95.3% AFP: 1/case FROC score of 0.9226
George et al,[184] 2018	Lung nodule detection	CT	YOLO	n = 880	Sensitivity:89% AFP: 6/case
Wang et al[185] 2020	Lung nodule detection	CT	FocalMix: semi-supervised learning	n = 400	Sensitivity:90.7% (average sensitivity)
Jiang et al,[186] 2017	Lung nodule detection	CT	CNN (4- channel input: image patches enhanced by the Frangi filter)	n = 1018 N = 1010	Sensitivity:90.1/94% AFP: 15.1/case
Huang et al,[187] 2017	Lung nodule detection	CT	Local Geometric-model-based filter to generate nodule candidate &CNN to differentiate nodule/nonnodule	N = 1010	Sensitivity:90% AFP: 5 cases

Study	Task	Modality	Method	N	Results
Ding et al,[188] 2017	Pulmonary nodule detection	CT	Faster R-CNN-based	N = 1018	Sensitivity:94.6% AFP: 15/case
Shin et al,[77] 2016	Thoraco-abdominal lymph node (LN) detection & interstitial lung disease (ILD) classification	CT	CifarNet, AlexNet, Overfeat, VGG16, and GoogleNet (transfer learning(from nonmedical images)	n = 905 N = 120	sensitivity: 85% False positive per patient: 3
Vivanti et al,[92] 2017	Automatic detection of new tumors and tumor burden evaluation in longitudinal liver CT scan	CT	CNN	No of tumors: 246 (97 new tumors, from (n = 37) longitudinal liver CT studies)	TP new tumors detection rate of 86% vs 72% with stand-alone detection, Tumor burden volume overlap error of 16%.
Ghesu et al,[93] 2017	Reformulating the detection problem as a behavior learning task	CT	Deep reinforcement learning in a multi-scale scheme.	n = 1487 N = 532	Accuracy (mm) = 4.192* *With no failures of clinical significance
Xie et al,[94] 2019	Automated pulmonary nodule detection	CT	2D CNN (faster R-CNN)	n = 1018	(pulmonary nodule) Sensitivity = 73.4% at 1/8 FPs/scan Sensitivity = 74.4% at 1/4 FPs/scan
Deng et al,[82] 2017	Recognition of sFEPU and detection of lymphoma	PET	Five FCNs in parallel.	n = 569	detection rate = 80.0% false positives per volume 3.2
Afshari et al,[83] 2017	Localization and detection normal active organs in 3D PET scan	PET	CNN (YOLO)	n = 479 N = 156	average organ detection precision of 75%–98%, recall of 94%–100%, mean IOU of up to 72%.
Kawakami et al,[189] 2020	Detection of abnormal and physiologic uptake region	PET	CNN (YOLO)	n = 3198 MIP N = 491	APs for physiologic uptakes were: Brain: 0.993 Liver: 0.913 Bladder: 0.879 mAP = .831 IoU threshold value 0.5. FPS: 31.60 ± 4.66. false-positive rate = 0.3704 ± 0.0213, false-negative rate = 0.1000 ± 0.0774

(continued on next page)

Table 1
(continued)

Study	Task	Modality	Method	# Of Scans (n) # Of Cases (N)	Results
Schwyzer et al,[104] 2018	Detection of lung cancer in FDG-PET imaging in the setting of standard and ultralow dose PET scan	PET	deep residual neural network (RNN)	N = 100	standard dose Sensitivity = 95.9% specificity = 98.1% ultralow dose $PET_{3.3\%}$ Sensitivity = 91.5% specificity = 94.2%
Blanc-Durand et al,[103] 2018	Lesion detection in gliomas	PET	CNN(3D U-net)	N = 37	sensitivity = 0.88 specificity = 0.99 positive predictive value = 0.78
Schwyzer et al,[104] 2018	Detection of lung cancer	PET	deep residual neural network (RNN)	N = 100	Sensitivity = 95.9% specificity = 98.1% ultralow dose $PET_{3.3\%}$ Sensitivity = 91.5% specificity = 94.2%
Bi et al,[81] 2017	Simultaneous classification of abnormalities and normal structures in lymphoma cases	PET-CT	CNN	N = 40	F-score = 91.73%
Xu et al,[100] 2018	Multiple myeloma lesion detection	PET/CT	W-net	N = 12	Sensitivity = 73.5 Specificity = 99.59 Precision = 72.46
Teramoto et al,[101] 2016	Detection of solitary pulmonary nodules	PET/CT	ACM + Thresholding (initial detection) CNN (feature extraction) Multi-step classifier (rule based and SVM)	N = 104	Sensitivity: 90.1% 4.9 FPs/case
Kumar et al,[102] 2019	Detection of nonsmall cell lung cancer (NSCLC) lesions	PET/CT	CNN	N = 50	Precision = 99.90 ± 0.11 Sensitivity = 97.94 ± 0.76 Specificity = 98.82 ± 1.33 Accuracy = 98.02 ± 0.71

Author	Aim	Modality	Model	N	Results
Borrelli et al,[106] 2021	Detection of the abnormal lung lesions and calculation of the total lesion glycolysis	PET/CT	CNNs for lung lesion detection in PET and CT images and organ segmentation in CT images.	N = 112	sensitivity = 90% missing lesions = 1 positive predictive values = 88% negative predictive values = 100%
Weisman et al,[190] 2020	Detection of diseased lymph nodes in lymphoma patients	PET/CT	CNN (ensemble of 3 DeepMedic)	N = 90 Hodgkin's (N = 63) diffuse large B-cell lymphoma (N = 27)	TPR: 85% 4 FPs/patient
Punithavathy et al,[191] 2019	Evaluation of the classification of lung cancer using a deep model (ResNet-18) on conventional CT and FDG PET/CT via transfer learning	PET/CT	ResNet-18	n = 359	Accuracy = 0.877 (CT data) Accuracy = 0.817 (CT data with metadata (SUVmax and lesion size)) Accuracy = 0.837 (CT of PET/CT data) Accuracy = 0.762 (CT of PET/CT data with metadata (SUVmax and lesion size))
Zhao et al,[108] 2020	Detection of pelvis bone and lymph node lesions	PET/CT (PSMA)	CNN (2.5D U-net)	N = 193	Bone lesion detection: Precision = 99% Recall = 99% F1 score = 99% Lymph node lesion detection: Precision: = 94%, Recall = 89% F1 score = 92%
Zhou et al,[192] 2019	Neuroendocrine tumor detection	PET-CT [68 Ga] DOTATATE	ML–based algorithm (random forests regression)	N = 19	Random Forests regression machine learning model is robust to generate parametric images

All the PET images are FDG PET except when it is indicated.
Abbreviations: AFP, average false positive; FCN, Fully Convolutional Neural Network; FP, false positive; IoU, Intersection over the Union; mAP, mean average precision; MIP, maximum intensity projection; TP, true positive.

high-response regions can reduce the FP rate by comparing the detection and thresholding masks.[87,88]

Computed tomography-only images as input

Most existing studies for detection in CT imaging applied DL (more specifically CNNs) in one of the following ways: (i) training CNNs from scratch or (ii) applying CNNs pretrained on natural or medical images via transfer learning. 3D networks for supervised learning require more training data, which is commonly a challenge in the field of medical imaging due to the relatively limited availability of labeled data. This is effectively a "curse of dimensionality" problem, resulting in overfitting of sparse data in 3D approaches.[89] Overall, detection based on 3D networks is nontrivial, and 2D or 2.5D networks (ie, using the information from only few adjacent slices) have been a commonly explored alternative given the sparsity of data. Unsupervised learning is also another noteworthy approach for detection; for example, Afifi and colleagues[90] used graph cuts, and iteratively estimated shape and intensity constraints for liver lesion detection in CT images.

Shin and colleagues[77] exploited a combination of training and transfer learning (from nonmedical images) to detect thoraco-abdominal lymph nodes and for interstitial lung disease classification in CT images. They used various CNN architectures (CifarNet, AlexNet, Overfeat, VGG16, and GoogleNet) with different numbers of layers and variation of parameters.. They specifically explorer the capability of 3 important approaches that use CNNs to medical image classification for detection and classification: (i) training the CNN from scratch, (ii) applying off-the-shelf pretrained CNN features, (iii) unsupervised CNN pretraining with supervised fine-tuning, (iv) transfer learning, that is, fine-tuning CNN models pretrained from natural image dataset to detection task. The results showed that the CNN model can be used for high-performance CADe systems.

A 3D approach for the localization of anatomic structures was proposed by de Vos and colleagues[91] based on the 2D detection scheme from orthogonal planes using independent CNNs. Their proposed method worked well for the localization of structures with clear boundaries. Vivanti and colleagues[92] proposed a detection method for liver tumors burden quantification in longitudinal liver CT images. Their proposed method detects new tumors in the follow-up scans and quantifies the tumor burden change using a CNN as a prior model without the need for large labeled training data. Ghesu and colleagues[93]

tried to solve the detection problem as a behavior learning task for an AI system. They defined a unified behavioral framework based on deep reinforcement learning in a multi-scale scheme. The network was trained to detect the anatomic object using an optimal navigation path to the target object in the 3D volume of data.

Xie and colleagues[94] suggested a detection framework based on 2D CNN for the pulmonary nodule in CT images. The Faster R-CNN was adjusted with 2 region proposal networks and a deconvolutional layer was used to detect the nodule candidates. Three models were trained for 3 kinds of slices to be fused in later stages. A boosting architecture based on 2D CNN was used to reduce the FP. The misclassified samples are then used to retrain a model to boost the sensitivity. The results of these networks were finally used to vote out the result. Their proposed detection framework is shown in **Fig. 5**.

Some of the AI models for cancer diagnosis applications can be interpretable by the determination of the most influential regions in the input images that determine the output of the model that is, saliency map.[95] Although most of the existing detection and segmentation networks, such as U-Net and Faster R-CNN need annotated data to be trained and such supervised models are prone to be biased to the distribution of the training data if they are not diverse enough. Weakly supervised techniques have gained much attention to overcome these limitations using only image-level annotations to locate ROIs in an image based on the saliency map that encodes the location of ROIs.[35,36] For instance, weakly supervised techniques have been applied for cancer detection in lung CT images.[96,97]

Combined positron emission tomography and computed tomography images as input

PET/CT imaging as a powerful tool for the accurate diagnostic of oncological patients is widely used for prognostication and therapy response assessment.[98] Some existing studies used the spatial information of CT and metabolic information of PET images to develop an automated detection framework. For example, to detect small lung nodules (<4 mm) in clinical workflow, the wait-and-see approach is suggested. Considering the risk of delayed treatment and biopsy, FDG PET/CT is recommended by the society of nuclear medicine recommends for diagnostic.[99] Tumor detection based on PET/CT images is performed generally by extracting the high SUV region and involving its information in the detection scheme based on CT images. Xu and colleagues[100] used 2 CNNs for multiple myeloma bone lesion detection and

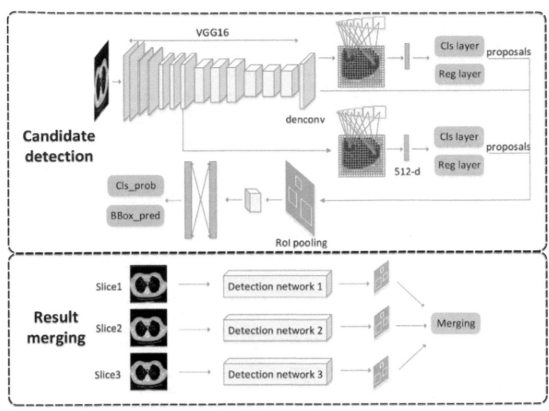

Fig. 5. The framework of the nodule candidate detection. The basic feature extraction network is VGG16 and a deconvolution layer is used to enlarge the feature map. Meanwhile 2 region proposal networks with designed 7 anciors are applied to obtain the proposals. Finally, ROI classified is used to get the candidates. (*Adapted from* Xie, H., D. Yang, N. Sun, et al., Automated pulmonary nodule detection in CT images using deep convolutional neural networks. Pattern Recognition, 2019. 85: p. 109-119.)

segmentation from ^{68}Ga-Pentixafor PET/CT. They used a 2-cascaded V-net that is, W-net; the first V-net model is fed by CT images and trained to learn the bone anatomic information. The output of the first V-net is a binary mask for the skeleton anatomic map. Both PET and CT data are fed into the second V-Net to detect the lesion. They showed that a W-net architecture, which combined the extracted features from the two-cascaded V-nets on PET and CT images, outperformed the V-nets on each modality for both lesion detection and segmentation tasks. Moreover, the CNNs outperformed conventional ML techniques such as random forest (RF), k-nearest neighbors (kNNs), and support vector machine (SVM).

Teramoto and colleagues[101] first located the candidate lung nodules separately by active contour model (ACM) and thresholding in CT and PET images. The results of these 2 streams are then combined using the logical OR function. An ensemble of (i) a multi-step classifier using 2 feature-extractor for CT and PET and (ii) a CNN followed by a two-step classifier and SVM were then applied. Their results revealed that the feature extracted by CNN (they used 3 convolution layers, 3 pooling layers, and 2 fully connected layers) help the FP reduction. Kumar and colleagues[102] used a CNN to facilitate the spatially varying fusion of complementary information of PET and CT images of nonsmall cell lung cancer (NSCLC) using an encoder for each modality, a colearning, and reconstruction components. The results showed the better performance of their proposed method than other CNN-based methods for bimodal detection of lungs, mediastinum, and tumors. Blanc-Durand and colleagues,[103] using amino-acids PET with ^{18}F-fluoro-ethyl-tyrosine (^{18}F-FET), show that a 3D U-net is able to successfully detect brain gliomas. Weisman and colleagues[70] used the multiresolution pathway CNN, DeepMedic for lesion detection in lymphoma patients. An ensemble of the 5-fold cross-validation model was applied and performance was assessed using the true-positive rate (TPR) and number of FP.

More recently, low-dose PET/CT has shown increasing potential for first-line screening. In a preliminary study, Schwyzer and colleagues[104] showed that using a transfer learning approach, a pretrained deep residual neural network (RNN) for binary classification can be used for fully automated lung cancer detection using FDG-PET scans with very low effective radiation doses (ultralow doses: 30-fold (PET3.3%)).[104] They also showed their network had the potential to aid in the detection of small FDG-avid pulmonary nodules (≤2 cm).[98] The results revealed that DL models could help in the detection of small ^{18}F-FDG-avid pulmonary nodules in PET/CT scans. Interestingly, they noted their DL method to perform significantly better on images with block sequential regularized expectation maximization (BSREM) reconstruction as compared with ordered subset expectation maximization (OSEM) reconstruction.[98]

Detection of malignant lesions in nonfluorodeoxyglucose positron emission tomography/computed tomography

Edenbrandt and colleagues[105] developed an AI tool using CNN for the detection and quantification of primary prostate tumors, bone metastases, and lymph nodes in PSMA PET/CT. They showed that using their AI tool decreased the influence of inter-reader variability. Borrelli and colleagues[106] used 2 CNNs for lung lesion detection in 18F-choline PET/CT images and organ segmentation in CT images. They used the segmented organs as an auxiliary input to the detection network (**Fig. 6**). They reported a sensitivity of 90% for their lesion detection approach. AI techniques have recently shown a very good potential to help detect metastases in ^{18}F-FACBC (fluciclovine), 68Ga-PSMA-11, and ^{18}F-choline PET/CT scans of patients with prostate cancer.[107–110] We will discuss more details of these studies in the classification section.

CLINICAL UTILITY OF ARTIFICIAL INTELLIGENCE-BASED CLASSIFICATION IN POSITRON EMISSION TOMOGRAPHY/COMPUTED TOMOGRAPHY: CURRENT STATUS

Classification is considered the most popular area in which CNNs have been used; for example, AlexNet, ResNet, DenseNet, VGG network, and others.[79] Similarly, in medical imaging, AI techniques have been widely used for the extraction of feature toward: (i) classification of suspicious lesions and tumor subtypes, as well as (ii) prediction/prognostication tasks, stratifying/classifying patients into risk groups.[111,112] We review both frontiers next.

Lesion classification in oncological positron emission tomography imaging

Lesion classification can be very challenging and has been conventionally attempted via thresholding. AI techniques seek to enhance such tasks. For instance, abnormal foci in ^{18}F-FACBC [fluciclovine] PET/CT images and the presence of recurrent or metastatic prostate cancer can be classified automatically using AI techniques.[107] **Table 2** lists several example studies using AI for classification. We review the application for both FDG and beyond.

Fluorodeoxyglucose positron emission tomography imaging

ML techniques such as RF can be used to classify the extracted ROIs into normal and abnormal.[113] Teramoto and Fujita and colleagues[114] developed an algorithm to characterize lung nodules by combining CT analysis and binarized PET images based on SUV thresholding. FPs among the leading candidates were eliminated using a rule-based classifier and 3 SVMs. Traditional ML techniques

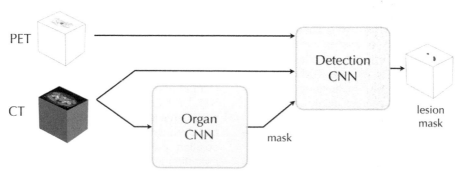

Fig. 6. The AI technique proposed by Borrelli and colleagues[106] based on 2 CNNs. The "Organ CNN" segments the lungs, vertebral bones, liver, and heart. The mask of the organs thus generated is used as an auxiliary input to the "Detection CNN", in addition to the PET and CT images. The output consists of lesion probabilities that can be thresholded to produce a lesion mask. (*Adapted from* Borrelli, P., J. Ly, R. Kaboteh, et al., AI-based detection of lung lesions in [18 F] FDG PET-CT from lung cancer patients. EJNMMI physics, 2021. 8(1): p. 1-11.)

Table 2
Selected studies on AI applications for classification in oncological PET and PET/CT imaging

Study	Task	Modality	Method	# Of Scans (n) # Of Cases (N)	Results
Lee et al,[107] 2020	Discriminating normal and abnormal scans	PET [18] F-FACBC	2D-CNN (ResNet-50) and a 3D-CNN (ResNet-14)	n = 251 N = 18	2D: Sensitivity = 85.7% specificity = 71.4% AUC = 0.750 3D: Sensitivity = 71.4% specificity = 71.4%, AUC = 0.699
Leung et al,[193] 2020	Classification of PCa lesions	PET (PSMA)	3D CNN	N = 267	Accuracy = 67.3%
Teramoto et al,[114] 2014	Classification of pulmonary nodules	PET/CT	a rule-based classifier and 3 support vector machines	N = 100	Sensitivity: 83% FP/case: 5
Sibille et al,[118] 2020	Classify uptake patterns in patients with lung cancer & lymphoma	PET, CT & PET MIPs	CNN	N = 629	Accuracy: CT: 78% PET: 97% PET/CT: 98% PET MIP: 98%
Kawauchi et al,[115] 2020	Classify whole-body FDG PET as 1) benign, 2) malignant or 3) equivocal.	PET/CT	CNN (ResNet)	N = 3485	Accuracy: Benign = 99.4% Malignant = 99.4% Equivocal = 87.5% probability of correct prediction: 97.3% (head-and-neck), 96.6% (chest), 92.8% (abdomen) and 99.6% (pelvic region)
Moitra et al,[116] 2020	Staging and grading of NSCLC	PET/CT	CNN	N = 211	Accuracy: T stage: 96% (2%) N stage: 94% (2%) M stage: 99% (2%) Grading: 95% (3%)
Perk et al,[110] 2018	Bone lesion classification	PET/CT	ML	N = 37	sensitivity = 88% specificity = 89%
Acar et al,[194] 2019	Differentiating metastatic and completely responded sclerotic bone lesion in prostate cancer	PET/CT PSMA	Decision tree, Discriminant analysis, SVM, kNN, ensemble classifier	N = 75	area under the curve (kNN): 0.76

Abbreviations: FP, false positive; kNN, k-nearest neighbor; MIP, maximum intensity projection; SVM, support vector machine; TLG, total lesion glycolysis

generally use domain-specific explicit features that require domain expertise whereas DL-based approaches, such as CNNs, can learn abstract features directly from the training data. Some studies evaluated different CNN configurations to classify the uptake patterns to suspicious and nonsuspicious for cancer from whole-body 18F-FDG PET/CT images. Kawauchi and colleagues[115] used a RES-net for whole-body FDG PET classification to benign, malignant, or equivocal.

The proper diagnosis of lung cancer is based on tumor staging and grading. For solid tumors, medical imaging is often used to determine the T (tumor), N (node), and M (metastasis) classification defining the stage of the disease. ML algorithms on PET/CT have been developed for lung cancers, notably T staging, using different methods including RF, SVM, and CNN. Moitra and colleagues[116] proposed a 1D CNN for lung cancer staging on a public (PET/CT) dataset in the cancer imaging archive (TCIA). The application of 1D CNN for staging and grading lung tumors is not frequent. Their 1D approach was applied to the extracted features from the segmented regions and the histopathological grade information. This 1D CNN approach could offer a lightweight solution that acts as a decision support system for oncologists and radiologists. Unlike the 2D and 3D networks that used the spatial attributes directly from the 2-D or 3-D images and generate huge resource-consuming architecture. Their proposed approach used the spatial information in a rank 2 tensor dataset (a CSV file) along with clinical staging and grading data for classification to classify the information. Capobianco and colleagues[117] used a prototype software (PET Assisted Reporting System [PARS]) to automatically detect and segment the high-uptake regions. The resulting ROIs were further processed by a CNN model to be classified as nonsuspicious or suspicious uptake. The CNN model was pretrained on an independent cohort consists of patients with lung cancer and different subtypes of lymphoma.[118,119] Sibille and colleagues[118] also proposed the use of the PARS algorithm to evaluate each extracted ROI independently and determine whether uptake is suspicious or benign. They used a combination of PET, CT, and PET MIPs, and atlas positions to classify uptakes in patients with lung cancer and lymphoma (**Fig. 7**). An example of the PARS system applied to lymphoma data is presented in **Fig. 8**.

Du and colleagues[120] investigated a variety of ML techniques for radiomics-based differentiation of local recurrence versus inflammation in posttreatment nasopharyngeal carcinoma posttherapy (NPC) PET/CT Images to be applicable for clinical decision making. They showed that the cross-combination fisher score (FSCR) + kNNs, FSCR + SVMs with radial basis function kernel (RBF-SVM), FSCR + RF, and minimum redundancy maximum relevance (MRMR) + RBF-SVM outperformed the other ML techniques and their combination. (see Seyed Mohammad H Gharavi and Armaghan Faghihimehr's article, "Clinical Application of AI in PET imaging of Head and Neck Cancer," in this issue)

Du and colleagues[121] also considered the discrimination power of the individualized radiomics nomogram in both the training and

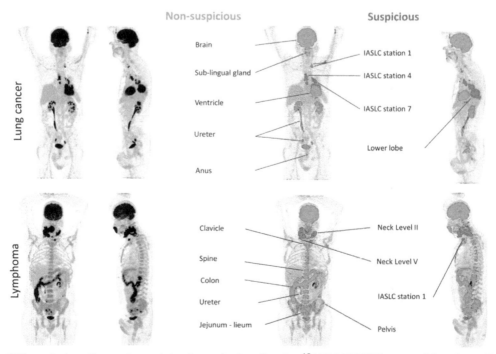

Fig. 7. CCN applied on the maximum intensity projection fluorine ¹⁸F-FDG PET/CT images of 2 patients. Patients with lung cancer and lymphoma with areas of uptake automatically color-coded by their classification and localization are shown. (IASLC=International Association for the Study of Lung Cancer). (*Adapted from* Sibille, L., R. Seifert, N. Avramovic, et al., 18F-FDG PET/CT uptake classification in lymphoma and lung cancer by using deep convolutional neural networks. Radiology, 2020. 294(2): p. 445–452.).

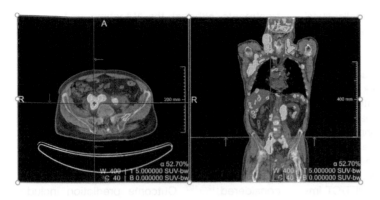

Fig. 8. A patient with diffuse large B-cell lymphoma (DLBCL). Green foci are classified as benign by the prototype software (PET Assisted Reporting System [PARS]) and red foci are classified as pathologic. Here, the algorithm has largely underestimated the pathology with an estimated volume in automated segmentation of 242 mL (SA) against 1270 mL in manual segmentation.

independent validation cohorts. They showed that considering PET, CT, and PET/CT diagnostic signatures, that the combination of metabolic characteristics of PET and anatomic information of CT improved diagnostic performance (**Fig. 9**). On the other hand,**Fig. 8** shows a model that uses radiomics and clinical semantic features in a radiomics nomogram outperformed the model that relied on PET only or CT only information.

Radiotracers beyond fluorodeoxyglucose

Although ^{18}F-FDG is the most widely used radiotracer in oncology and nuclear medicine, it is not as suitable for certain cancers, although the data access for tracers much less common than FDG, is limited. As an example, prostate adenocarcinomas, the most common cancer in men, can be imaged using other tracers such as radiolabeled choline, ^{18}F-Fluciclovine, and ^{18}F-Piflufolastat (targeting prostate-specific membrane antigen (PSMA)) or similar radiotracers such as ^{68}Ga-PSMA.[122] Promising results of VISION trial[123] closed the evidence gap in prostate cancer radiopharmaceutical therapy with ^{177}Lu-PSMA. At the dawn of this new era, the development of new imaging biomarkers for retreatment patient selection is on the horizon. Theranostic radio-isotope pairs for diagnosis (^{18}F, ^{68}Ga) versus therapy (^{177}Lu, [225]Ac) provide us with the possibility of having diagnostic and therapeutic radiopharmaceuticals with relatively similar biodistributions and kinetics. Several studies have already investigated the contribution of AI techniques to the analysis of PSMA PET/CT scans [see Ma and colleagues' article, "Clinical Application of AI in PET imaging of

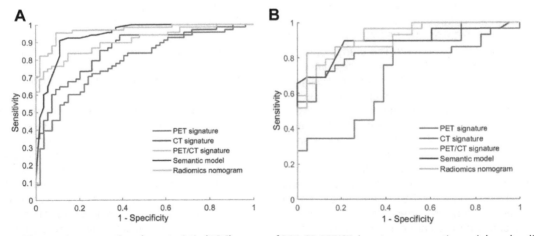

Fig. 9. The receiver operating characteristic (ROC) curves of PET, CT, PET/CT signatures, semantic model, and radiomics nomogram for (*A*) training and (*B*) validation cohorts. Compared with the CT signature, the PET/CT signature significantly improved AUC for the training cohort. Combining the PET/CT features with the semantic features in a radiomics nomogram significantly improves the diagnostic performance with respect to the semantic model alone or PET/CT signature alone in training cohort, whereas did not significantly improve the performance in the validation cohort. The DeLong test method was used for the statistical comparison of ROC curves. (*Adapted from Du, D., J. Gu, X. Chen, and colleagues, Integration of PET/CT radiomics and semantic features for differentiation between active pulmonary tuberculosis and lung cancer. Molecular Imaging and Biology, 2021. 23(2): p. 287–298.*)

Prostate Cancer" and Brosch-Lenz and colleagues' article, "Role of AI in Theranostics: Towards Routine Personalized Radiopharmaceutical Therapies," articles].

Zhao and colleagues[108] in a pilot study focused on the pelvis, developed a framework to characterize the local and secondary prostate tumors in the lymph nodes and bones and to facilitate the optimization of PSMA directed radionuclide therapy by using a 2.5D U-net architecture. . Polymeri and colleagues[109] used a CNN to segment prostate cancer and prostate volume based on ^{18}F-choline and found the derived features from PET/CT images were significantly associated with overall survival. They found that the other common clinical features including age, prostate-specific antigen, and Gleason score did not affect the overall survival. Leung and colleagues[124] developed a 3D CNN to automatically classify the PCa lesions in ^{18}F-DCFPyL PSMA PET images by PSMA-RADS score prediction for lesion classification. The 3D PET images were cropped to yield varied size cubic volumes-of-interest (VOIs) around the center of each lesion as the input to the 3D CNN along with the manual segmentation. This classification approach showed promising results.

Perk and colleagues[110] developed an automated bone lesion classification by using ML techniques to classify lesions in ^{18}F-NaF PET/CT images, as bone metastases can be confounded by tracer uptake in benign diseases, such as osteoarthritis. Acar and colleagues[106] used ML techniques including decision tree, discriminant analysis, SVM, kNN, and ensemble classifier on the textural features to distinguish the lesions imaged via ^{68}Ga-PSMA PET/CT as metastatic and completely responded. The study population contains patients with known bone metastasis and previously treated patients and the weighted kNN outperformed the other classifiers. As it is considered in the above-mentioned studies, it has been shown that using the hybrid information of CT and PET images statistically significantly improved the lesion classification accuracy.

Lee and colleagues[107] used a 2D-CNN (ResNet-50) and a 3D-CNN (ResNet-14) to discriminate normal and abnormal PET scans based on the presence of tumor recurrence and/or metastases in patients with prostate cancer and biochemical recurrence in ^{18}F-FACBC (fluciclovine) images. They reported that a 2D slice-based approach depicted better results than 2D or 3D case-based approaches. [^{68} Ga]DOTATATE PET/CT scans have shown significant value for imaging neuroendocrine tumors (NETs), improving detection, and characterization, grading, staging, and predicting/monitoring the responses to treatments, although the AI techniques for detection have not been explored.

Prediction/prognosis in oncological positron emission tomography imaging

Prognostic tasks provide information about the patient outcome, regardless of therapy, whereas predictive tasks consider the effect of therapeutic interventions.[125] The prognostic value of pretreatment ^{18}F-FDG-PET/CT images for treatment planning and decision support has been extensively considered.[126,127] Outcome prediction includes the extraction of radiomics feature from PET and CT images, combined with any valuable clinical indicators, to predict survival, for example, recurrence-free, metastasis-free, progression-free, and/or overall survival.[127–129]

Cottereau and colleagues[130] showed that "lesion dissemination" is a strong prognosticator of progression-free survival (PFS) and overall survival (OS) in diffuse large B-cell lymphoma (DLBCL) cases. Their work emphasizes that outcome prediction can consist of finding links among tumors. They showed that the largest distance between 2 lesions (Dmax) that indicates the spread of the disease is independent and complementary to metabolic tumor volume (MTV)) for outcome prediction in DLBCL patients. Desseroit and colleagues[131] considered features in 4 categories: (1) clinical variables, (2) volume and standard metrics, (3) PET heterogeneity, and (4) CT heterogeneity (Fig. 10). They showed that tumor heterogeneity quantified with textural features on the CT and PET components of ^{18}F-FDG PET/CT images can provide complementary prognostic value in NSCLC. They designed a four-variable nomogram that outperformed the standard clinical staging.

The hope is that AI methods can enable robust risk-stratification, thus enabling improved the staging of patients. In this subsection, we consider the important applications of AI in the prognosis of cancer recurrence rates, outcome prediction for response assessment and clinical decision-making. Effective prognostic signatures include both clinical and imaging features by integrating quantitative voxel-wise features and valuable clinical information. The increasing availability of high-throughput omics datasets from large patient cohorts has facilitated the development of AI techniques to classify patients according to survival or disease recurrence. Specifically, for the stratification of patients with cancer, their death or other survival information (eg, progression-free survival) are considered endpoints.

Existing predictive modeling frameworks may perform: (1) statistical survival analysis on explicit

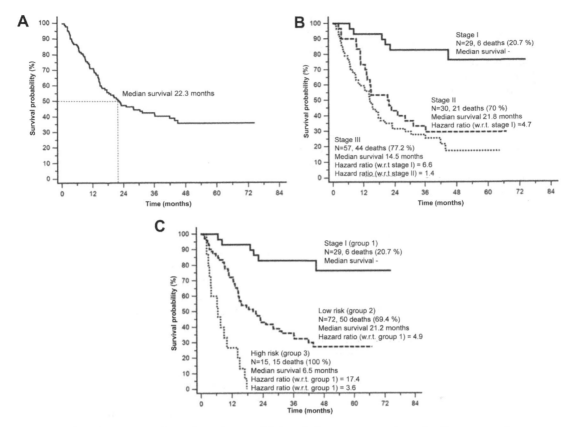

Fig. 10. Kaplan–Meier curves for a the cohort and b in relation to stage only, and c the proposed nomogram (w.r.t. in the figures means with respect to). (*A*) The goal of this study is to build a nomogram combining the best features of each category to improve the stratification provided by stage alone. (*B*) Patients with stage III disease had worse survival than those with stage II disease. (*C*) The best stratification was obtained by including all four parameters in the model. (*Adapted from* Desseroit, M.-C., D. Visvikis, F. Tixier, et al., Development of a nomogram combining clinical staging with 18 F-FDG PET/CT image features in non-small-cell lung cancer stage I–III. European journal of nuclear medicine and molecular imaging, 2016. 43(8): p. 1477–1485.)

features; (2) ML-based techniques applied to explicit and/or deep features; and (3) DL (CNN) models for outcome prediction. In addition to deep feature extraction, NNs can model nonlinear survival data by classifications and estimation of the risk of failure as the nonlinear extension of Cox proportional hazards.[132] Recent studies have shown the superiority of ML techniques over statistical analyses in terms of discriminant power using a feature selection scheme based on complementary features.[44,133] Prognostication (prognostic stratification) has been primarily determined based on semantic tumor staging, leading to relatively coarse, and discrete stratification.[134] As such, direct outcome prediction without the intermediate stages of image/tumor classification has gained increasing attention. CNNs are able to learn the prognostically relevant features of the images directly by bypassing the intermediate steps for the identification of predictive

biomarkers. Explicit feature-based ML techniques for outcome prediction usually suffer from the feature selection step that is, often unstable given the high-dimensional features (curse of dimensionality), though there is ongoing research on using dimensionality reduction algorithms (feature selection or extraction algorithms).[135] It has been shown that CNNs have enhanced predictive power than explicit features.[136,137]

Ypsilantis and colleagues[138] considered both of the above-mentioned frameworks that is, ML and CNN approaches to predict outcome in patients with esophageal cancer. The first approach included feature extraction and using ML classifiers such as linear regression (LR), gradient boosting, RFs, and SVMs. The second approach applied CNNs on image data and corresponding segmented region that had higher average accuracy. Pereira and colleagues[139] suggested a pipeline for response to treatment evaluation and stratification into a 5-classe Deauville scale using different CNN architectures on patient data with Hodgkin's lymphoma. An AI method suggested by Capobianco and colleagues[140] can generate a TMTV value prognostic of outcome in a large series of patients with non-Hodgkin's lymphoma (ie, DLBCL). On a database of 97 patients, Bizzego and colleagues[66] showed that the analysis of PET tumor images with a 3D CNN produced very promising results to predict treatment response in esophageal cancer, and outperformed 2D CNN architectures, as well as explicit feature extraction with RF classifiers. The hybrid—explicit and deep feature approach was the most accurate. The same authors proposed to carry out internal transfer-learning based on the prediction of the grade of the disease to improve the prediction of their prognostic model and have shown a better classification accuracy using this transfer learning approach. On the other hand, Wang and colleagues[141] showed that CNN results were not superior to explicit radiomics for mediastinal lymph nodes classification in nonsmall lung cancer data. They concluded that explicit features are sometimes preferred, as they are user-friendly and can be applied with less amount of data and are less affected by feature selection bias.

FUTURE DIRECTIONS AND OPEN QUESTIONS
Temporal changes in radiomics features: dynamic-radiomics and delta-radiomics

Radiomics signatures of medical images are usually derived from static images. It has been shown that temporal changes for example in tracer uptake of PET scans can also reveal new aspects of tumor biology.[142–145] Analysis of features extracted from the temporal analysis of dynamic PET scans can be referred to as "dynamic-radiomics" (microscale temporal changes). By contrast, "delta-radiomics" refer to the analysis of features derived from the comparison of a study with prior images (to capture macro-scale temporal changes). Clinical experience highlights the importance of temporal changes as one of the most important characteristics of the lesion.[146] Fave and colleagues[144] showed the utility of CT delta-radiomics for the prediction of patient outcome in lung cancer.[144] Later, numerous groups expanded the use of CT-based delta-radiomics to other cancers such as gastric cancer,[147] and also the detection of treatment side-effects such as radiation-induced xerostomia[148,149] and pneumonitis.[148] MR-based delta-radiomics is also widely used in various cancers, including prostate cancer,[150] sarcoma,[151] colorectal cancer,[152] and rectal cancer.[152] It has been suggested that delta-radiomics may increase

multicentric reproducibility.[153] As such, delta radiomics frameworks are being developed (for example, using pre, intra, and/or post-therapy scans in combination. Such a framework also has potentially significant value when applying to theranostics paradigms in the context of radiopharmaceutical therapies [see Yousefirizi and colleagues' article, "Towards High-throughput AI-based Segmentation in Oncological PET Imaging," in this issue] *Efforts to Translate* artificial intelligence *technique to routine clinical usage*

Translating AI techniques into routinely used clinical workflows requires collaboration between AI researchers, radiologists, and oncologists, and predefined frameworks for evaluating these techniques to be integrated into clinical applications and accepted by the oncology community.[112] The decisions made by nuclear medicine physicians and radiologists are not based on 2D slices of PET or CT scans. Some of the existing studies suggested the AI techniques applied on the limited 2D slices for detection tasks that can be very prone to errors and considering the advanced 3D AI techniques, it should be reconsidered in future studies in the field of PET oncology.

Explainable AI techniques such based on attention or saliency maps are demanded especially for clinical decision support systems.[31,154,155] The explanations is needed to: (i) verify the model's output to the physicians, (ii) increase the trustworthiness of AI techniques, and (iii) identify the potential biases.[156,157] Consequently, explainable AI techniques facilitate the communication between the "black-box" DL models and physicians.

Reproducible measurements made by AI methods for lesion evaluation in oncology reports have been shown to be helpful for reducing the reporting errors and increasing the workflow efficiency.[158] Considering the lower FPs and high sensitivity of DL based methods than traditional ML techniques for detection, DL based methods can be clinically feasible if they showed similar performance in the extensive clinical trials.

AI frameworks have the potential to be used as a "second reader" for radiologists to improve diagnostic accuracy and efficiency.[111,112] It is worth noting that AI-based solutions (considering the superior performance of DL approaches) can be used as the decision support tools while they have been mostly considered as the replacement of clinicians in clinical practice that is, far from reality.[159] In fact, AI techniques try to mimic and augment the clinicians' work instead of replacing them.[160] Freeman and colleagues[161] showed that the promising results of AI techniques in smaller studies of breast cancer screening programs are not replicated in larger studies.

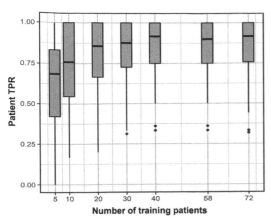

Fig. 11. Considering the impact of the number of training patients on detection performance. The detection performance was not improved when training was done on more than 40 subjects. No significant differences (P > .05) were observed in the performance of the model trained on N = 40 subjects compared to the model trained with 58 subjects. Likewise, model performance did not significantly improve when training with 72 subjects (using the validation cohort as additional training subjects). Boxplots show the median and interquartile range of patient-level true-positive rate (TPR) across all 90 patients as a function of training patient number, operating at an average of four false-positive findings per patient. Dots represent outliers, which are determined by points lying further than 1.5 times the interquartile range from the edge of the box. *(Adapted from Weisman, A.J., M.W. Kieler, S.B. Perlman, et al., Convolutional Neural Networks for Automated PET/CT Detection of Diseased Lymph Node Burden in Patients with Lymphoma. Radiology: Artificial Intelligence, 2020. 2(5): p. e200016.)*

Most studies to date on radiomics signature have involved a limited number of cases (<100 prone to overfitting), retrospective (selection bias), and monocentric (less likely to be generalized); the last limitation refers to the fact that most of the developed models were never evaluated on external datasets.[162] Furthermore, it has been demonstrated that despite the growing number of developed frameworks for disease severity classification (estimation), the existing models have been reported to be largely dependent on the demographics and clinical history of the patient.[163]

Challenges with existing AI techniques include the limited interpretability of the resulting networks and the high dependency on large datasets in supervised techniques. Weisman and colleagues[70] investigated the impact of the number of training subjects on detection performance; their results showed that it is not always the case that using a much larger dataset can improve the performance of supervised AI techniques and that the performance of the DL model is limited by the consistency of the labels (**Fig. 11**). In the other words,

sample size, data quality, and diversity are all important.[164] New AI techniques that need a lower amount of annotation are highly demanded, for example, semisupervised and weakly supervised techniques that use sparse and weak annotations showed acceptable performances. Using the annotations made by multiple experts for every scan was proposed to produce limited data with high-quality annotations that are not achieved usually.[31] The platforms for "crowd-sourced" image labeling can help in this regard.[165]

The number of cases needed for developing a radiomics signature model is highly dependent on the complexity of the problem.[166] In addition to the use of unsupervised and weakly supervised techniques, using DL models pretrained on different pathologies can also be helpful.[167] Capobianco and colleagues[168] showed that using transfer learning the CNN network trained for tumor detection in ^{18}F-FDG PET/CT can be applied for tumor assessment in ^{68}Ga-PSMA-11 PET/CT images.

The nuclear medicine community is now aware of the impact of image acquisition and reconstruction parameters on handcrafted radiomic features (and on the performance of models combining them) but this issue has been less discussed and reported in deep radiomics whereas there is no guarantee that the effect is not as strong and more difficult to detect.

Several problems need to be tackled for the clinical application of DL-based techniques. For instance, the performance of the model is highly affected by the curse of hyper-parameters[169] (a range of parameters to optimize such as learning rate, number of epochs, activation functions, and so forth that usually are chosen arbitrarily). The lack of the explainable model for an AI-based decision support system in clinical application is another issue that prevents rapid translation of AI techniques into clinical workflow.[170]

Application of natural language processing for labeling

The extracted information from clinical reports can be used to develop AI techniques that can help to report in clinics. Although there are guidelines for diagnostic imaging reports and label extraction, most of these reports are composed of free-text.[171] Rule-based[172] or recurrent NNs [173] for natural language processing (NLP) are used for information extraction from radiology reports. In the field of NLP, nonexperts mostly do manual labeling; this approach is not applicable in the field of medical image segmentation especially for advanced modalities that is, CT and PET. Recently, reporting that contains hypertexts,[174] labeling before the radiologist that is, prospective labeling[175] and interactive reporting[176] are considered as potential solutions to cope up with the problem of limited ground truth. As an example, Ryoo and colleagues[177] for interpreting brain perfusion SPECT trained a long short-term memory (LSTM) network on the unstructured text reports to predict abnormalities of basal perfusion and vascular reserve for each vascular territory. Using this trained LSTM model, the structured information of the text reports can be extracted. They developed a 3D CNN model with AUC 0.83 for basal perfusion and 0.89 for vascular reserve. This model can be used as a support system to identify the perfusion abnormalities and the quantitative scores of abnormalities.

Neuro-symbolic artificial intelligence models for detection and classification

AI techniques for detection and classification should not be trained only on the images, incorporating the complementary clinical information of the patients improves the performance and generalization of the developed AI models. Neuro-symbolic AI models involve the integration of complementary approaches that is, NN (connectionist) and rule-based (symbolist) frameworks. Especially see Toosi and colleagues [Toos and colleagues' article, "A Brief History of Artificial Intelligence (Past, Present, and Future), and What Can Prevent Another 'Winter'" in this issue] for discussions of these 2 frameworks. Symbolic AI integrates contextual knowledge and generalizable rules into the AI framework. The rules that have been previously extracted (considering the decision made by physicians) can be used for feature prediction in new images. In the other words, these rules make the (deep) NN biased toward the physicians' decision. Rule-based AI attracted significant attention in the early decades of AI research, but was later superseded by NN approaches,[170] and integration of the 2 seems to be on the horizon to significantly improve the performance and generalizability of AI-based models.

Clinicians often use a set of conditions, different image modalities for a patient, treatment and surgery history, as well as biological and physiologic conditions to decide about a suspicious lesion based on their experiences.[178] By incorporating these "rules" into the AI models for detection, classification, and segmentation, we can move forward to neuro-symbolic NNs and explainable AI techniques for detection and segmentation.[179]

SUMMARY

Considering the strength of AI techniques in performing effective image phenotyping including robust identification of patterns beyond visual assessments, there is significant potential for use in accelerating and automating detection and classification tasks in medical imaging and as an example oncologic PET imaging, as reviewed in the present work. AI techniques can also link radiomics signatures and biological properties extracted by radiologists and nuclear medicine physicians in the routine clinical workflow. Having access to appropriate labeled data is vital for supervised AI techniques in the derivation and validation of reliable detection and classification workflows. Alternatively, weakly- and unsupervised techniques along with transfer learning from different pathologies can be helpful in this regard. Considering the large existing database of electronic health records, applying NLP has shown potential to help tackle the labor-intensive task of labeling for supervised techniques. Besides, new insight into rule-based NNs, that is, neuro-symbolic networks, can obtain clues from decisions made by the physicians, with potential for further enhanced and generalizable AI clinical decision support systems.

CLINICS CARE POINTS

- Stratification of cancer into reliably distinct risk subgroups enables personalization of treatment.
- Detection of organs or lesions as regions of interests (ROIs) or volumes of interests (VOIs) is an important step towards classification.
- Classification tasks for identification and characterization of lesions have significant potential in clinical workflows. Classification in the context of prediction/prognosis also enables risk stratification.
- Radiomics mines for potentially significant quantitative information beyond what is nowadays captured in routine clinical evaluations.
- AI techniques can perform quantitative high-throughput image phenotyping (extracting numerous image-based features) and identifying important discriminative features that, individually or in combination, form effective radiomics signatures for detection, classification and prediction/prognosis.
- Integration of AI techniques into routine clinical workflows require collaboration between AI researchers and clinicians, and standardized evaluation frameworks.

ACKNOWLEDGEMENTS

This project was in part supported by the Natural Sciences and Engineering Research Council of Canada (NSERC) Discovery Grant RGPIN-2019-06467, and the Canadian Institutes of Health Research (CIHR) Project Grant PJT-173231.

DISCLOSURE

Authors do not have anything to disclose regarding conflict of interest with respect to this article.

REFERENCES

1. Langlotz CP. RadLex: a new method for indexing online educational materials. Radiographics 2006; 26(6):1595–7.

2. Chernyak V, Sirlin CB. LI-RADS: future directions. Clin Liver Dis 2021;17(3):149.

3. Bruno MA, Walker EA, Abujudeh HH. Understanding and confronting our mistakes: the epidemiology of error in radiology and strategies for error reduction. Radiographics 2015;35(6):1668–76.

4. Daniel K. Thinking, fast and slow 2017.

5. Kim YW, Mansfield LT. Fool me twice: delayed diagnoses in radiology with emphasis on perpetuated errors. Am J roentgenology 2014;202(3):465–70.

6. Zhaoping L, Li Z. Understanding vision: theory, models, and data. USA: Oxford University Press; 2014.

7. Zhaoping L. A new framework for understanding vision from the perspective of the primary visual cortex. Curr Opin Neurobiol 2019;58:1–10.

8. Riesenhuber M, Poggio T. Hierarchical models of object recognition in cortex. Nat Neurosci 1999; 2(11):1019–25.

9. DiCarlo JJ, Cox DD. Untangling invariant object recognition. Trends Cognitive Sciences 2007; 11(8):333–41.

10. DiCarlo JJ, Zoccolan D, Rust NC. How does the brain solve visual object recognition? Neuron 2012;73(3):415–34.

11. Bar M. A cortical mechanism for triggering top-down facilitation in visual object recognition. J Cogn Neurosci 2003;15(4):600–9.

12. Kim JU, Kim ST, Kim ES, et al. Towards high-performance object detection: Task-specific design considering classification and localization separation. in ICASSP 2020-2020 IEEE International Conference on Acoustics, Speech and Signal Processing (ICASSP). 4-8 May 2020. Barcelona, Spain: IEEE.

13. Murray NM, Unberath M, Hager GD, et al. Artificial intelligence to diagnose ischemic stroke and identify large vessel occlusions: a systematic review. J neurointerventional Surg 2020;12(2): 156–64.

14. Chamberlin J, Kocher MR, Waltz J, et al. Automated detection of lung nodules and coronary artery calcium using artificial intelligence on low-dose CT scans for lung cancer screening: accuracy and prognostic value. BMC Med 2021;19(1):1–14.

15. Kim H-E, Kim HH, Han B-K, et al. Changes in cancer detection and false-positive recall in mammography using artificial intelligence: a retrospective, multireader study. Lancet Digital Health 2020;2(3): e138–48.

16. Winkel DJ, Heye T, Weikert TJ, et al. Evaluation of an AI-based detection software for acute findings in abdominal computed tomography scans: toward an automated work list prioritization of routine CT examinations. Invest Radiol 2019; 54(1):55–9.

17. Food U, Administration D. Computer-assisted detection devices applied to radiology images and radiology device data—Premarket notification [510 (k)] submissions. Silver spring: Food and Drug Administration; 2012.

18. Center for Devices, & Radiological Health. (n.d.). Clinical Performance Assessment: Considerations for CAD Devices. Available at: https://www.fda. gov/regulatory-information/search-fda-guidance-documents/clinical-performance-assessment-con siderations-computer-assisted-detection-devices-applied-radiology. Accessed October 19, 2021.

19. Zhou SK, Rueckert D, Fichtinger G. Handbook of medical image computing and computer assisted intervention. Academic Press; 2019.

20. Cho JS, Shrestha S, Kagiyama N, et al. A network-based "phenomics" approach for discovering patient subtypes from high-throughput cardiac imaging data. JACC: Cardiovasc Imaging 2020;13(8): 1655–70.

21. Houle D, Govindaraju DR, Omholt S. Phenomics: the next challenge. Nat Rev Genet 2010;11(12):855–66.

22. Hoyles L, Fernandez-Real J-M, Federici M, et al. Molecular phenomics and metagenomics of hepatic steatosis in non-diabetic obese women. Nat Med 2018;24(7):1070–80.

23. Zbuk KM, Eng C. Cancer phenomics: RET and PTEN as illustrative models. Nat Rev Cancer 2007;7(1):35–45.

24. Bizhanova A, Kopp P. Genetics and phenomics of Pendred syndrome. Mol Cell Endocrinol 2010; 322(1–2):83–90.

25. Bourdais G, Burdiak P, Gauthier A, et al. Large-scale phenomics identifies primary and fine-tuning roles for CRKs in responses related to oxidative stress. PLoS Genet 2015;11(7):e1005373.

26. Kafkas Ş, Althubaiti S, Gkoutos GV, et al. Linking common human diseases to their phenotypes;

development of a resource for human phenomics. J Biomed semantics 2021;12(1):1–15.

27. Seifert R, Weber M, Kocakavuk E, et al. Artificial intelligence and machine learning in nuclear medicine: future Perspectives. Semin Nucl Med 2021; 51(2):170–7.

28. Hatt M, Tixier F, Visvikis D, et al. Radiomics in PET/CT: more than meets the eye? J Nucl Med 2017; 58(3):365–6.

29. Orlhac F, Nioche C, Klyuzhin I, et al. Radiomics in PET imaging: a practical guide for newcomers. PET Clin 2021;16(4):597–612.

30. Horvat N, Bates DD, Petkovska I. Novel imaging techniques of rectal cancer: what do radiomics and radiogenomics have to offer? A literature review. Abdom Radiol 2019;44(11):3764–74.

31. Langlotz CP, Allen B, Erickson BJ, et al. A roadmap for foundational research on artificial intelligence in medical imaging: from the 2018 NIH/RSNA/ACR/The Academy Workshop. Radiology 2019;291(3): 781–91.

32. Al-shamasneh ARM, Obaidellah UHB. Artificial intelligence techniques for cancer detection and classification: review study. Eur Scientific J 2017; 13(3):342–70.

33. D'Amore B, Smolinski-Zhao S, Daye D, et al. Role of machine learning and artificial intelligence in interventional oncology. Curr Oncol Rep 2021;23(6):1–8.

34. Visvikis D, Le Rest CC, Jaouen V, et al. Artificial intelligence, machine (deep) learning and radio (geno) mics: definitions and nuclear medicine imaging applications. Eur J Nucl Med Mol Imaging 2019;46(13):2630–7.

35. Oquab M, Bottou L, Laptev I, et al. Is object localization for free?-weakly-supervised learning with convolutional neural networks. in Proceedings of the IEEE conference on computer vision and pattern recognition. Boston, USA: 7-12 June 2015.

36. Zhou B, Khosla A, Lapedriza A, et al. Learning deep features for discriminative localization. in Proceedings of the IEEE conference on computer vision and pattern recognition. Los Vegas, USA: June 26th - July 1st 2016.

37. Gillies RJ, Kinahan PE, Hricak H. Radiomics: images are more than Pictures, they are data. Radiology 2016;278(2):563–77.

38. El Naqa I, Grigsby PW, Apte A, et al. Exploring feature-based approaches in PET images for predicting cancer treatment outcomes. Pattern recognition 2009;42(6):1162–71.

39. Vallieres M, Kay-Rivest E, Perrin LJ, et al. Radiomics strategies for risk assessment of tumour failure in head-and-neck cancer. Scientific Rep 2017;7(1):1–14.

40. Kidd EA, El Naqa I, Siegel BA, et al. FDG-PET-based prognostic nomograms for locally advanced cervical cancer. Gynecol Oncol 2012;127(1): 136–40.

41. Vallières M, Freeman CR, Skamene SR, et al. A radiomics model from joint FDG-PET and MRI texture features for the prediction of lung metastases in soft-tissue sarcomas of the extremities. Phys Med Biol 2015;60(14):5471.

42. Vaidya M, Creach KM, Frye J, et al. Combined PET/CT image characteristics for radiotherapy tumor response in lung cancer. Radiother Oncol 2012; 102(2):239–45.

43. Frood R, Burton C, Tsoumpas C, et al. Baseline PET/CT imaging parameters for prediction of treatment outcome in Hodgkin and diffuse large B cell lymphoma: a systematic review. Eur J Nucl Med Mol Imaging 2021;1–23.

44. Parmar C, Grossmann P, Bussink J, et al. Machine learning methods for quantitative radiomic biomarkers. Scientific Rep 2015;5(1):1–11.

45. Kotrotsou A, Zinn PO, Colen RR. Radiomics in brain tumors: an emerging technique for characterization of tumor environment. Magn Reson Imaging Clin 2016;24(4):719–29.

46. Li X, Yin G, Zhang Y, et al. Predictive power of a radiomic signature based on 18F-FDG PET/CT images for EGFR mutational status in NSCLC. Front Oncol 2019;9:1062.

47. Lartizien C, Rogez M, Niaf E, et al. Computer-aided staging of lymphoma patients with FDG PET/CT imaging based on textural information. IEEE J Biomed Health Inform 2013;18(3):946–55.

48. Avanzo M, Wei L, Stancanello J, et al. Machine and deep learning methods for radiomics. Med Phys 2020;47(5):e185–202.

49. Kebir S, Khurshid Z, Gaertner FC, et al. Unsupervised consensus cluster analysis of [18F]-fluoroethyl-L-tyrosine positron emission tomography identified textural features for the diagnosis of pseudoprogression in high-grade glioma. Oncotarget 2017;8(5): 8294.

50. Afshar P, Mohammadi A, Plataniotis KN, et al. From handcrafted to deep-learning-based cancer radiomics: challenges and opportunities. IEEE Signal Process. Mag 2019;36(4):132–60.

51. Van Griethuysen JJ, Fedorov A, Parmar C, et al. Computational radiomics system to decode the radiographic phenotype. Cancer Res 2017; 77(21):e104–7.

52. Nioche C, Orlhac F, Boughdad S, et al. LIFEx: a freeware for radiomic feature calculation in multimodality imaging to accelerate advances in the characterization of tumor heterogeneity. Cancer Res 2018;78(16):4786–9.

53. Ashrafinia S, DiGianvittorio M, Rowe S, et al. Reproducibility and reliability of radiomic features in 18F-DCFPyL PET/CT imaging of prostate cancer. J Nucl Med 2017;58(supplement 1):503.

54. Deasy JO, Blanco AI, Clark VH. CERR: a computational environment for radiotherapy research. Med Phys 2003;30(5):979–85.

55. Zwanenburg A, Vallières M, Abdalah MA, et al. The image biomarker standardization initiative: standardized quantitative radiomics for high-throughput image-based phenotyping. Radiology 2020;295(2):328–38.

56. Ashrafinia S, Dalaie P, Sadaghiani MS, et al. Radiomics analysis of clinical Myocardial perfusion stress SPECT images to identify Coron Artery Calcification. medRxiv, 2021.

57. Zhang Y, Oikonomou A, Wong A, et al. Radiomics-based prognosis analysis for non-small cell lung cancer. Scientific Rep 2017;7(1):1–8.

58. Rizzo S, Botta F, Raimondi S, et al. Radiomics: the facts and the challenges of image analysis. Eur Radiol Exp 2018;2(1):1–8.

59. Lohmann P, Bousabarah K, Hoevels M, et al. Radiomics in radiation oncology—basics, methods, and limitations. Strahlenther Onkol 2020;196(10): 848–55.

60. Oktay O, Schlemper J, Folgoc LL, et al., Attention u-net: Learning where to look for the pancreas. arXiv preprint arXiv:1804.03999, 2018.

61. Khalvati F, Zhang J, Chung AG, et al. MPCaD: a multi-scale radiomics-driven framework for automated prostate cancer localization and detection. BMC Med Imaging 2018;18(1):1–14.

62. Geirhos R, Rubisch P, Michaelis C, et al. ImageNet-trained CNNs are biased towards texture; increasing shape bias improves accuracy and robustness. arXiv preprint arXiv:1811.12231, 2018.

63. Islam MA, Kowal M, Esser P, et al. Shape or texture: understanding discriminative features in CNNs. arXiv preprint arXiv:2101.11604, 2021.

64. Klyuzhin IS, Xu Y, Ortiz A, et al. Testing the Ability of Convolutional Neural Networks to Learn Radiomic Features. medRxiv, 2020.

65. Kim J, Seo S, Ashrafinia S, et al. Training of deep convolutional neural nets to extract radiomic signatures of tumors. J Nucl Med 2019;60(supplement 1):406.

66. Bizzego, A., N. Bussola, D. Salvalai, et al. Integrating deep and radiomics features in cancer bioimaging. in 2019 IEEE Conference on Computational Intelligence in Bioinformatics and Computational Biology (CIBCB). 9-11 July 2019. Siena, Italy: IEEE.

67. Peng H, Dong D, Fang M-J, et al. Prognostic value of deep learning PET/CT-based radiomics: potential role for future individual induction chemotherapy in advanced nasopharyngeal carcinoma. Clin Cancer Res 2019;25(14):4271–9.

68. Rizzo A, Triumbari EKA, Gatta R, et al. The role of 18F-FDG PET/CT radiomics in lymphoma. Clin Translational Imaging 2021;1–10.

69. Domingues I, Pereira G, Martins P, et al. Using deep learning techniques in medical imaging: a systematic review of applications on CT and PET. Artif Intelligence Rev 2020;53(6):4093–160.

70. Weisman AJ, Kieler MW, Perlman SB, et al. Convolutional neural networks for automated PET/CT detection of diseased lymph node burden in patients with lymphoma. Radiol Artif Intelligence 2020;2(5):e200016.

71. Gruetzemacher R, Gupta A, Paradice D. 3D deep learning for detecting pulmonary nodules in CT scans. J Am Med Inform Assoc 2018;25(10): 1301–10.

72. Barbu A, Suehling M, Xu X, et al. Automatic detection and segmentation of lymph nodes from CT data. IEEE Trans Med Imaging 2011; 31(2):240–50.

73. Cherry KM, Wang S, Turkbey EB, et al. Abdominal lymphadenopathy detection using random forest. in Medical imaging 2014: computer-Aided diagnosis. Int Soc Opt Photon 2014.

74. Topol EJ. High-performance medicine: the convergence of human and artificial intelligence. Nat Med 2019;25(1):44–56.

75. Gaonkar B, Beckett J, Attiah M, et al. Eigenrank by committee: Von-Neumann entropy based data subset selection and failure prediction for deep learning based medical image segmentation. Med Image Anal 2021;67:101834.

76. Karimi D, Dou H, Warfield SK, et al. Deep learning with noisy labels: Exploring techniques and remedies in medical image analysis. Med Image Anal 2020;65:101759.

77. Shin H-C, Roth HR, Gao M, et al. Deep convolutional neural networks for computer-aided detection: CNN architectures, dataset characteristics and transfer learning. IEEE Trans Med Imaging 2016;35(5):1285–98.

78. Vauclin S, Doyeux K, Hapdey S, et al. Development of a generic thresholding algorithm for the delineation of 18FDG-PET-positive tissue: application to the comparison of three thresholding models. Phys Med Biol 2009;54(22):6901.

79. Hellwig D, Graeter TP, Ukena D, et al. 18F-FDG PET for mediastinal staging of lung cancer: which SUV threshold makes sense? J Nucl Med 2007; 48(11):1761–6.

80. Wahl RL, Jacene H, Kasamon Y, et al. From RECIST to PERCIST: evolving considerations for PET response criteria in solid tumors. J Nucl Med 2009;50(Suppl 1):122S–50S.

81. Bi L, Kim J, Kumar A, et al. Automatic detection and classification of regions of FDG uptake in whole-body PET-CT lymphoma studies. Comput Med Imaging Graphics 2017;60:3–10.

82. DENG C-L, JIANG H-Y, LI H-M. Automated high uptake regions recognition and lymphoma

detection based on fully convolutional networks on chest and abdomen PET image. DEStech Trans Biol Health 2017 (icmsb).

83. Afshari S, BenTaieb A, Hamarneh G. Automatic localization of normal active organs in 3D PET scans. Comput Med Imaging Graphics 2018;70:111-8.

84. Kawakami M, Hirata K, Furuya S, et al. Development of combination methods for detecting malignant uptakes based on physiological uptake detection using object detection with PET-CT MIP images. Front Med 2020;7.

85. Redmon J, Divvala S, Girshick R, et al. You only look once: Unified, real-time object detection. in Proceedings of the IEEE conference on computer vision and pattern recognition. 2016.

86. Bi L, Kim J, Kumar A, et al. Synthesis of positron emission tomography (PET) images via multi-channel generative adversarial networks (GANs), in molecular imaging, reconstruction and analysis of moving body organs, and stroke imaging and treatment. Springer; 2017. p. 43–51.

87. Ben-Cohen A, Klang E, Raskin SP, et al. Cross-modality synthesis from CT to PET using FCN and GAN networks for improved automated lesion detection. Eng Appl Artif Intelligence 2019;78:186–94.

88. Wei L, El Naqa I. AI for response evaluation with PET/CT. In Seminars in nuclear medicine. Elsevier; 2020.

89. Roth HR, Lu L, Liu J, et al. Improving computer-aided detection using convolutional neural networks and random view aggregation. IEEE Trans Med Imaging 2015;35(5):1170–81.

90. Afifi, A. and T. Nakaguchi. Unsupervised detection of liver lesions in CT images. in 2015 37th Annual International Conference of the IEEE Engineering in Medicine and Biology Society (EMBC). 25-29 Aug 2015. Milan, Italy: IEEE.

91. de Vos BD, Wolterink JM, de Jong PA, et al. ConvNet-based localization of anatomical structures in 3-D medical images. IEEE Trans Med Imaging 2017;36(7):1470–81.

92. Vivanti R, Szeskin A, Lev-Cohain N, et al. Automatic detection of new tumors and tumor burden evaluation in longitudinal liver CT scan studies. Int J Comput Assist Radiol Surg 2017;12(11):1945–57.

93. Ghesu F-C, Georgescu B, Zheng Y, et al. Multi-scale deep reinforcement learning for real-time 3D-landmark detection in CT scans. IEEE Trans pattern Anal machine intelligence 2017;41(1):176–89.

94. Xie H, Yang D, Sun N, et al. Automated pulmonary nodule detection in CT images using deep convolutional neural networks. Pattern Recognition 2019;85:109–19.

95. Shen Y, Wu N, Phang J, et al. An interpretable classifier for high-resolution breast cancer screening images utilizing weakly supervised localization. Med image Anal 2021;68:101908.

96. Feng X, Yang J, Laine AF, et al. Discriminative localization in CNNs for weakly-supervised segmentation of pulmonary nodules. in International conference on medical image computing and computer-assisted intervention. Springer; 2017.

97. Schlemper J, Oktay O, Chen L, et al. Attention-gated networks for improving ultrasound scan plane detection. arXiv preprint arXiv:1804.05338, 2018.

98. Schwyzer M, Martini K, Benz DC, et al. Artificial intelligence for detecting small FDG-positive lung nodules in digital PET/CT: impact of image reconstructions on diagnostic performance. Eur Radiol 2020;30(4):2031–40.

99. Gu D, Liu G, Xue Z. On the performance of lung nodule detection, segmentation and classification. Comput Med Imaging Graphics 2021;89:101886.

100. Xu L, Tetteh G, Lipkova J, et al. Automated whole-body bone lesion detection for multiple myeloma on 68Ga-Pentixafor PET/CT imaging using deep learning methods. Contrast media Mol Imaging 2018;2391925.

101. Teramoto A, Fujita H, Yamamuro O, et al. Automated detection of pulmonary nodules in PET/CT images: ensemble false-positive reduction using a convolutional neural network technique. Med Phys 2016;43(6Part1):2821–7.

102. Kumar A, Fulham M, Feng D, et al. Co-learning feature fusion maps from PET-CT images of lung cancer. IEEE Trans Med Imaging 2019;39(1):204–17.

103. Blanc-Durand P, Van Der Gucht A, Schaefer N, et al. Automatic lesion detection and segmentation of 18F-FET PET in gliomas: a full 3D U-Net convolutional neural network study. PLoS One 2018;13(4):e0195798.

104. Schwyzer M, Ferraro DA, Muehlematter UJ, et al. Automated detection of lung cancer at ultralow dose PET/CT by deep neural networks–initial results. Lung Cancer 2018;126:170–3.

105. Edenbrandt L, Borrelli P, Ulen J, et al. Automated analysis of PSMA-PET/CT studies using convolutional neural networks. medRxiv, 2021.

106. Borrelli P, Ly J, Kaboteh R, et al. AI-based detection of lung lesions in [18 F] FDG PET-CT from lung cancer patients. EJNMMI Phys 2021;8(1):1–11.

107. Lee JJ, Yang H, Franc BL, et al. Deep learning detection of prostate cancer recurrence with 18 F-FACBC (fluciclovine, Axumin®) positron emission tomography. Eur J Nucl Med Mol Imaging 2020;47(13):2992–7.

108. Zhao Y, Gafita A, Vollnberg B, et al. Deep neural network for automatic characterization of lesions on 68 Ga-PSMA-11 PET/CT. Eur J Nucl Med Mol Imaging 2020;47(3):603–13.

109. Polymeri E, Sadik M, Kaboteh R, et al. Deep learning-based quantification of PET/CT prostate gland uptake: association with overall survival. Clin Physiol Funct Imaging 2020;40(2):106–13.

110. Perk T, Bradshaw T, Chen S, et al. Automated classification of benign and malignant lesions in 18F-NaF PET/CT images using machine learning. Phys Med Biol 2018;63(22):225019.

111. Rattan R, Kataria T, Banerjee S, et al. Artificial intelligence in oncology, its scope and future prospects with specific reference to radiation oncology. BJR| Open 2019;1(xxxx):20180031.

112. Cheung H, Rubin D. Challenges and opportunities for artificial intelligence in oncological imaging. Clin Radiol 2021;76(10):728–36.

113. Grossiord E, Talbot H, Passat N, et al. Automated 3D lymphoma lesion segmentation from PET/CT characteristics. in 2017 IEEE 14th international symposium on biomedical imaging (ISBI 2017). 18-21 April 2017. Melbourne, VIC, Australia: IEEE.

114. Teramoto A, Fujita H, Takahashi K, et al. Hybrid method for the detection of pulmonary nodules using positron emission tomography/computed tomography: a preliminary study. Int J Comput Assist Radiol Surg 2014;9(1):59–69.

115. Kawauchi K, Furuya S, Hirata K, et al. A convolutional neural network-based system to classify patients using FDG PET/CT examinations. BMC cancer 2020;20(1):1–10.

116. Moitra D, Mandal RK. Classification of non-small cell lung cancer using one-dimensional convolutional neural network. Expert Syst Appl 2020;159:113564.

117. Capobianco N, Meignan M, Cottereau A-S, et al. Deep-learning 18F-FDG uptake classification enables total metabolic tumor volume estimation in diffuse large B-cell lymphoma. J Nucl Med 2021; 62(1):30–6.

118. Sibille L, Seifert R, Avramovic N, et al. 18F-FDG PET/CT uptake classification in lymphoma and lung cancer by using deep convolutional neural networks. Radiology 2020;294(2):445–52.

119. Sibille L, Avramovic N, Spottiswoode B, et al. PET uptake classification in lymphoma and lung cancer using deep learning. Soc Nucl Med 2018.

120. Du D, Feng H, Lv W, et al. Machine learning methods for optimal radiomics-based differentiation between recurrence and inflammation: application to nasopharyngeal carcinoma post-therapy PET/CT images. Mol Imaging Biol 2020;22(3): 730–8.

121. Du D, Gu J, Chen X, et al. Integration of PET/CT radiomics and semantic features for differentiation between active pulmonary tuberculosis and lung cancer. Mol Imaging Biol 2021;23(2):287–98.

122. Lawhn-Heath C, Salavati A, Behr SC, et al. Prostate-specific membrane antigen PET in prostate cancer. Radiology 2021;299(2):248–60.

123. Sartor O, de Bono J, Chi KN, et al. Lutetium-177–PSMA-617 for metastatic Castration-Resistant prostate cancer. N Engl J Med 2021;385(12): 1091–103.

124. Leung K, Ashrafinia S, Sadaghiani MS, et al. A fully automated deep-learning based method for lesion segmentation in 18F-DCFPyL PSMA PET images of patients with prostate cancer. J Nucl Med 2019; 60(supplement 1):399.

125. Oldenhuis C, Oosting S, Gietema J, et al. Prognostic versus predictive value of biomarkers in oncology. Eur J Cancer 2008;44(7):946–53.

126. Lambin P, Roelofs E, Reymen B, et al. Rapid Learning health care in oncology'–an approach towards decision support systems enabling customised radiotherapy. Radiother Oncol 2013;109(1):159–64.

127. Martens RM, Koopman T, Noij DP, et al. Predictive value of quantitative 18 F-FDG-PET radiomics analysis in patients with head and neck squamous cell carcinoma. EJNMMI Res 2020;10(1):1–15.

128. Wang X, Lu Z. Radiomics analysis of PET and CT components of 18F-FDG PET/CT imaging for prediction of progression-free survival in advanced high-grade serous Ovarian cancer. Front Oncol 2021;11.

129. Lv W, Ashrafinia S, Ma J, et al. Multi-level multi-modality fusion radiomics: application to PET and CT imaging for prognostication of head and neck cancer. IEEE J Biomed Health Inform 2019;24(8): 2268–77.

130. Cottereau A-S, Meignan M, Nioche C, et al. Risk stratification in diffuse large B-cell lymphoma using lesion dissemination and metabolic tumor burden calculated from baseline PET/CT. Ann Oncol 2021;32(3):404–11.

131. Desseroit M-C, Visvikis D, Tixier F, et al. Development of a nomogram combining clinical staging with 18 F-FDG PET/CT image features in non-small-cell lung cancer stage I–III. Eur J Nucl Med Mol Imaging 2016;43(8):1477–85.

132. Katzman JL, Shaham U, Cloninger A, et al. Deep-Surv: personalized treatment recommender system using a Cox proportional hazards deep neural network. BMC Med Res Methodol 2018;18(1):1–12.

133. Desbordes P, Ruan S, Modzelewski R, et al. Predictive value of initial FDG-PET features for treatment response and survival in esophageal cancer patients treated with chemo-radiation therapy using a random forest classifier. PLoS One 2017;12(3): e0173208.

134. Hosny A, Parmar C, Coroller TP, et al. Deep learning for lung cancer prognostication: a retrospective multi-cohort radiomics study. PLoS Med 2018;15(11):e1002711.

135. Salmanpour MR, Shamsaei M, Rahmim A. Feature selection and machine learning methods for optimal identification and prediction of subtypes

in Parkinson's disease. Computer Methods Programs Biomed 2021;206:106131.

136. Paul R, Hawkins SH, Balagurunathan Y, et al. Deep feature transfer learning in combination with traditional features predicts survival among patients with lung adenocarcinoma. Tomography 2016; 2(4):388–95.

137. Lao J, Chen Y, Li Z-C, et al. A deep learning-based radiomics model for prediction of survival in glioblastoma multiforme. Scientific Rep 2017; 7(1):1–8.

138. Ypsilantis P-P, Siddique M, Sohn H-M, et al. Predicting response to neoadjuvant chemotherapy with PET imaging using convolutional neural networks. PloS one 2015;10(9):e0137036.

139. Pereira G. Deep Learning techniques for the evaluation of response to treatment in Hogdkin Lymphoma. 2018, Universidade de Coimbra.2018.

140. Capobianco N, Meignan MA, Cottereau A-S, et al. Deep learning FDG uptake classification enables total metabolic tumor volume estimation in diffuse large B-cell lymphoma. J Nucl Med 2020;120: 242412.

141. Wang H, Zhou Z, Li Y, et al. Comparison of machine learning methods for classifying mediastinal lymph node metastasis of non-small cell lung cancer from 18 F-FDG PET/CT images. EJNMMI Res 2017;7(1): 1–11.

142. Noortman WA, Vriens D, Slump CH, et al. Adding the temporal domain to PET radiomic features. PloS one 2020;15(9):e0239438.

143. Carvalho S, Leijenaar R, Troost E, et al. Early variation of FDG-PET radiomics features in NSCLC is related to overall survival-the "delta radiomics" concept. Radiother Oncol 2016;118:S20–1.

144. Fave X, Zhang L, Yang J, et al. Delta-radiomics features for the prediction of patient outcomes in non–small cell lung cancer. Scientific Rep 2017;7(1):1–11.

145. Nasief H, Zheng C, Schott D, et al. A machine learning based delta-radiomics process for early prediction of treatment response of pancreatic cancer. NPJ precision Oncol 2019;3(1):1–10.

146. Chelala L, Hossain R, Kazerooni EA, et al. Lung-RADS version 1.1: challenges and a Look Ahead, from the AJR special series on radiology reporting and data systems. Am J Roentgenology 2021; 216(6):1411–22.

147. Mazzei MA, Di Giacomo L, Bagnacci G, et al. Delta-radiomics and response to neoadjuvant treatment in locally advanced gastric cancer—a multicenter study of GIRCG (Italian Research Group for Gastric Cancer). Quantitative Imaging Med Surg 2021;11(6):2376.

148. Wang L, Gao Z, Li C, et al. Computed tomography–based delta-radiomics analysis for discriminating radiation pneumonitis in patients with esophageal

cancer after radiation therapy. Int J Radiat Oncol Biol Phys 2021;111(2):443–55.

149. Liu Y, Shi H, Huang S, et al. Early prediction of acute xerostomia during radiation therapy for nasopharyngeal cancer based on delta radiomics from CT images. Quantitative Imaging Med Surg 2019; 9(7):1288.

150. Sushentsev N, Rundo L, Blyuss O, et al. Comparative performance of MRI-derived PRECISE scores and delta-radiomics models for the prediction of prostate cancer progression in patients on active surveillance. Eur Radiol 2021;1–10.

151. Peeken JC, Asadpour R, Specht K, et al. MRI-based Delta-Radiomics predicts pathologic complete response in high-grade soft-tissue sarcoma patients treated with neoadjuvant therapy. Radiother Oncol 2021.

152. Shayesteh S, Nazari M, Salahshour A, et al. Treatment response prediction using MRI-based pre-, post-, and delta-radiomic features and machine learning algorithms in colorectal cancer. Med Phys 2021.

153. Nardone V, Reginelli A, Guida C, et al. Delta-radiomics increases multicentre reproducibility: a phantom study. Med Oncol 2020;37(5):1–7.

154. Jin W, Fatehi M, Abhishek K, et al. Artificial intelligence in glioma imaging: challenges and advances. J Neural Eng 2020;17(2):021002.

155. He J, Baxter SL, Xu J, et al. The practical implementation of artificial intelligence technologies in medicine. Nat Med 2019;25(1):30–6.

156. Zhang, Y., Q.V. Liao, and R.K. Bellamy. Effect of confidence and explanation on accuracy and trust calibration in AI-assisted decision making. in Proceedings of the 2020 Conference on Fairness, Accountability, and Transparency. Barcelona Spain: January 27 - 30, 2020.

157. Jin W, Li X, Hamarneh G. Hamarneh, One map does not Fit all: evaluating saliency map explanation on multi-modal medical images. arXiv preprint arXiv:2107.05047, 2021.

158. Zaharchuk G, Davidzon G. Artificial intelligence for optimization and interpretation of PET/CT and PET/MR images. Semin Nucl Med 2020;51(2):134–42.

159. Arabi H, AkhavanAllaf A, Sanaat A, et al. The promise of artificial intelligence and deep learning in PET and SPECT imaging. Physica Med 2021;83:122–37.

160. Langlotz CP. Will artificial intelligence replace radiologists? 2019. Radiological Soc North America 2019;1(3):e190058.

161. Freeman K, Geppert J, Slinton C, et al. Use of artificial intelligence for image analysis in breast cancer screening programmes: systematic review of test accuracy. bmj 2021;374.

162. Hatt M, Le Rest CC, Antonorsi N, et al. Radiomics in PET/CT: current status and future AI-based Evolutions. Semin Nucl Med 2020;51(2):126–33.

163. Shakir H, Deng Y, Rasheed H, et al. Radiomics based likelihood functions for cancer diagnosis. Scientific Rep 2019;9(1):1–10.

164. Papanikolaou N, Matos C, Koh DM. How to develop a meaningful radiomic signature for clinical use in oncologic patients. Cancer Imaging 2020;20(1):1–10.

165. Krishna R, Zhu Y, Groth O, et al. Visual genome: Connecting language and vision using crowdsourced dense image annotations. Int J Comput Vis 2017;123(1):32–73.

166. Kumar V, Gu Y, Basu S, et al. Radiomics: the process and the challenges. Magn Reson Imaging 2012;30(9):1234–48.

167. Kersting D, Weber M, Umutlu L, et al. Using a lymphoma and lung cancer trained neural network to predict the outcome for breast cancer on FDG PET/CT data. Nuklearmedizin 2021;60(02):V74.

168. Capobianco N, Gafita A, Platsch G, et al. Transfer learning of AI-based uptake classification from 18F-FDG PET/CT to 68Ga-PSMA-11 PET/CT for whole-body tumor burden assessment. J Nucl Med 2020;61(supplement 1):1411.

169. Wu J, Chen X-Y, Zhang H, et al. Hyperparameter optimization for machine learning models based on Bayesian optimization. J Electron Sci Technology 2019;17(1):26–40.

170. Sundar LKS, Muzik O, Buvat I, et al. Potentials and caveats of AI in hybrid imaging. Methods 2021; 188:4–19.

171. (ESR), E.S.o.R., ESR paper on structured reporting in radiology. Insights into imaging 2018;9:1–7.

172. Lakhani P, Kim W, Langlotz CP. Automated extraction of critical test values and communications from unstructured radiology reports: an analysis of 9.3 million reports from 1990 to 2011. Radiology 2012;265(3):809–18.

173. Lipton ZC, Berkowitz J, Elkan C. A critical review of recurrent neural networks for sequence learning. arXiv preprint arXiv:1506.00019, 2015.

174. Folio LR, Machado LB, Dwyer AJ. Multimedia-enhanced radiology reports: concept, components, and challenges. RadioGraphics 2018; 38(2):462–82.

175. Do H, Farhadi F, Xu Z, et al. AI radiomics in a monogenic autoimmune disease: deep learning of routine radiologist annotations correlated with pathologically verified lung findings. Oak Brook, III: Radiological Society of North America; 2019.

176. Willemink MJ, Koszek WA, Hardell C, et al. Preparing medical imaging data for machine learning. Radiology 2020;295(1):4–15.

177. Ryoo HG, Choi H, Lee DS. Deep learning-based interpretation of basal/acetazolamide brain perfusion SPECT leveraging unstructured reading reports. Eur J Nucl Med Mol Imaging 2020;47(9): 2186–96.

178. Manhaeve R, Dumancic S, Kimmig A, et al. Deepproblog: neural probabilistic logic programming. Adv Neural Inf Process Syst 2018;31:3749–59.

179. Došilović FK, Brčić M, Hlupić N. Explainable artificial intelligence: a survey. in 2018 41st International convention on information and communication technology, electronics and microelectronics (MIPRO). Opatija, Croatia: IEEE; 2018.

180. Cai J, Harrison AP, Zheng Y, et al. Lesion-harvester: iteratively mining unlabeled lesions and hard-negative examples at scale. IEEE Trans Med Imaging 2020;40(1):59–70.

181. Huang X, Sun W, Tseng T-LB, et al. Fast and fully-automated detection and segmentation of pulmonary nodules in thoracic CT scans using deep convolutional neural networks. Comput Med Imaging Graphics 2019;74:25–36.

182. Zhu W, Liu C, Fan W, et al. Deeplung: Deep 3d dual path nets for automated pulmonary nodule detection and classification. in 2018 IEEE Winter Conference on Applications of Computer Vision (WACV). 12-15 March 2018. Lake Tahoe, NV, USA: IEEE; pp. 673-81.

183. Xie Z. 3D Region Proposal U-Net with Dense and Residual Learning for Lung Nodule Detection. LUNA16, 2017.

184. George J, Skaria S, Varun V. Using YOLO based deep learning network for real time detection and localization of lung nodules from low dose CT scans. in Medical Imaging 2018: computer-Aided Diagnosis. Int Soc Opt Photon 2018.

185. Wang, D., Y. Zhang, K. Zhang, et al. Focalmix: Semi-supervised learning for 3d medical image detection. in Proceedings of the IEEE/CVF Conference on Computer Vision and Pattern Recognition. Seattle, WA, USA: 13-19 June 2020.

186. Jiang H, Ma H, Qian W, et al. An automatic detection system of lung nodule based on multigroup patch-based deep learning network. IEEE J Biomed Health Inform 2017;22(4):1227–37.

187. Huang X, Shan J, Vaidya V. Lung nodule detection in CT using 3D convolutional neural networks. in 2017 IEEE 14th International Symposium on Biomedical Imaging (ISBI 2017). 18-21 April 2017. 18-21 April 2017: IEEE.

188. Ding J, Li A, Hu Z, et al. Accurate pulmonary nodule detection in computed tomography images using deep convolutional neural networks. in International Conference on Medical Image Computing and Computer-Assisted Intervention. 2017. Springer.

189. Kawakami M, Sugimori H, Hirata K, et al. Evaluation of automatic detection of abnormal uptake by deep

learning and combination technique in FDG-PET images. Soc Nucl Med 2020.

190. Weisman A, Kieler M, Perlman S, et al. Ensemble 3D convolutional neural networks for automated detection of diseased lymph nodes. Soc Nucl Med 2020.

191. Punithavathy K, Poobal S, Ramya M. Performance evaluation of machine learning techniques in lung cancer classification from PET/CT images. FME Trans 2019;47(3):418–23.

192. Zhou Y, Yu J, Liu M, et al. A machine learning-based parametric imaging algorithm for noninva-sive quantification of dynamic [68Ga] DOTATATE PET-CT. Soc Nucl Med 2019.

193. Leung K, Sadaghiani MS, Dalaie P, et al. A deep learning-based approach for lesion classification in 3D 18F-DCFPyL PSMA PET images of patients with prostate cancer. Soc Nucl Med 2020.

194. Acar E, Leblebici A, Ellidokuz BE, et al. Machine learning for differentiating metastatic and completely responded sclerotic bone lesion in prostate cancer: a retrospective radiomics study. Br J Radiol 2019;92(1101):20190286.

Moving?

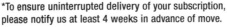

Make sure your subscription moves with you!

To notify us of your new address, find your **Clinics Account Number** (located on your mailing label above your name), and contact customer service at:

Email: journalscustomerservice-usa@elsevier.com

800-654-2452 (subscribers in the U.S. & Canada)
314-447-8871 (subscribers outside of the U.S. & Canada)

Fax number: 314-447-8029

Elsevier Health Sciences Division
Subscription Customer Service
3251 Riverport Lane
Maryland Heights, MO 63043

*To ensure uninterrupted delivery of your subscription, please notify us at least 4 weeks in advance of move.